Care for the Term Newborn

Editors

ANUP C. KATHERIA
LISA MARIE STELLWAGEN

CLINICS IN PERINATOLOGY

www.perinatology.theclinics.com

Consulting Editor
LUCKY JAIN

September 2021 • Volume 48 • Number 3

ELSEVIER

1600 John F. Kennedy Boulevard • Suite 1800 • Philadelphia, Pennsylvania, 19103-2899

http://www.theclinics.com

CLINICS IN PERINATOLOGY Volume 48, Number 3
September 2021 ISSN 0095-5108, ISBN-13: 978-0-323-89688-7

Editor: Kerry Holland
Developmental Editor: Karen Solomon

Clinics in Perinatology (ISSN 0095-5108) is published quarterly by Elsevier Inc., 360 Park Avenue South, New York, NY 10010-1710. Months of issue are March, June, September, and December. Business and Editorial Offices: 1600 John F. Kennedy Blvd., Ste. 1800, Philadelphia, PA 19103-2899. Customer Service Office: 3251 Riverport Lane, Maryland Heights, MO 63043. Periodicals postage paid at New York, NY and additional mailing offices. Subscription prices are $321.00 per year (US individuals), $788.00 per year (US institutions), $365.00 per year (Canadian individuals), $835.00 per year (Canadian institutions), $435.00 per year (international individuals), $835.00 per year (international institutions), $100.00 per year (US and Canadian students), and $195.00 per year (International students). International air speed delivery is included in all Clinics subscription prices. All prices are subject to change without notice. **POSTMASTER:** Send address changes to *Clinics in Perinatology*, Elsevier Health Sciences Division, Subscription Customer Service, 3251 Riverport Lane, Maryland Heights, MO 63043. **Customer Service: Telephone: 1-800-654-2452** (U.S. and Canada); **1-314-447-8871** (outside U.S. and Canada). **Fax: 1-314-447-8029. E-mail: journalscustomerservice-usa@elsevier.com** (for print support); **journalsonlinesupport-usa@elsevier.com** (for online support).

Reprints. For copies of 100 or more, of articles in this publication, please contact the Commercial Reprints Department, Elsevier Inc., 360 Park Avenue South, New York, NY 10010-1710. Tel. 212-633-3874; Fax: 212-633-3820; E-mail: reprints@elsevier.com.

Clinics in Perinatology is also published in Spanish by McGraw-Hill Interamericana Editores S.A., P.O. Box 5-237, 06500 Mexico D.F., Mexico.

Clinics in Perinatology is covered in *MEDLINE/PubMed (Index Medicus) Current Contents, Excepta Medica, BIOSIS and ISI/BIOMED.*

Contributors

CONSULTING EDITOR

LUCKY JAIN, MD, MBA
George W. Brumley Jr Professor and Chairman, Department of Pediatrics, Emory University School of Medicine, Chief Academic Officer, Children's Healthcare of Atlanta, Executive Director, Emory + Children's Pediatric Institute, Atlanta, Georgia, USA

EDITORS

ANUP C. KATHERIA, MD, FAAP
Adjunct Assistant Professor, Department of Pediatrics, Loma Linda University, Loma Linda, California, USA; Director, Neonatal Research Institute, Sharp Mary Birch Hospital for Women and Newborns, San Diego, California, USA

LISA MARIE STELLWAGEN, MD, FAAP
Clinical Professor, Department of Pediatrics, UC San Diego School of Medicine, San Diego, California, USA; Executive Director, University of California Health Milk Bank, UC San Diego Health, San Diego, California, USA

AUTHORS

WANDA J. ABREU, MD
Assistant Professor of Pediatrics, Well Baby Nursery Medical Director, Columbia University Vagelos College of Physicians and Surgeons, New York, New York, USA

OLA ANDERSSON, MD, PhD
Associate Professor, Department of Clinical Sciences, Lund, Pediatrics, Lund University, Department of Neonatology, Skåne University Hospital, Sweden

WILLIAM E. BENITZ, MD
Professor of Pediatrics (Emeritus), Division of Neonatal and Developmental Medicine, Department of Pediatrics, Stanford University School of Medicine, Palo Alto, California, USA

SONIA LOMELI BONIFACIO, MD, FAAP
Clinical Professor of Pediatrics, Associate Medical Director, NeuroNICU, Division of Neonatal and Developmental Medicine, Stanford University, Palo Alto, California, USA

MAYA BUNIK, MD, MPH
Professor, Pediatrics, University of Colorado Anschutz Medical Campus, Children's Hospital Colorado, Aurora Colorado, USA

VALERIAN CATANZARITE, MD, PhD
San Diego Perinatal Center, Rady Children's Specialists of San Diego, San Diego, California, USA

LORI FELDMAN-WINTER, MD, MPH
Children's Regional Hospital at Cooper University Healthcare, Cooper Medical School of Rowan University, Camden, New Jersey, USA

VALERIE FLAHERMAN, MD, MPH
Departments of Pediatrics, and Epidemiology and Biostatistics, University of California, San Francisco, San Francisco, California, USA

ADAM FRYMOYER, MD
Clinical Associate Professor of Pediatrics, Division of Neonatal and Developmental Medicine, Department of Pediatrics, Stanford University School of Medicine, Palo Alto, California, USA

CATHY HAMMERMAN, MD
Department of Neonatology, Shaare Zedek Medical Center, The Faculty of Medicine of the Hebrew University, Jerusalem, Israel

WILLIAM W. HAY Jr. MD
Retired Professor of Pediatrics, Retired, University of Colorado, Denver, Colorado, USA

EUSTRATIA M. HUBBARD, MD
Clinical Professor of Pediatrics, UC San Diego School of Medicine, UC San Diego Health, La Jolla, California, USA

SHANDEE HUTSON, MD, FAAP
Department of Neonatology, Co-director, NICN, Sharp Mary Birch Hospital for Women and Newborns, San Diego, California, USA

KATHRYN A. JOHNSON, MD, MS
Associate Clinical Professor, University of California, San Diego, La Jolla, California, USA

MICHAEL KAPLAN, MBChB
The Faculty of Medicine of the Hebrew University, Department of Neonatology, Shaare Zedek Medical Center (Emeritus), Jerusalem, Israel

ANN KELLAMS, MD, IBCLC
Department of Pediatrics, University of Virginia, Charlottesville, Virginia, USA

SATYAN LAKSHMINRUSIMHA, MD, FAAP
Professor and Dennis & Nancy Marks Chair of Pediatrics, Pediatrician-in-Chief, Department of Pediatrics, UC Davis Children's Hospital, UC Davis Health, Sacramento, California, USA

MICHELLE LEFF, MD, IBCLC, FAAP
Associate Professor, Department of Pediatrics, University of California San Diego, San Diego, California, USA

TINA A. LEONE, MD
Associate Professor of Pediatrics, Neonatal-Perinatal Medicine Training Program Director, Columbia University Vagelos College of Physicians and Surgeons, New York, New York, USA

JASPREET LOYAL, MD, MS
Associate Professor, Department of Pediatrics, Yale School of Medicine, New Haven, Connecticut, USA

JUDITH S. MERCER, PhD, CNM
Neonatal Research Institute at Sharp Mary Birch Hospital for Women and Newborns, San Diego, California, USA; University of Rhode Island, Kingston, Rhode Island, USA

TORRI D. METZ, MD, MS
Associate Professor, Department of Obstetrics and Gynecology, University of Utah Health, Salt Lake City, Utah, USA

AMARAN MOODLEY, MD
Associate Clinical Professor, Department of Pediatrics, Division of Infectious Diseases, Rady Childrens Hospital, University of California San Diego, San Diego, California, USA

SAGORI MUKHOPADHAY, MD, MMSc
Assistant Professor of Pediatrics, Division of Neonatology, Department of Pediatrics, Children's Hospital of Philadelphia, Department of Pediatrics, University of Pennsylvania Perelman School of Medicine, Philadelphia, Pennsylvania, USA

KURLEN S.E. PAYTON, MD
Associate Professor of Pediatrics, David Geffen School of Medicine at University of California Los Angeles, Division of Neonatology, Cedars-Sinai Medical Center, Los Angeles, California, USA

KAREN M. PUOPOLO, MD, PhD
Associate Professor of Pediatrics, Division of Neonatology, Department of Pediatrics, Children's Hospital of Philadelphia, Chief, Section on Newborn Medicine, Pennsylvania Hospital, Department of Pediatrics, University of Pennsylvania Perelman School of Medicine, Philadelphia, Pennsylvania, USA

YOGEN SINGH MD, MA (Cantab), FRCPCH
Professor of Pediatrics, Department of Pediatrics – Division of Neonatology, Loma Linda University Children's Hospital and Loma Linda University School of Medicine, California, USA; Department of Pediatrics – Neonatology and Pediatric Cardiology, Cambridge University Hospitals, Cambridge, United Kingdom

COURTNEY TOWNSEL, MD, MSc
Assistant Professor, Department of Obstetrics and Gynecology, University of Michigan, Ann Arbor, Michigan, USA

ISABELLE VON KOHORN, MD, PhD
Department of Pediatrics, Holy Cross Health, Silver Spring, Maryland, USA; Department of Pediatrics, The George Washington University School of Medicine and Health Sciences, Washington, DC, USA

Contents

Foreword: Newborn Care is a Team Sport **xvii**

Lucky Jain

Preface: The Term Infant **xxi**

Anup C. Katheria and Lisa Marie Stellwagen

The Term Newborn: Delivery Room Triage and Transitions of Care **431**

Tina A. Leone and Wanda J. Abreu

Term newborn infants without significant medical problems usually transition from fetal to newborn life without medical assistance. Infants requiring therapy often need care in a neonatal intensive care unit as opposed to a well-baby unit. Infants with unclear physiologic status or disease that may require therapies in the immediate newborn period may benefit from a period of observation with close monitoring before admission to a well-baby unit. Whenever possible, providing care for a newborn infant in an area that provides care for the newborn and mother together in the same room facilitates adaptation to the extra-uterine environment, bonding and breastfeeding for those electing to do so.

Cord Management of the Term Newborn **447**

Ola Andersson and Judith S. Mercer

Keeping the umbilical cord intact after delivery facilitates transition from fetal to neonatal circulation and allows a placental transfusion of a considerable amount of blood. A delay of at least 3 minutes improves neurodevelopmental outcomes in term infants. Although regarded as common sense and practiced by many midwives, implementation of delayed cord clamping into practice has been unduly slow, partly because of beliefs regarding theoretic risks of jaundice and lack of understanding regarding the long-term benefits. This article provides arguments for delaying cord clamping for a minimum of 3 minutes.

The Term Newborn: Early-Onset Sepsis **471**

Karen M. Puopolo, Sagori Mukhopadhay, Adam Frymoyer, and William E. Benitz

The changing epidemiology of early-onset neonatal sepsis among term infants has required reappraisal of approaches to management of newborn infants at potential risk. As this is now a rare disease, new strategies for reduction in diagnostic testing and empirical treatment have been developed. Adoption and refinement of these strategies should be a priority for all facilities where babies are born.

The Term Newborn: Congenital Infections 485

Amaran Moodley and Kurlen S.E. Payton

Maternal pathogens can be transmitted to the fetus resulting in congenital infection with sequelae ranging from asymptomatic infection to severe debilitating disease and still birth. The TORCH pneumonic (toxoplasmosis, rubella, cytomegalovirus, and herpes simplex virus) is used widely, but it provides a limited description of the expanding list of pathogens associated with congenital infection. This article focuses on the evaluation and management of infants with common congenital infections such as cytomegalovirus, and infections that warrant early diagnosis and treatment to prevent serious complications, such as toxoplasmosis, human immunodeficiency virus, and syphilis. Zika virus and Chagas disease remain uncommon.

Human Milk for the Term Newborn 513

Isabelle Von Kohorn and Valerie Flaherman

Human milk provides optimal nutrition for term newborns, but the prevalence of its use is below target, and risks have been identified. Infants of black mothers as well as term newborns admitted to the neonatal intensive care unit are at risk for not receiving human milk. To improve human milk intake, multiple individual-level interventions have been shown to be effective, but some popular system-level interventions are ineffective or harmful. Expressed milk and donor milk may be less beneficial than direct breastfeeding. Nuanced public policies can help support lactation while promoting individual choice and equity.

Hyperbilirubinemia in the Term Infant: Re-evaluating What We Think We Know 533

Cathy Hammerman and Michael Kaplan

This article attempts to highlight contemporary issues relating to term neonatal hyperbilirubinemia and to focus attention on controversial issues and concepts with the potential to effect change in clinical approach. On the one hand, the focus is bilirubin neurotoxicity, which is now known to encompass a wide, diverse spectrum of features. The various aspects of this spectrum are outlined and defined. On the other hand, bilirubin also possesses antioxidant properties. As such, mild hyperbilirubinemia is suggested as actually offering the neonate some protective advantage.

The Term Newborn: Postnatal Screening and Testing 555

Kathryn A. Johnson and Valerian Catanzarite

Prenatal genetic screening, including evaluation for inherited genetic disorders, aneuploidy risk assessment, and sonographic assessment, combined with a thorough newborn examination and standard newborn screening, including blood, hearing, and congenital heart disease screening, can reveal conditions requiring further evaluation after delivery. Abnormal prenatal or newborn screening results should prompt additional diagnostic testing guided by maternal fetal medicine, perinatal genetics, or pediatric specialists.

Understanding the perinatal cardiovascular physiology is essential for timely diagnosis and management of congenital heart defects (CHDs) in neonatal period. The incidence of CHDs is reported in 7 to 9 out of 1000 live births, with around 25% of them being critical congenital heart disease, defined as a congenital heart condition needing surgery/intervention or leading to death within 1 month after birth. Around 50% to 60% of the critical CHDs are detected on fetal anomaly screening. The signs and symptoms of critical congenital heart defects are often nonspecific during early neonatal period. The routine newborn physical examination often fails to detect many of these critical CHDs during the transitional circulation because of lack of signs soon after birth. While routine pulse oximetry screening typically performed at 24 to 48 hours after birth may help in detecting cyanotic heart conditions, noncyanotic CHDs such as coarctation of aorta may go undetected on pulse oximetry screening in asymptomatic infants. Some infants may deteriorate early while waiting for pulse oximetry screening, and this risk is much higher if the pulse oximetry screening is not performed to detect congenital heart conditions. There should be high degree of suspicion of critical CHDs in infants presenting with shock or hypoxia. Delay in diagnosis of CHDs has been reported to be associated with poor outcomes, and hence, it is extremely important to detect them in asymptomatic well-infants. Timely recognition and therapy with prostaglandin E1 infusion can be lifesaving in neonatal cardiac emergencies, and they should be urgently discussed with a pediatric cardiologist. This article reviews diagnosis and management of CHD in the delivery room and before surgery in the NICU.

Persistent pulmonary hypertension of the newborn (PPHN) is a disorder of circulatory transition resulting in high pulmonary vascular resistance with extrapulmonary right-to-left shunts causing hypoxemia. There has been substantial gain in understanding of pathophysiology of PPHN over the past 2 decades, and biochemical pathways responsible for abnormal vasoconstriction of pulmonary vasculature are now better understood. Easy availability of bedside echocardiography helps in establishing early definitive diagnosis, understanding the pathophysiology and hemodynamic abnormalities, monitoring the disease process, and response to therapeutic intervention. There also has been significant advancement in specific management of PPHN targeted at deranged biochemical pathways and hemodynamic instability.

Sudden unexpected infant death is a leading cause of death in infancy. Both safe sleep practices and breastfeeding can help decrease the risk, although the current practice of educating parents about the recommendations has not resulted in universal adherence. Prenatal counseling provides opportunities to discuss recommendations as well as troubleshoot common barriers to breastfeeding and safe infant sleep with goals to gradually change attitudes, address social norms, and prepare new parents. A conversational, motivational approach to discussions about the importance of safe sleep and continued breastfeeding, with explanations as to the reasoning behind these recommendations, can help parents incorporate optimal practices into their lifestyles in a way that is sustainable for adherence.

The Term Newborn: Prenatal Substance Exposure **631**

Courtney Townsel, Torri D. Metz, and Maya Bunik

Care for pregnant patients with substance use disorder must be provided in a nonjudgmental manner with recognition of addiction as a chronic medical illness in order to establish a therapeutic relationship and improve outcomes. All pregnant patients should be screened for substance use during prenatal care. Screening can be accomplished through several validated screening tools. Patients who screen positive need to be evaluated and referred for treatment as appropriate. This article reviews specific adverse perinatal outcomes associated with the use of a variety of substances and provides guidance on exposure with continued breastfeeding.

The Term Newborn: Alternative Birth Practices, Refusal, and Therapeutic Hesitancy **647**

Michelle Leff and Jaspreet Loyal

The care of late preterm and term newborns delivered in hospital settings in the United States is largely standardized with many routine interventions and screenings that are evidence-based and serve to protect newborn's and the public's health. Refusals of various aspects of routine newborn care are uncommon but can be challenging for clinicians who care for newborns to navigate for many reasons. In this article, we describe the spectrum of refusal. We review suggested approaches that clinicians can take starting with increasing their own awareness of what specific components of newborn care are refused and why.

The Term Newborn: Hypoglycemia **665**

Eustratia M. Hubbard and William W. Hay Jr.

This review provides an update on neonatal hypoglycemia in the term infant, including discussion of glucose metabolism, definitions of hypoglycemia, identification of infants commonly at risk, and the screening, treatment, and potential neurological outcomes of postnatal hypoglycemia. Neonatal hypoglycemia is a common metabolic condition that continues to plague clinicians because there is no clear relationship between low glucose concentrations or their duration that determines adverse neurological outcomes. However, severely low, prolonged, recurrent low glucose concentrations in infants who also have marked symptoms such as seizures, flaccid hypotonia with apnea, and coma clearly are associated with permanent brain damage. Early identification of at-risk infants, early and continued breastfeeding augmented with oral dextrose gel, monitoring prefeed glucose concentrations, treating symptomatic infants who have very low and recurrent low glucose concentrations, and identifying and aggressively managing infants with persistent hyperinsulinemia and metabolic defects may help prevent neuronal injury.

The Term Newborn: Evaluation for Hypoxic-Ischemic Encephalopathy **681**

Sonia Lomeli Bonifacio and Shandee Hutson

Neonatal encephalopathy due to perinatal hypoxia-ischemia (hypoxic-ischemic encephalopathy [HIE]) occurs at a rate of 1 to 3 per 1000 live births. Therapeutic hypothermia is the standard of care and the only currently available therapy to reduce the risk of death or disability in newborns with moderate to severe HIE. Hypothermia therapy needs to be initiated within 6 hours after birth in order to provide the best chance for neuroprotection. All pediatricians and delivery room attendants should be trained to recognize encephalopathy and understand the eligibility criteria for treatment. The modified Sarnat examination is the most frequently used tool to assess the degree of encephalopathy and has six categories, each of which can have mild, moderate, severe abnormalities. Apart from historical and biochemical criteria, a neonate must have 3 of 6 categories scored in the moderate or severe range in order to qualify for hypothermia as was done in the randomized trials. Whether an infant qualifies or there is concern that an infant might have HIE, transfer to a center that can perform treatment should be initiated immediately. Hypothermia significantly reduces the risk of death or moderate to severe impairments at 2 years and at school age. On average, only 7 neonates need to be treated for one neonate to benefit. Although easy in concept, implementation of hypothermia does require expertise and should be carried out under the guidance of a neonatologist. If infants are passively cooled prior to transport, core temperature needs to be closely monitored with a target of 33.5°C $\pm$ 0.5°C. Maintenance of homeostasis is important in order to prevent conditions that may result in additional brain injury. Seizures are common in neonates with HIE, but electrographic seizures are rare in the first few hours after birth if the insult occurred during labor and delivery. Prophylactic antiepileptic drugs should not be administered. Brain monitoring in the form of electroencephalogram (EEG) and or amplitude-integrated EEG should be implemented as soon as possible to help with prognosis and to accurately diagnose seizures.

PROGRAM OBJECTIVE

The goal of *Clinics in Perinatology* is to keep practicing perinatologists, neonatologists, obstetricians, practicing physicians and residents up to date with current clinical practice in perinatology by providing timely articles reviewing the state of the art in patient care.

TARGET AUDIENCE

Perinatologists, neonatologists, obstetricians, practicing physicians, residents and healthcare professionals who provide patient care utilizing findings from *Clinics in Perinatology*.

LEARNING OBJECTIVES

Upon completion of this activity, participants will be able to:

1. Review arguments for delaying cord clamping; the benefits and risks of human milk for the term newborn; diagnosis and management of congenital heart defects in the delivery room; and the pathophysiology and hemodynamic changes that occur in persistent pulmonary hypertension of the newborn.
2. Discuss determining the appropriate level of care for newborns at the time of birth; the current epidemiology and recommended approaches to the management of early onset sepsis among term infants; screening for substance use in pregnancy; and refusal of routine newborn care.
3. Recognize approaches to reduce incidences of the sudden infant death syndrome as well as updates to screening and treatment of neonatal hypoglycemia.

ACCREDITATION

The Elsevier Office of Continuing Medical Education (EOCME) is accredited by the Accreditation Council for Continuing Medical Education (ACCME) to provide continuing medical education for physicians.

The EOCME designates this journal-based CME activity for a maximum of 14 *AMA PRA Category 1 Credit*(s)™. Physicians should claim only the credit commensurate with the extent of their participation in the activity.

All other health care professionals requesting continuing education credit for this enduring material will be issued a certificate of participation.

DISCLOSURE OF CONFLICTS OF INTEREST

The EOCME assesses conflict of interest with its instructors, faculty, planners, and other individuals who are in a position to control the content of CME activities. All relevant conflicts of interest that are identified are thoroughly vetted by EOCME for fair balance, scientific objectivity, and patient care recommendations. EOCME is committed to providing its learners with CME activities that promote improvements or quality in healthcare and not a specific proprietary business or a commercial interest.

The planning committee, staff, authors and editors listed below have identified no financial relationships or relationships to products or devices they or their spouse/life partner have with commercial interest related to the content of this CME activity:

Wanda Abreu, MD; Ola Andersson, MD, PhD; William E. Benitz, MD; Sonia Lomeli Bonifacio, MD, FAAP; Maya Bunik, MD, MPH; Valerian Catanzarite, MD, PhD; Regina Chavous-Gibson, MSN, RN; Lori Feldman-Winter, MD, MPH; Valerie Flaherman, MD, MPH; Adam Frymoyer, MD; Cathy Hammerman, MD; William W. Hay, Jr, MD; Shandee Hutson, MD, FAAP; Lucky Jain, MD, MBA; Kathryn A. Johnson, MD, MS; Michael Kaplan, MBChB; Anup C. Katheria, MD, FAAP; Ann Kellams, MD, IBCLC; Satyan Lakshminrusimha, MD; Michelle Leff, MD, IBCLC, FAAP; Tina A. Leone, MD; Jaspreet Loyal, MD, MS; Judith S. Mercer, CNM, PhD; Torri D. Metz, MD, MS; Amaran Moodley, MD; Sagori Mukhopadhay, MD, MMSc; Kurlen S.E. Payton, MD; Karen M. Puopolo, MD, PhD; Yogen Singh, MBBS, MD; Lisa Marie Stellwagen, MD, FAAP; Jeyanthi Surendrakumar; Courtney Townsel, MD, MSc; Isabelle Von Kohorn, MD, PhD

The planning committee, staff, authors and editors listed below have identified financial relationships or relationships to products or devices they or their spouse/life partner have with commercial interest related to the content of this CME activity:

Eustratia M. Hubbard, MD: Research support: Dexcom, Inc.

UNAPPROVED/OFF-LABEL USE DISCLOSURE

The EOCME requires CME faculty to disclose to the participants:

1. When products or procedures being discussed are off-label, unlabelled, experimental, and/or investigational (not US Food and Drug Administration [FDA] approved); and

2. Any limitations on the information presented, such as data that are preliminary or that represent ongoing research, interim analyses, and/or unsupported opinions. Faculty may discuss information about pharmaceutical agents that is outside of FDA-approved labelling. This information is intended solely for CME and is not intended to promote off-label use of these medications. If you have any questions, contact the medical affairs department of the manufacturer for the most recent prescribing information.

TO ENROLL

To enroll in the *Clinics in Perinatology* Continuing Medical Education program, call customer service at 1-800-654-2452 or sign up online at http://www.theclinics.com/home/cme. The CME program is available to subscribers for an additional annual fee of USD 265.00.

METHOD OF PARTICIPATION

In order to claim credit, participants must complete the following:

1. Complete enrolment as indicated above.
2. Read the activity.
3. Complete the CME Test and Evaluation. Participants must achieve a score of 70% on the test. All CME Tests and Evaluations must be completed online.

CME INQUIRIES/SPECIAL NEEDS

For all CME inquiries or special needs, please contact elsevierCME@elsevier.com.

CLINICS IN PERINATOLOGY

FORTHCOMING ISSUES

December 2021
Advances in Respiratory Management
Manuel Sánchez Luna, *Editor*

March 2022
Current Controversies in Neonatology
Robert M. Kliegman and Susan Cohen, *Editors*

June 2022
Neonatal and Perinatal Nutrition
Akhil Maheshwari and Jonathan R. Swanson, *Editors*

RECENT ISSUES

June 2021
Perinatal and Neonatal Infections
Joseph B. Cantey and Andi L. Shane, *Editors*

March 2021
Neonatal Malignant Disorders
Daniel S. Wechsler, *Editor*

December 2020
Advances in Maternal Fetal Medicine
Cynthia Gyamfi-Bannerman and Russell Miller, *Editors*

SERIES OF RELATED INTEREST

Pediatric Clinics of North America
https://www.pediatric.theclinics.com/
Obstetrics and Gynecology Clinics of North America
https://www.obgyn.theclinics.com/

Foreword

Newborn Care is a Team Sport

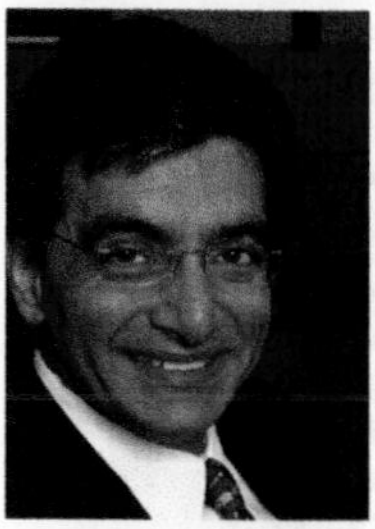

Lucky Jain, MD, MBA,
Consulting Editor

The birth of a healthy newborn is truly a miracle! Increasingly, well-informed parents are looking for a perfect outcome of a pregnancy and delivery that is much anticipated and planned. This puts an added burden on a team that is often operating with imperfect information and a general lack of evidence-based guidelines. Practitioners struggle with various aspects of delivery: optimal time (gestational age), mode (vaginal, cesarean), site (home, hospital), management of labor (induction, augmentation), and so on. Equally confusing are guidelines and practices related to normal newborn transition, early feeding practices, management of jaundice, and other newborn issues. Indeed, it takes a village for the successful transition of a fetus to a healthy thriving newborn (**Fig. 1**).[1]

Yet, a significant number of newborns fail to make a smooth transition and suffer from newborn complications. A 2010 publication by Black et al[2] showed that an estimated 4 million newborns, equal to nearly all births in the United States each year, die worldwide of birth asphyxia alone.[2,3] A more recent publication from Ethiopia found that more than one-third of the neonatal deaths in one of the neonatal intensive care units were from birth asphyxia, and most of these were preventable.[4] The spectrum of childbirth and newborn care needs is wide, and it is easy to see how gaps appear in inadequately resources environments.

There is also a need to focus on what matters most to women during childbirth and how those experiences influence the newborn. A systemic qualitative review published in 2018 showed that safety and psychosocial well-being were equally valued by most healthy childbearing women who want a healthy experience.[5] Similarly, evidence clearly demonstrates that newborns are sentient beings and readily influenced by the physical environment and routine care provided to them.[6]

In this issue of the *Clinics in Perinatology*, Drs Katheria and Stellwagen have brought together well-known experts, who have covered key aspects of normal newborn care. The authors point to the need for a uniform approach to early care. As always, I am

Clin Perinatol 48 (2021) xvii–xix
https://doi.org/10.1016/j.clp.2021.06.002

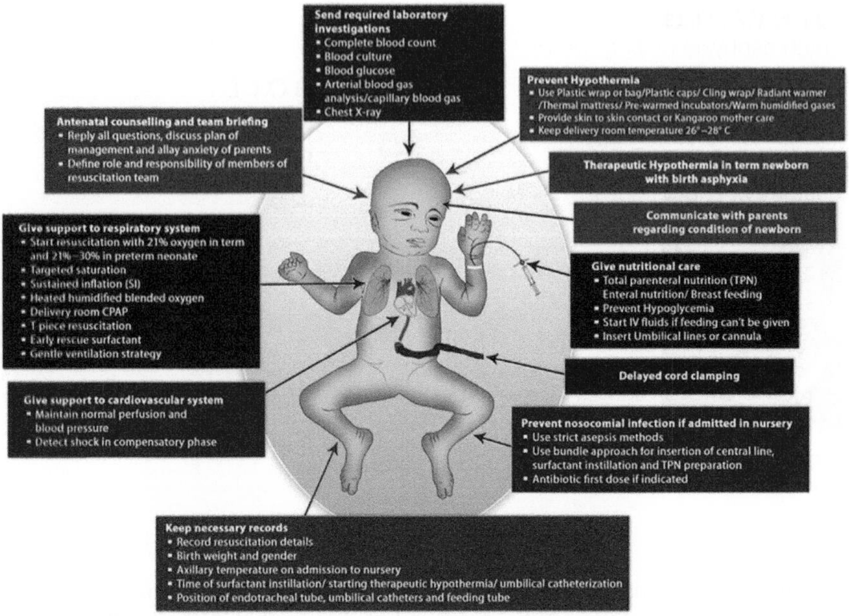
Send required laboratory investigations
• Complete blood count
• Blood culture
• Blood glucose
• Arterial blood gas analysis/capillary blood gas
• Chest X-ray
Prevent Hypothermia
• Use Plastic wrap or bag/Plastic caps/ Cling wrap/ Radiant warmer /Thermal mattress/ Pre-warmed incubators/Warm humidified gases
• Provide skin to skin contact or Kangaroo mother care
• Keep delivery room temperature 26°–28° C
Antenatal counselling and team briefing
• Reply all questions, discuss plan of management and allay anxiety of parents
• Define role and responsibility of members of resuscitation team
Therapeutic Hypothermia in term newborn with birth asphyxia
Communicate with parents regarding condition of newborn
Give support to respiratory system
• Start resuscitation with 21% oxygen in term and 21%–30% in preterm neonate
• Targeted saturation
• Sustained inflation (SI)
• Heated humidified blended oxygen
• Delivery room CPAP
• T piece resuscitation
• Early rescue surfactant
• Gentle ventilation strategy
Give nutritional care
• Total parenteral nutrition (TPN) Enteral nutrition/ Breast feeding
• Prevent Hypoglycemia
• Start IV fluids if feeding can't be given
• Insert Umbilical lines or cannula
Delayed cord clamping
Give support to cardiovascular system
• Maintain normal perfusion and blood pressure
• Detect shock in compensatory phase
Prevent nosocomial infection if admitted in nursery
• Use strict asepsis methods
• Use bundle approach for insertion of central line, surfactant instillation and TPN preparation
• Antibiotic first dose if indicated
Keep necessary records
• Record resuscitation details
• Birth weight and gender
• Axillary temperature on admission to nursery
• Time of surfactant instillation/ starting therapeutic hypothermia/ umbilical catheterization
• Position of endotracheal tube, umbilical catheters and feeding tube

Fig. 1. Golden hour interventions to be done at the time of preterm and term newborn birth. CPAP, continuous positive airway pressure. (*From* Sharma D. Golden hour of neonatal life: Need of the hour. Maternal Health, Neonatology, and Perinatology. 2017;3:16 (pages 1-21, figure from page 2).)

grateful to the publishing staff at Elsevier, including Kerry Holland and Karen Justine Solomon, for their support in bringing this important publication to you.

Lucky Jain, MD, MBA
Department of Pediatrics
Emory University School of Medicine
Children's Healthcare of Atlanta
1760 Haygood Drive, W409
Atlanta, GA 30322, USA

E-mail address:
ljain@emory.edu

REFERENCES

1. Sharma D. Golden hour of neonatal life: need of the hour. Matern Health Neonatol Perinatol 2017;3:16.

2. Black RE, Cousens S, Johnson HL, et al. Child Health Epidemiology Reference Group of WHO UNICEF: global, regional, and national causes of child mortality in 2008: a systemic analysis. Lancet 2010;375:1969–87.

3. Jain L. Birth asphyxia and the inextricable intersection of fetal and neonatal physiology. Clin Perinatol 2016;43:xv–xvii.

4. Bayih WA, Yitbarek GY, Aynalem YA, et al. Prevalence and associated factors of birth asphyxia among live births at Debre Tabor General Hospital, North Central Ethiopia. BMC Pregnancy Childbirth 2020;20:653.
5. Downe S, Finlayson K, Oladapo O, et al. What matters to women during childbirth: a systematic qualitative review. PLoS One 2018;13(4):e0194906.
6. Andre V, Henry S, Lemasson A, et al. The human newborn's umwelt: unexplored pathways and perspectives. Psychon Bull Rev 2018;25:350–69.

Preface

The Term Infant

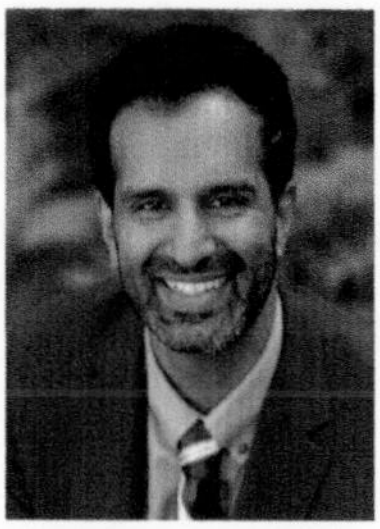

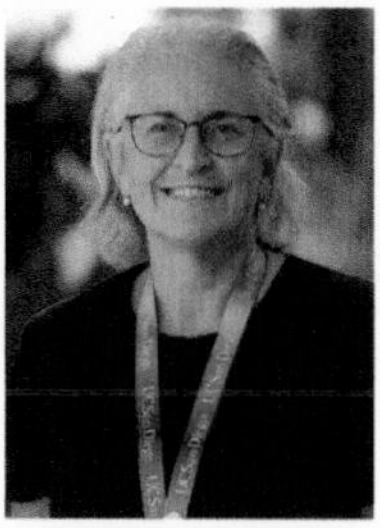

Anup C. Katheria, MD, FAAP Lisa Marie Stellwagen, MD, FAAP
Editors

Reproduction, pregnancy, and lactation are all processes that are mandatory for the survival of our species. Evolution has put an enormous amount of energy into the survival of the newborn; and they are, as a rule, robust little beings. However, the transition of the infant at the time of delivery is one of the most amazing and complex physiologic transitions that humans undergo. How the infant manages that transition is key to their survival.

The care of the newborn had been in the hands of the delivering physician, and over time, pediatricians with specialized training formed the practice of Neonatal Perinatal Medicine. Recently, there has been a surge in the number of Newborn Hospitalists who care for the well newborn and those with mild illness who can be managed in the nursery or family-centered care unit. Looking at infant health and illness from both perspectives can be helpful as we work on evidenced-based practices, improving infant outcomes, and promoting family-centered care.

In part, based on these observations, this issue of the *Clinics in Perinatology* addresses some of the major clinical problems from both perspectives. We have asked experts in the field to review these transitions, illnesses, and care practices and to provide an update in the evidence-based knowledge on their subjects, hot topics, and practical recommendations. The sections are all written by at least two authors with different perspectives due to their training (ie, hospitalist vs a neonatologist, perinatologist vs a pediatrician). As editors (a neonatologist and a newborn hospitalist), we aim to address each topic from these perspectives. Each article is a review of the latest

Clin Perinatol 48 (2021) xxi–xxii
https://doi.org/10.1016/j.clp.2021.06.001
0095-5108/21/© 2021 Published by Elsevier Inc.

literature and is written to provide guidance for managing common issues that arise in the care of the term newborn.

Anup C. Katheria, MD, FAAP
Sharp Mary Birch Hospital for
Women and Newborns
3003 Health Center Drive
San Diego, CA 92123, USA

Lisa Marie Stellwagen, MD, FAAP
UC San Diego School of Medicine
9500 Gilman Drive
La Jolla, CA 92093, USA

E-mail addresses:
Anup.Katheria@sharp.com (A.C. Katheria)
lstellwagen@health.ucsd.edu (L.M. Stellwagen)

The Term Newborn

Delivery Room Triage and Transitions of Care

Tina A. Leone, MD[a,*], Wanda J. Abreu, MD[b]

KEYWORDS

• Newborn • Term • Delivery room • Triage • Levels of care

KEY POINTS

- Determining the appropriate level of care for newborn infants at the time of birth can affect the health and well-being of infants and their families.
- Infants requiring ongoing therapy after initial stabilization at birth are likely to require neonatal intensive care unit care.
- Infants who are healthy and can perform the necessary newborn functions of daily living (breathing, feeding, and maintaining euthermia) without medical therapy benefit from routine well-baby care provided with the family's presence.

INTRODUCTION

The triage of the newborn in the delivery room and immediate postpartum period involves differentiating those newborns who have transient issues related to the transition from the fetal to extrauterine environment and those that require more urgent resuscitation or complex diagnostic or treatment plans. Often, these decisions must be made in the crucial first minutes of life and can have critical consequences for the health of the newborn. The keys to appropriate diagnosis and management are a thorough maternal, gestational, and delivery history, as well as a thorough physical examination. This information may or may not be readily available in the delivery room, but every effort to obtain the prenatal history should be made. Obvious congenital deformities or dysmorphic features should alert the clinician and may lead to immediate decisions for transfer to a neonatal intensive care unit (NICU) or continued monitoring in a well-baby area. Although encouraging maternal-infant interactions by caring for the mother and infant together is preferred whenever possible, some clinical situations require separation of the mother and the baby for increased monitoring or therapy. Although some newborns clearly require resuscitation and neonatal intensive care, others are not readily identified as critical and pose the true challenge to clinicians.

The authors have no conflicts of interest to disclose.

[a] Columbia University Vagelos College of Physicians and Surgeons, 622 West 168th Street, PH 17-302, New York, NY 10032, USA; [b] Columbia University Vagelos College of Physicians and Surgeons, 622 West 168th Street, VC-402A, New York, NY 10032, USA
* Corresponding author.
E-mail address: tal2132@cumc.columbia.edu

Clin Perinatol 48 (2021) 431–445
https://doi.org/10.1016/j.clp.2021.05.001

The classification of newborn levels of care has been defined by the American Academy of Pediatrics (AAP) and is summarized in **Table 1**.[1] Level I care can be provided with a variety of different care models. These models range from a standard newborn nursery where many babies are cared for in a single room separate from their mothers (the newborn nursery) to a full family-centered care model where newborns and their mothers are cared for in the same room. The latter model has variably been termed couplet care, rooming-in, or family-centered care and requires a significant level of involvement of the family to care for the baby. There are institutions that uniformly provide care either in the newborn nursery or in couplet care, and others that can provide routine well-baby care using a combination of these options. Over the last 20 years, the number of hospitals that routinely provide care for mothers and babies in the same room has increased steadily.[2] This article refers to all of these models of well-baby care as level I units or level I care. The decision to admit to a level I unit or NICU (levels II–IV) varies depending on the model of level I care used at the facility and must always be carefully considered. Additional guidance on the scope of practice for level I units has been outlined by the Newborn Nursery Special Interest Group of the Academic Pediatrics Association.[3] Consideration of the training and comfort level of ancillary health care staff as well as the geographic area in which you practice will affect your decision making. Rural areas may require a significant lead time in the event of need for transfer. Gestational age also plays a significant role in where infants are admitted because this often affects their morbidity and mortality. However, this article focuses on full-term infants and their optimal level of care.

POSTRESUSCITATION CARE

Although it is clear that those newborn infants resuscitated after birth who continue to need any form of respiratory or cardiovascular support must be admitted to the NICU, it is less clear whether infants treated with brief positive pressure ventilation (PPV) or other transient interventions may be cared for in a level I unit. The need for

Table 1
Levels of newborn care

Level of Nursery	Patient Population
Level I: basic newborn care	Healthy full-term infants and late preterm infants (35–37 wk gestation) who are stable
Level II: advanced newborn care	Infants who are more than 32 wk gestation and have birthweight more than 1500 g with moderate level of illness. Level II nurseries can care for newborns who are recovering from intensive care. They can provide ventilation for up to 24 h and more significantly ill newborns before transport to higher level of care
Level III: subspecialty NICU care	Critically ill newborn infants of all gestational ages who may require varied types of ventilatory support, diagnostic modalities, and access to many pediatric subspecialists
Level IV: regional NICU	Critically ill newborn infants of all gestational ages, including those who require surgical interventions in the newborn period and all types of pediatric subspecialists. These NICUs provide transport services and support to other local NICUs

Data from AAP policy statement: Levels of Neonatal Care. *Pediatrics.* 2012;130:587-597.

resuscitation has been associated with hypoglycemia, hypothermia, and poor feeding. The need for resuscitation may also be a sign of prior hypoxic-ischemic insult that may lead to encephalopathy as well as multiorgan failure. Infants with moderate to severe encephalopathy may benefit from therapeutic hypothermia and should be transferred to an NICU that can provide that support as early as possible but certainly before 6 hours of age.[4] However, for infants who have undergone brief, transient resuscitation interventions such as PPV, the decision about where to provide ongoing newborn care is less clear. Frazier and Werthammer[5] attempted to determine whether PPV for at least 1 minute was associated with complications after birth. They found that complications occurred in 61% of the infants receiving PPV for more than 1 minute compared with 3% in a group of matched controls. The complications identified in these infants included hypoglycemia, transient tachypnea of the newborn, meconium aspiration syndrome, pneumothorax, and hypermagnesemia. Even for infants who received PPV for less than 1 minute after birth, Akinloye and colleagues[6] found that nearly 60% of infants developed complications requiring treatment for more than 1 day in a special care (level II or III) nursery. By contrast, approximately 7% of infants who did not receive PPV after birth required treatment in a special care nursery for at least 1 day. Late preterm infants are at even higher risk than full-term infants for complications following resuscitation. Spillane and colleagues[7] found that late preterm infants treated with continuous positive airway pressure alone during resuscitation were significantly more likely to need transfer to the NICU after initial stabilization. It is therefore important to have a higher level of suspicion and a system of monitoring any infant who has needed any form of positive pressure after birth, regardless of the duration. Whether this type of monitoring is done in a level I unit, a special observation unit, or an NICU depends on the resources of the hospital.

The need for resuscitation that involves at least some form of positive pressure after birth is one marker for risk of complications after birth. Other possible markers of risk include low Apgar scores or acidosis identified on umbilical cord gases. Although any one infant may not develop a complication at any given level of acidosis, the risk of complications requiring NICU admission increases with increasing level of acidosis as measured by pH or base deficit.[8–11]

RESPIRATORY DISEASES

Respiratory distress remains a common cause for admission to the NICU. Transitioning from the intrauterine to extrauterine environment happens seamlessly for most newborns. However, the physiologic changes that must occur in the perinatal period are extensive and can lead to transient or even more prolonged respiratory symptoms.[12,13] Signs of respiratory distress in newborns include tachypnea, grunting, nasal flaring, retractions, and cyanosis or hypoxemia. In some infants, these signs are transient and resolve as the newborn adapts to the postnatal environment. However, approximately 7% of term newborn infants go on to require admission to the NICU for further observation and intervention.[14]

The most common diagnoses leading to NICU admission for respiratory causes in term infants include transient tachypnea of the newborn, meconium aspiration syndrome, respiratory distress syndrome, pneumothorax, and persistent pulmonary hypertension of the newborn. Congenital anomalies such as congenital pulmonary and airway malformations, congenital diaphragmatic hernia, trachea-esophageal fistula, and nonrespiratory illnesses such as sepsis can all present with signs of respiratory distress. Undiagnosed congenital heart disease might also present as respiratory distress or cyanosis. The management and complications of these different causes vary; thus, establishing a differential diagnosis also requires consideration of the timing and type of symptoms in addition to diagnostic studies.

It is important to reexamine the prenatal and delivery history to aid in establishing a cause. Information that should be obtained on initial assessment includes gestational age, type of delivery, maternal group B *Streptococcus* (GBS) colonization, presence of chorioamnionitis, and whether the amniotic fluid was clear versus meconium stained. In addition, any prenatal ultrasonography scans or fetal echocardiograms should be reviewed to identify potential anomalies that may cause newborn symptoms.

For infants with tachypnea, mild increased work of breathing or hypoxemia as determined by oxyhemoglobin saturation levels less than the target for time after birth, clinicians may consider a trial of therapy with continuous positive airway pressure or blow-by oxygen and a brief observational period. If the symptoms do not resolve within 20 to 30 minutes, the infant should be admitted to the NICU for further observation, evaluation, and treatment.

NEONATAL HYPOGLYCEMIA

Hypoglycemia presents frequently in the evaluation and management of newborns and is the primary cause for NICU admission in approximately 5% to 10% of term infant NICU admissions.[15,16] The burden of hypoglycemia can cause significant distress to families, and increases the number of interventions to the infant and the burden of care on the nursing staff. Hypoglycemia occurs when glucose delivery cannot meet the glucose demand and can occur at a wide range of values depending on the status of the infant. Following an uneventful pregnancy and delivery, routine monitoring is not recommended in infants who are term gestational age.[17] A physiologic low glucose level is expected in most infants shortly after birth, but most healthy infants stabilize their blood glucose levels between 50 and 60 mg/dL over the first 12 hours of life.[18] A key to screening newborns for hypoglycemia lies in identifying which infants are at an increased risk. Every level I unit should have protocols in place for identifying, monitoring, and treating at-risk infants. These protocols include infants that are small for gestational age (SGA), defined as less than 10% on the appropriate growth curve; large for gestational age (LGA), defined as more than 90% on the appropriate growth curve; infants of diabetic mothers (IDM); and late preterm (LPT) infants. Other categories that might cause a baby to have neonatal hypoglycemia include polycythemia with hematocrit more than 65%, maternal use of β-blockers or oral hypoglycemic medications such as metformin, and evidence of fetal stress such as low Apgar scores or need for significant resuscitation in the delivery room. It is recommended that SGA and LPT infants have their glucose levels monitored every 3 hours for 24 hours, whereas infants that are LGA or IDM should have their glucose monitored every 3 hours for 12 hours.[17]

Although many infants with hypoglycemia are asymptomatic, it is important to be aware of the different minor and major symptoms that may occur in relation to hypoglycemia. Major symptoms, such as seizures, apnea, lethargy, hypotonia, and cyanosis, require immediate treatment and transfer to the NICU. Infants showing minor symptoms, including irritability, exaggerated Moro reflex, tremulousness, poor feeding, and a high-pitched cry, require close monitoring and oral treatments.

Infants who have symptoms of hypoglycemia should be tested regardless of risk factors because this can be an indication of an unknown problem. In an infant without risk factors, additional causes must be considered, such as inborn errors of metabolism, maternal tocolytics, endocrine disorders, hemolytic disease of the newborn, and sepsis.

In the setting of asymptomatic hypoglycemia, the treatment plan should be discussed with the family so as not to interfere with their preferred feeding practice unless necessary. Infants should feed on demand with a minimum interval of 2 to 3 hours in the at-risk population. If a family has chosen to breastfeed an at-risk infant, they should receive early education and instruction to support successful breastfeeding.

At-risk infants who experience asymptomatic hypoglycemia may be treated with 40% glucose gel orally. Oral glucose gel has been shown to decrease the need for invasive intravenous dextrose, decrease NICU admissions, and therefore decrease separation of mothers and babies.[19–21] Use of glucose gel should be in conjunction with oral feedings. The decrease in separation has the potential to increase bonding time as well as limit the need for formula supplementation and support exclusive breastfeeding practices.

Infants who show minor symptoms during episodes of hypoglycemia may also benefit from glucose gel in conjunction with feedings as long as they are clinically stable. In these instances, the physician should be notified, and intravenous (IV) dextrose considered. Infants who remain symptomatic or have persistent or recurrent hypoglycemia may require IV dextrose. In these instances, an IV bolus of D10W (dextrose 10% in water) at a dose of 2 mL/kg (200 mg/kg) is delivered over 5 to 15 minutes followed by a continuous infusion of dextrose. Plasma glucose concentration should be measured 30 to 45 minutes after the initiation of parental therapy.[20] Symptomatic hypoglycemia can result in brain injury and may lead to impaired neurodevelopmental outcomes in childhood and beyond.[22] Therefore, our treatment goal is to avoid potential cognitive, motor, or neurodevelopmental deficits caused by severe hypoglycemia.

CARDIOVASCULAR DISEASES

Fetal ultrasonography and echocardiography identify infants with congenital heart disease in 30% to 90% of cases.[23,24] Those with critical congenital heart disease who will require prostaglandin to maintain ductal patency clearly must be cared for in the NICU. However, fetal echocardiograms also identify infants with congenital heart disease that will not require intervention in the newborn period. Infants with lesions such as mild tetralogy of Fallot, balanced atrioventricular septal defect, and ventricular septal defects are expected to be discharged from the hospital after birth and followed by a pediatrician and a cardiologist as outpatients.[24] Providers must determine which of these infants can safely be cared for in a level I unit. Although many of these babies are asymptomatic in the newborn period, these congenital heart diseases can also lead to symptoms that require more intensive monitoring and treatment. A reasonable approach for any infant diagnosed with a noncritical congenital heart disease on fetal echocardiogram is to have an early evaluation in the NICU or a similar observation unit after birth. The evaluation would include a careful physical examination, oxygen saturation monitoring, blood pressure monitoring, and electrocardiogram. An echocardiogram and cardiology consultation are also useful if available. If this evaluation reveals an infant with stable physiology who is unlikely to require treatment before hospital discharge, early transfer to the level I unit would be appropriate. Any infants who are cared for in the level I unit who develop concerning signs of disease, such as tachypnea, cyanosis, or poor perfusion, should be reevaluated and transferred to the NICU.

Fetal echocardiograms can also be inconclusive and may not identify all lesions. For those that have a question of a lesion, which is often the case for coarctation of the aorta, the diagnosis of disease versus normal variant may not be apparent until the ductus arteriosus closes. For such cases of uncertainty, each hospital must determine the appropriate location for the level of monitoring required to identify critical illness. Coarctation of the aorta and other aortic arch anomalies are among the most frequently missed diagnoses on fetal echocardiogram.[25,26] For those that are possibly abnormal but inconclusive, postnatal monitoring should include serial physical examinations, preductal and postductal oxyhemoglobin saturation monitoring, serial 4-extremity blood pressure monitoring, and serial echocardiograms until the ductus arteriosus closes or the infant develops signs of inadequate systemic blood flow. At the time the ductus arteriosus closes, an undiagnosed critical coarctation of the aorta can lead to circulatory collapse and multiorgan system failure, leading to significant morbidities and even mortality.[25] It is therefore necessary to ensure that adequate sequential follow-up and monitoring can be performed in the newborn period. For infants with normal fetal ultrasonography and echocardiograms, critical congenital heart disease may still be identified by physical examination findings or pulse oximetry screening.

Fetal evaluations can also identify arrhythmias that will require NICU care or further evaluation after birth. The range of rhythm abnormalities identified in the fetus include premature atrial contractions, premature ventricular contractions, supraventricular tachycardias, and varying grades of heart block. Clearly, infants with ongoing serious arrhythmias such as supraventricular tachycardia or complete heart block require evaluation and treatment in the NICU. However, isolated premature atrial or ventricular contractions can mostly be cared for in a level I unit if the immediate newborn examination is otherwise normal. Evaluation after birth includes careful physical examination and 12-lead electrocardiogram. Echocardiogram is likely to be performed if available in the birth hospital or after discharge if unavailable in the birth hospital and the infant is otherwise physiologically stable. Consultation with cardiology and planning according to local resources is necessary.

INFECTIOUS DISEASES

Several infectious diseases can affect newborn infants at the time of birth significantly enough to require immediate evaluation and intensive care for monitoring and systemic therapy. There are also diseases that are not obvious but for which identification from review of maternal history is critical for initiation of early therapy. Diseases such as human immunodeficiency virus ,[27] hepatitis B virus,[28] and COVID-19 (coronavirus disease 2019)[29] do not require separation of the mother and infant but do require early initiation of therapy, prophylactic interventions, or appropriate infection prevention and control measures in order to prevent newborn illness. Others that may require NICU care are discussed further later. It is critical that clinicians present at the time of birth be aware of these potential problems, determine the appropriate level of care, and address the newborn needs in a timely manner.

Early-Onset Sepsis

Early-onset sepsis (EOS), infection within the first 72 hours of life, remains a significant concern in the triage of late preterm and term newborns. Although the incidence of EOS has decreased dramatically to 0.5 per 1000 live-born infants with the implementation of universal GBS screening and administration of intrapartum antibiotic prophylaxis for colonized mothers, GBS remains the leading cause of EOS.[30] Physicians continue to face the conundrum of identifying which infants are truly infected and require treatment compared with those that are healthy and can be observed during newborn care. This decision is made more difficult because laboratory testing in well-appearing infants can be nonspecific. The treatment of infants with antibiotics carries risks because it affects the microbiome, can lead to antibiotic resistance as well as separation of newborns from their parents, and evaluation involves painful interventions. Recent guidance published jointly by the AAP and American College of Obstetricians and Gynecologists (ACOG) provides updated recommendations on the management of infants at risk for EOS.[31] While providing 3 approaches to risk assessment (**Table 2**), the approach favored by many institutions at this time is the EOS calculator.[32,33] This tool calculates the likelihood of EOS based on risk factors as well as the infant's clinical status. The risk factors considered are gestational age, highest maternal temperature, duration of rupture of membranes, maternal GBS status, and whether the mother received adequate intrapartum antibiotics. Meta-analysis of studies evaluating the use of the sepsis calculator found that use of the calculator decreased the use of empiric antibiotics with limited data on safety.[34] Regardless of which strategy is used to identify infants with possible EOS, it is critical to remember that clinical signs of infection are among the most important factors in determining need for antibiotic therapy.

Table 2
Risk assessment models for early-onset sepsis

Model	Factors Assessed	Threshold for Empiric Antibiotic Treatment
Categorical risk factor assessment	• Clinical appearance of newborn • Maternal diagnosis of chorioamnionitis • Laboratory testing for those with GBS colonization without adequate IAP plus: ◦ ROM>18 h ◦ Birth<37 wk GA • Clinical observation for at least 48 h for those who are GBS colonized without adequate IAP and no other risk factors	• Clinical signs of illness in newborn • Diagnosis of chorioamnionitis • Abnormal laboratory values
Multivariable risk assessment (EOS calculator)	• GA • Highest maternal intrapartum temperature • GBS colonization status • Duration of ROM • Type and duration of IAP • Clinical appearance of newborn[a]	• Clinical signs of illness in newborn • EOS risk estimate ≥3/1000 live births
Newborn clinical condition	• Clinical appearance of newborn (intervals of objective observation determined by hospital)	• Clinical signs of illness in newborn

Abbreviation: GA, gestational age; IAP, intrapartum antibiotic prophylaxis; ROM, rupture of membranes.

[a] Increase frequency of objective observations of newborn and obtain laboratory testing if EOS risk estimate is greater than or equal to 1/1000 live births.

Data from Puopolo KM, et al. Management of neonates born at ≥35 0/7 weeks' gestation with suspected or proven early-onset bacterial sepsis. *Pediatrics.* 2018;142:e20182894.

Herpes Simplex Virus

Herpes simplex virus (HSV) remains an infection of critical concern during triage of newborns. The risk and postnatal screening and treatment recommendations are based on multiple factors, such as the type of maternal infection (primary vs recurrent), the antibody status of the mother, type of delivery, integrity of skin and mucosa, duration of rupture of membranes, and gestational age. Women who have primary genital HSV infections who are shedding HSV at delivery are 10 to 30 times more likely to transmit the virus to their newborn infants than women with a recurrent infection.[35] The AAP has developed an algorithm for the evaluation of asymptomatic neonates after vaginal or cesarean delivery to women with active genital herpes lesions.[36] Newborns exposed to HSV during birth should be monitored carefully and consultation with a pediatric infectious disease specialist considered. In following the current guidelines, specimen collection when recommended includes conjunctivae, nasopharynx, mouth, rectum, any skin lesions, and in some cases cerebrospinal fluid. These specimens should be collected at approximately 24 hours of life for culture and/or polymerase chain reaction (PCR) testing. This testing is important because a positive HSV culture from a sample collected 12 to 24 hours after delivery is evidence of virus replication from the infant, whereas, if done earlier, this may indicate maternal contamination.[37] Infants born to mothers who have active primary infection and are asymptomatic or any infant who is symptomatic should receive acyclovir with treatment duration determined by the results of the laboratory evaluation and clinical course.

Neonatal Syphilis

There has been a significant increase in the rates of syphilis throughout the world, including the United States, in recent years.[38] Congenital syphilis can have devastating consequences to newborns and is preventable with prompt recognition of maternal infection and treatment with penicillin. Congenital syphilis can be associated with miscarriage, stillbirth, and neonatal death. Infants with congenital syphilis may have bone or blood abnormalities, meningitis, or neurologic disabilities.

One of the most crucial factors for newborn providers is identifying mothers who were diagnosed with syphilis during pregnancy but were not adequately treated. A recent Centers for Disease Control and Prevention (CDC) report showed that half of US congenital syphilis cases in 2018 occurred because of gaps in testing and treatment during prenatal care.[39] For a case of congenital syphilis to be categorized as resulting from a missed opportunity, a pregnant person (1) needs to have evidence of a diagnosis of syphilis during pregnancy with syphilis testing performed greater than or equal to 30 days before delivery, and (2) needs to have not received adequate treatment of syphilis. Those who did not receive adequate treatment had no treatment at all, only received 1 dose when 3 doses were indicated based on maternal staging, received the doses at improper intervals, received the first dose of treatment less than 30 days before delivery, or were treated with a nonpenicillin regimen.[39]

Suspicion for congenital syphilis should arise if a neonate presents with snuffles, lymphadenopathy, acral rash, thrombocytopenia, anemia, nonimmune hydrops, or pneumonia, although most cases are asymptomatic.[39] All newborns born to mothers with reactive nontreponemal and treponemal test results should be evaluated with a quantitative nontreponemal serologic test (rapid plasma reagin or venereal disease research laboratory) performed on the newborn's serum. Infants born to mothers with no or inadequate therapy and infants whose mothers received therapy less than 4 weeks before delivery need further evaluation, including cerebrospinal fluid evaluation, to aid in management decisions, including type and duration of penicillin therapy.

Cytomegalovirus

Cytomegalovirus (CMV) is a common virus of the herpes virus family, and most people acquire this infection at some time in their lives.[40] Transmission is through body fluids, typically from direct contact with the saliva or urine of babies and young children, sexual contact, via breastmilk to nursing infants, or organ transplants and blood transfusion. Exposure during pregnancy can lead to fetal transmission with serious health effects. The risk of transmission is greater later in pregnancy but it tends to be less severe than when acquired during early pregnancy. Although most infants are asymptomatic and experience no health problems, approximately 10% have identifiable effects at birth.[41] At present, CMV testing is not part of the routine testing of pregnancy. However, if any clinical suspicion of infection is present, then testing the mother and the newborn is appropriate. Prenatal testing can pose a challenge because mothers can have primary infections or reactivation. Primary infection during pregnancy is associated with a higher risk to the fetus.

Clinical manifestations of congenital CMV include intrauterine growth restriction, low birthweight, prematurity, microcephaly, rash, hepatomegaly with unconjugated hyperbilirubinemia and transaminitis, and thrombocytopenia. Neurologic manifestations may include microcephaly, intracerebral calcifications, chorioretinitis and sensorineural hearing loss. This condition can lead to long-term sequelae such as neurodevelopmental disabilities, progressive sensorineural hearing loss, vision loss, and seizures. Long-term sequelae are frequent in children who had symptoms noted at birth but also occur in up to 15% of children who were asymptomatic at birth.[42]

The standard test for diagnosing congenital CMV infection is PCR of saliva, with urine collected and tested for confirmation. Confirmation with urine should be performed, because CMV can be shed by the mother via breastmilk and lead to a false-positive result of salivary samples. In order to diagnose congenital CMV as opposed to postnatally acquired infection, it must be detected before 3 weeks of age. The timing is important because intrapartum and early postpartum infection, although common, do not result in long-term sequelae.

Randomized controlled trials support antiviral treatment of symptomatic congenital CMV with neurologic involvement.[43,44] Treatment options include ganciclovir and valganciclovir for up to 6 months. However, because of the risk of side effects from antiviral therapy, the decision should be made on an individual basis in conjunction with an infectious disease specialist.

HEMATOLOGIC DISEASES

Although anti-D immune globulin therapy has significantly decreased the incidence of severe hemolytic disease of the fetus and newborn (HDFN), 0.4% to 1% of pregnancies continue to be affected by alloimmunization.[45,46] Infants with HDFN at highest risk for invasive therapy may benefit from immediate care after birth in the NICU to monitor and prevent severe hyperbilirubinemia, as opposed to routine care in a level I unit. Infants at highest risk for HDFN requiring neonatal therapy are born to mothers who have Rhesus or Kell alloimmunization identified during pregnancy. In these severe cases, hemolysis begins during fetal life and can lead to fetal anemia, fetal hydrops, and fetal death if not treated. Intrauterine transfusion for fetal anemia can prevent the significant fetal morbidities and mortality associated with HDFN. However, despite fetal therapy, hemolysis continues after birth and can lead to anemia, severe hyperbilirubinemia, and kernicterus if untreated. Neonatal treatments can include phototherapy, red blood cell transfusion, exchange transfusion, and intravenous immunoglobulin therapy. In a study that evaluated the neonatal outcomes for all pregnancies treated with intrauterine transfusion, among those with alloimmunization, 78% of the newborn infants were treated in an NICU.[47] Almost all were treated with phototherapy, most of which was considered intensive. More than half of the subjects were treated with a blood transfusion and more than one-third were treated with an exchange transfusion. This study suggests that newborn providers should consider early NICU admission after birth for infants who required fetal therapy with intrauterine blood transfusion. In addition, others with alloimmunization and positive direct antibody test should be closely monitored for hyperbilirubinemia and transferred to the NICU if needed.

Many other infants at risk for hyperbilirubinemia can safely be observed, monitored, and treated for hyperbilirubinemia in a level I unit. Infants in this category include most babies with ABO blood group incompatibilities and infants with nonimmune causes of indirect hyperbilirubinemia. In these cases, infants can then be transferred to the NICU for more intensive phototherapy, intravenous immunoglobulin treatment, or even exchange transfusion if the bilirubin levels increase to the point of concern.

Fetal and neonatal alloimmune thrombocytopenia (FNAIT) has a pathogenesis similar to HDFN but is caused by maternal platelet antibodies directed against paternally derived platelet antigens. FNAIT is less common than HDFN and can be more difficult to identify because routine screening is not recommended. Therefore, cases may not present until the newborn develops a bleeding complication of thrombocytopenia. Although intracranial hemorrhage often occurs before birth, it may not come to attention until after birth. Infants with FNAIT may not be identified until after admission to a level I unit unless a bleeding complication was identified during the pregnancy or the mother has a history or a prior child with FNAIT. When infants with FNAIT, suspected FNAIT, or suspected intracranial hemorrhage are identified at the time of birth, a prompt platelet count must be assessed and platelet transfusion administered if the platelet count is below threshold or bleeding is present.[48]

NEUROLOGIC DISEASES

Infants presenting with acute hypotonia associated with encephalopathy at the time of birth should undergo a careful evaluation to assess indications for therapeutic hypothermia (**Table 3**). As discussed earlier, infants with neonatal encephalopathy are usually identified by the need for resuscitation at the time of birth. Hypotonia without encephalopathy may also present in the newborn period and lead to a diagnostic evaluation for the cause of hypotonia. The decision about whether these infants should be evaluated in the NICU or a level I unit can most likely be made based on the ability of the infant to perform the appropriate functions of daily living needed at birth, such as the ability to feed and breathe adequately. Depending on the level of hypotonia and other associated findings, clinicians may choose to observe the infant for a period of time in an NICU or may admit directly to a level I unit.

Infants at risk for neonatal abstinence syndrome (NAS) pose another dilemma for clinicians determining the best location for care of the newborn after birth. Care practices for NAS, including the location of observation for onset of symptoms, vary significantly among hospitals.[49] Often infants exposed to opiate substances in utero are admitted to a level I unit and transferred to the NICU if signs of NAS develop. Some hospitals may be unable to consistently use scoring systems to identify NAS in the level I unit and admit all at-risk infants to the NICU. On the other end of the spectrum are hospitals that allow treatment of NAS in a rooming-in environment.[50] Clinicians must consider additional factors regarding the appropriate location and level of care for infants with possible NAS, such as other medical conditions, other substance exposures, and ability of the mother to participate in the baby's care when

Table 3
Indications for therapeutic hypothermia

Category	Indication for Therapy
History	Acute perinatal event such as abnormal fetal heart rate monitoring, cord prolapse, uterine rupture, maternal trauma, hemorrhage, or maternal cardiac arrest
Metabolic acidosis	pH $\leq$ 7.0 or base deficit $\geq$16 on umbilical cord gas or blood gas obtained in the first hour of life
Need for resuscitation	• Assisted ventilation initiated at birth and continued for at least 10 min Or • Apgar score $\leq$5 at 10 min
Neurologic examination consistent with moderate to severe encephalopathy	• Signs of encephalopathy on a standardized examination that may include: ○ Lethargy or altered consciousness ○ Hypotonia ○ Abnormal posturing ○ Decreased spontaneous activity ○ Weak or absent suck ○ Incomplete or absent Moro reflex ○ Abnormal pupillary reflexes ○ Bradycardia ○ Periodic breathing or apnea
Amplitude integrated EEG or EEG[a]	• Abnormal background activity or seizures

Based on criteria from several large randomized controlled trials.
Abbreviation: EEG, electroencephalogram.
[a] Amplitude integrated EEG or EEG are not required criteria for initiating therapeutic hypothermia (although institutions practicing head cooling may include this as a required criterion).

determining the best location of care. In the absence of other factors requiring NICU care, rooming-in may decrease the use of pharmacotherapy for NAS and decrease the hospital length of stay.[51] Ultimately, each clinician must determine where to care for an individual newborn based on both the clinical factors and the hospital policies.

With the continuing advancement in fetal ultrasonography imaging, the identification of infants with differing degrees of ventriculomegaly has become common. When these findings are severe or associated with other anomalies, the need for NICU care is often clear. However, for infants with isolated mild ventriculomegaly, care and further evaluation in a level I unit is likely appropriate. Although an evaluation for additional associated neurologic or systemic anomalies and genetic conditions is often performed prenatally, postnatal evaluation with additional imaging, physical examination, genetic evaluation, and further neurologic evaluation is warranted. Much of this can be performed in the level I unit if the infant is physiologically stable and able to perform the appropriate newborn functions of daily living.

SPECIAL CIRCUMSTANCES

Among the most common genetic syndromes encountered at the time of birth, trisomy 21 offers a unique challenge in providing uniform care guidelines. Although level I care (specifically rooming-in) would be ideal for infant-family bonding and education, infants with trisomy 21 frequently have physiologic reasons to require increased levels of monitoring and intervention in the immediate newborn period. In a recent evaluation of the immediate postnatal care for infants with Down syndrome, Martin and colleagues[52] found that 55% of infants in their population were admitted to the NICU directly after birth and, altogether, 87% were cared for in the NICU at some point in the birth hospitalization. They found that the most common reason for admission to the NICU was hypoxemia, followed by poor feeding. Infants with trisomy 21 are known to have higher rates of pulmonary hypertension after birth and a high incidence of congenital heart disease. Both of these findings may require NICU care. Additional anomalies that may occur in infants with trisomy 21, such as intestinal atresias and Hirschsprung disease, are also potential causes of NICU admission. In many cases, trisomy 21 is diagnosed before birth and the parents have received some initial preparation. However, when a baby appears to have Down syndrome at the time of birth without a prenatal diagnosis, a sensitive conversation with the parents and diagnostic evaluation must take place either in the NICU or the level I unit as appropriate for the infant's physiologic needs.[53]

Another congenital anomaly that may lead to NICU admission is cleft lip and palate. However, infants with isolated cleft lip and palate, cleft lip alone, or cleft palate alone are likely able to be cared for appropriately in the level I unit. In these infants, establishing adequate feeding is the most important factor to ensure a safe discharge from the hospital. Establishing feeding may be done effectively with the involvement of the parents in the level I unit if there is also support from individuals knowledgeable about best feeding practices for infants with cleft lip and palate.[54] Support from feeding specialists and use of specialized feeding devices may be critical in establishing effective feeding that will lead to adequate weight gain in the newborn period. These infants require multidisciplinary follow-up after discharge, which should be established during the birth hospitalization.

SUMMARY

The decision of where to care for a newborn infant after birth depends on both the needs of the infant and the resources available in the birth hospital. Unless there is a medical need, the goal for all term infants is to allow care with the mother at all times to encourage parental-infant bonding, breastfeeding, and education about newborn care. A thorough history and physical examination at the time of birth can help determine whether a medical need for NICU care exists.

CLINICS CARE POINTS

- A newborn's risk of complications after birth increases with the need of PPV (Positive Pressure Ventilation), low APGAR scores and acidosis.
- Routine glucose screening is not necessary in healthy term newborns; however, it is recommended in at risk infants. It is critical to avoid severe and prolonged hypoglycemia as it can result in brain injury and impaired neurodevelopmental outcomes.
- Critical congenital heart defects have a high mortality rate if left untreated. Though there has been significant advancement in fetal ultrasonography and echocardiography, one must also perform thorough clinical exams, vital sign and pulse oximetry measurements.
- Infants presenting with acute hypotonia associated with encephalopathy at the time of birth should undergo careful evaluation to assess indications for therapeutic hypothermia.
- Early NICU admission should be considered for infants with hemolytic disease of the fetus and newborn who required fetal therapy with intrauterine blood transfusion.
- Different approaches to the evaluation of newborn sepsis exist, however, it is critical to remember that clinical signs of infection are the principal factors in determining the need for antibiotic therapy.

- Congenital infections can cause significant morbidity and mortality in the newborn. For prompt interventions to occur, it is critical to identify risks as early as possible and requires effective communication and collaboration between the obstetrical and newborn teams.

REFERENCES

1. Barfield WD, Papile LA, Baley JE, et al. Levels of neonatal care. Pediatrics 2012;130(3):587–97.
2. Barrera CM, Nelson JM, Boundy EO, et al. Trends in rooming-in practices among hospitals in the United States, 2007-2015. Birth 2018;45(4):432–9.
3. Chung EK, Gable EK, Golden WC, et al. Current scope of practice for newborn care in non-intensive hospital settings. Hosp Pediatr 2017;7(8):471–82.
4. Jacobs SE, Berg M, Hunt R, et al. Cooling for newborns with hypoxic ischaemic encephalopathy. Cochrane Database Syst Rev 2013;(1). https://doi.org/10.1002/14651858.CD003311.pub3.
5. Frazier MD, Werthammer J. Post-resuscitation complications in term neonates. J Perinatol 2007;27(2):82–4.
6. Akinloye O, O'Connell C, Allen AC, et al. Post-resuscitation care for neonates receiving positive pressure ventilation at birth. Pediatrics 2014;134(4):e1057–62.
7. Spillane NT, Chivily C, Andrews T. Short term outcomes in term and late preterm neonates admitted to the well-baby nursery after resuscitation in the delivery room. J Perinatol 2019;39(7):983–9.
8. Victory R, Penava D, Da Silva O, et al. Umbilical cord pH and base excess values in relation to adverse outcome events for infants delivering at term. Am J Obstet Gynecol 2004. https://doi.org/10.1016/j.ajog.2004.04.026.
9. Yeh P, Emary K, Impey L. The relationship between umbilical cord arterial pH and serious adverse neonatal outcome: analysis of 51 519 consecutive validated samples. BJOG 2012;119(7):824–31.
10. Sabol BA, Caughey AB. Acidemia in neonates with a 5-minute Apgar score of 7 or greater – what are the outcomes? Am J Obstet Gynecol 2016. https://doi.org/10.1016/j.ajog.2016.05.035.
11. De Bernardo G, De Santis R, Giordano M, et al. Predict respiratory distress syndrome by umbilical cord blood gas analysis in newborns with reassuring Apgar score. Ital J Pediatr 2020;46(1):1–7.
12. Chowdhury N, Giles BL, Dell SD. Full-term neonatal respiratory distress and chronic lung disease. Pediatr Ann 2019;48(4):e175–81.
13. Hooper SB, Te Pas AB, Kitchen MJ. Respiratory transition in the newborn: a three-phase process. Arch Dis Child Fetal Neonatal Ed 2016;101(3):F266–71.
14. Hibbard J, Wilkins I, Sun L, et al. Respiratory morbidity in late preterm infants. JAMA 2010;304(4):419–25.
15. Harding JE, Hegarty J, Crowther CA, et al. Evaluation of oral dextrose gel for prevention of neonatal hypoglycemia (hPOD): a multicenter, double blind, randomized controlled trial. PLoS Med 2021;1–16. https://doi.org/10.1371/journal.pmed.1003411.
16. Fradkin EC, Lafferty MA, Greenspan JS, et al. Neonatal intensive care unit admissions before and after the adoption of the baby friendly hospital initiative. J Matern Fetal Neonatal Med 2020;1–6. https://doi.org/10.1080/14767058.2020.1730796.
17. Adamkin DH, Papile LA, Baley JE, et al. Clinical report - postnatal glucose homeostasis in late-preterm and term infants. Pediatrics 2011;127(3):575–9.

18. Harris DL, Weston PJ, Gamble GD, et al. Glucose profiles in healthy term infants in the first 5 days: the Glucose in Well Babies (GLOW) Study. J Pediatr 2020;223: 34–41.e4.
19. Makker K, Alissa R, Dudek C, et al. Glucose gel in infants at risk for transitional neonatal hypoglycemia. Am J Perinatol 2018;35(11):1050–6.
20. Harris DL, Weston PJ, Signal M, et al. Dextrose gel for neonatal hypoglycaemia (the Sugar Babies Study): a randomised, double-blind, placebo-controlled trial. Lancet 2013;382(9910):2077–83.
21. Weston PJ, Harris DL, Battin M, et al. Oral dextrose gel for the treatment of hypoglycaemia in newborn infants. Cochrane Database Syst Rev 2016;(5). https://doi.org/10.1002/14651858.CD011027.pub2.
22. Shah R, Harding J, Brown J, et al. Neonatal glycaemia and neurodevelopmental outcomes: a systematic review and meta-analysis. Neonatology 2019;115(2): 116–26.
23. Friedberg MK, Silverman NH, Moon-Grady AJ, et al. Prenatal detection of congenital heart disease. J Pediatr 2009;155(1):26–31.e1.
24. Donofrio MT, Moon-Grady AJ, Hornberger LK, et al. Diagnosis and treatment of fetal cardiac disease: a scientific statement from the American Heart Association. Circulation 2014;129(21):2183–242.
25. Lannering K, Bartos M, Mellander M. Late diagnosis of coarctation despite prenatal ultrasound and postnatal pulse oximetry. Pediatrics 2015;136(2):e406–12.
26. Kailin JA, Santos AB, Yilmaz Furtun B, et al. Isolated coarctation of the aorta in the fetus: a diagnostic challenge. Echocardiography 2017;34(12):1768–75.
27. Hurst SA, Appelgren KE, Kourtis AP. Prevention of mother-to-child transmission of HIV Type 1: the role of neonatal and infant prophylaxis. Expert Rev Anti Infect Ther 2015;13(2):169–81.
28. AAP Committee on Infectious Diseases, AAP Committee on Fetus and Newborn. Elimination of perinatal hepatitis B: providing the first vaccine dose within 24 hours of birth. Pediatrics 2017;140(3):e20171870. Available at: www.aappublications.org/news.
29. Saiman L, Acker KP, Dumitru D, et al. Infection prevention and control for labor and delivery, well baby nurseries, and neonatal intensive care units. Semin Perinatol 2020;44(7):151320.
30. Stoll BJ, Puopolo KM, Hansen NI, et al. Early-onset neonatal sepsis 2015 to 2017, the rise of Escherichia coli, and the need for novel prevention strategies. JAMA Pediatr 2020;174(7):1–12.
31. Puopolo KM, Benitz WE, Zaoutis TE, COFN, COID. Management of neonates born at >35 0/7 weeks' gestation with suspected or proven early-onset bacterial sepsis. Pediatrics 2018;142(6):e20182894.
32. Kuzniewicz MW, Walsh EM, Li S, et al. Development and implementation of an early-onset sepsis calculator to guide antibiotic management in late preterm and term neonates. Jt Comm J Qual Patient Saf 2016;42(5):232–9.
33. Kaiser_Permanente _Department _of_Research. Neonatal early onset sepsis calculator. Available at: https://neonatalsepsiscalculator.kaiserpermanente.org/InfectionProbabilityCalculator.aspx. Accessed April 10, 2021.
34. Achten NB, Klingenberg C, Benitz WE, et al. Association of use of the neonatal early-onset sepsis calculator with reduction in antibiotic therapy and safety: a systematic review and meta-analysis. JAMA Pediatr 2019;173(11):1032–40.
35. Brown ZA, Wald A, Morrow RA, et al. Effect of serologic status and cesarean delivery on transmission rates of herpes simplex virus from mother to infant. J Am Med Assoc 2003;289(2):203–9.

36. Kimberlin DW, Baley J. Guidance on management of asymptomatic neonates born to women with active genital herpes lesions. Pediatrics 2013;131(2). https://doi.org/10.1542/peds.2012-3216.
37. Turner R, Shehab Z, Osborne K, et al. Shedding and survival of herpes simplex virus from "fever blisters. Pediatrics 1982;70(4):547–9.
38. Ghanem KG, Ram S, Rice PA. The modern epidemic of syphilis. N Engl J Med 2020;382(9):845–54.
39. Kimball A, Torrone E, Miele K, et al. Missed opportunities for prevention of congenital syphilis -United States, 2018. Pediatr Infect Dis J 2020;39(11):1062.
40. Gantt S, Bitnun A, Renaud C, et al. Diagnosis and management of infants with congenital cytomegalovirus infection. Paediatr Child Health 2017;22(2):72–4.
41. Nicloux M, Peterman L, Parodi M, et al. Outcome and management of newborns with congenital cytomegalovirus infection. Arch Pediatr 2020;27(3):160–5.
42. Dollard SC, Grosse SD, Ross DS. New estimates of the prevalence of neurological and sensory sequelae and mortality associated with congenital cytomegalovirus infection. Rev Med Virol 2007;17(5):355–63.
43. Kimberlin DW, Jester PM, Sánchez PJ, et al. Valganciclovir for symptomatic congenital cytomegalovirus disease. N Engl J Med 2015;372(10):933–43.
44. Kimberlin DW, Lin C-Y, Sanchez PJ, et al. Effect of ganciclovir therapy on hearing in symptomatic. J Pediatr 2003;143(1):16–25.
45. Lieberman L, Callum J, Cohen R, et al. Impact of red blood cell alloimmunization on fetal and neonatal outcomes: a single center cohort study. Transfusion 2020. https://doi.org/10.1111/trf.16061.
46. Bollason G, Hjartardottir H, Jonsson T, et al. Red blood cell alloimmunization in pregnancy during the years 1996-2015 in Iceland: a nation-wide population study. Transfusion 2017. https://doi.org/10.1111/trf.14262.
47. Garabedian C, Rakza T, Thomas D, et al. Neonatal outcome after fetal anemia managed by intrauterine transfusion. Eur J Pediatr 2015;174(11):1535–9.
48. Lieberman L, Greinacher A, Murphy MF, et al. Fetal and neonatal alloimmune thrombocytopenia: recommendations for evidence-based practice, an international approach. Br J Haematol 2019;185(3):549–62.
49. MacMillan KDL. Neonatal abstinence syndrome: review of epidemiology, care models, and current understanding of outcomes. Clin Perinatol 2019;46(4):817–32.
50. Holmes AV, Atwood EC, Whalen B, et al. Rooming-In to treat neonatal abstinence syndrome: improved family-centered care at lower cost. Pediatrics 2016;137(6). https://doi.org/10.1542/peds.2015-2929.
51. MacMillan KDL, Rendon CP, Verma K, et al. Association of rooming-in with outcomes for neonatal abstinence syndrome: a systematic review and meta-analysis. JAMA Pediatr 2018;172(4):345–51.
52. Martin T, Smith A, Breatnach CR, et al. Infants born with Down syndrome: burden of disease in the early neonatal period. J Pediatr 2018;193:21–6.
53. Bull MJ, Saal HM, Braddock SR, et al. Clinical report - health supervision for children with Down syndrome. Pediatrics 2011;128(2):393–406.
54. Lewis CW, Jacob LS, Lehmann CU. The primary care pediatrician and the care of children with cleft lip and/or cleft palate. Pediatrics 2017;139(5). https://doi.org/10.1542/peds.2017-0628.

Cord Management of the Term Newborn

Ola Andersson, PhD, MD[a,b,*], Judith S. Mercer, PhD, CNM[c,d,1]

KEYWORDS

• Placental transfusion • Umbilical cord clamping • Term • Resuscitation • Delivery

KEY POINTS

- Keeping the umbilical cord intact by delaying cord clamping for at least 3 minutes improves iron stores during infancy and supports health and development for the growing child. In preterm infants, delayed cord clamping reduces mortality by approximately 30%.
- Many midwives prefer to delay cord clamping until pulsations cease or until the placenta is ready to deliver and experience good results.
- To warn for risk of jaundice and need for phototherapy after delayed cord clamping is not evidence based.
- A multidisciplinary approach is critical to implement guidelines, training, and education with scheduled audits to increase compliance with delayed cord clamping.
- Intact cord resuscitation has been practiced for centuries at midwifery births, and has shown physiologic improvements in animal and human trials.

INTRODUCTION

Leaving the umbilical cord intact after birth has ensured our survival for millennia. Early cord clamping (CC) has emerged in modern society as a concern in the past century. Recent research has reestablished the value of delayed CC, which many regard as common sense and most midwives experience in their practice.

In the mid twentieth century, with the advance of modern medicine, delayed CC was replaced with the efficiency and expedieny of immediate CC without testing for its safety. Practice was guided by expert opinion and delayed CC at birth was discarded from mainstream practice.[1] For term infants, the focus of this article, early CC decreases hematocrit, blood pressure, blood volume, and iron stores, increases anemia,

[a] Department of Clinical Sciences, Lund, Pediatrics, Lund University, SE-221 85 Lund, Sweden; [b] Department of Neonatology, Skåne University Hospital, Jan Waldenströms gata 47, Malmö SE-214 28, Sweden; [c] Neonatal Research Institute at Sharp Mary Birch Hospital for Women and Newborns, San Diego, CA, USA; [d] University of Rhode Island, Kingston, RI, USA
[1] Present address: 670 Front Street, Marion, MA 02738.
* Corresponding author.
E-mail address: ola.andersson@med.lu.se

Clin Perinatol 48 (2021) 447–470
https://doi.org/10.1016/j.clp.2021.05.002 perinatology.theclinics.com

and seems to result in less brain myelin and poorer neurodevelopmental skills compared with keeping the cord intact for at least 3 minutes (**Fig. 1**).[2–7]

This article focuses on the physiologic effects of placental transfusion on term neonates; the current evidence; benefits and potential risks from immediate and delayed CC; practice recommendations, including special cases such as shoulder dystocia and nuchal cord; and a discussion of further needed research.

PHYSIOLOGY OF PLACENTAL TRANSFUSION

Fetal and Neonatal Blood Volume

Throughout pregnancy, the fetal-placental blood volume is approximately 110 to 115 mL/kg of fetal weight.[8] Waiting to clamp the cord results in a net transfer of blood from the placenta to the neonate.[8,9] The volume of the transfusion can be estimated by comparing birth weight,[10] by measurement of the residual placental blood volume (RPBV),[11,12] and by serial weights on individuals directly after birth.[13] In the Cochrane analysis in 2013, including 12 trials and 3139 infants, birth weight was ~100 g higher in the delayed CC group, compared with early CC.[2] In a study on serial measurements on individual neonates, weight after delayed CC increased by ~87 g.[13]

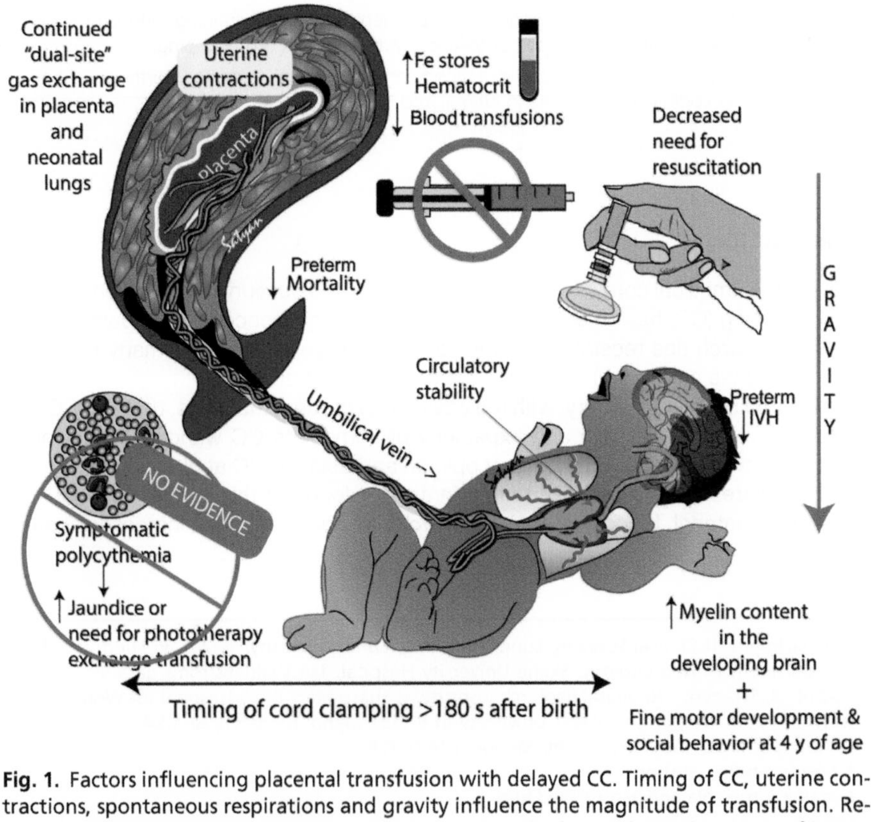
Continued "dual-site" gas exchange in placenta and neonatal lungs
Uterine contractions
placenta
↑Fe stores
Hematocrit
↓ Blood transfusions
Decreased need for resuscitation
↓ Preterm Mortality
Circulatory stability
Umbilical vein
NO EVIDENCE
Symptomatic polycythemia
↑ Jaundice or need for phototherapy exchange transfusion
Preterm ↓IVH
G R A V I T Y
↑Myelin content in the developing brain
+
Fine motor development & social behavior at 4 y of age
Timing of cord clamping >180 s after birth

Fig. 1. Factors influencing placental transfusion with delayed CC. Timing of CC, uterine contractions, spontaneous respirations and gravity influence the magnitude of transfusion. Reported long-term benefits are shown. IVH, intraventricular hemorrhage. (*Courtesy of* Satyan Lakshminrusimha; with permission.)

Circulation

After receiving only 8% of the cardiac output during pregnancy, the pulmonary circulation must increase at birth to 40% to 55% of the cardiac output. An unclamped umbilical cord allows the newborn to equilibrate blood volume, oxygen levels, and pH through ongoing placental exchange.[14,15] Closure of the umbilical arteries occurs later than previously thought,[16] whereas the remaining uterine contractions may help to squeeze additional blood through the umbilical vein.[17,18]

Timing of cord clamping

Extending the time of CC after birth results in an increase in placental transfusion (**Fig. 2**).[11,18]

Farrar and colleagues[13] estimated placental transfusion by measuring infant weight gain while the cord was left intact. The mean amount of placental transfusion was 81 mL or 25 mL/kg. In a randomized control trial (RCT), Chen and colleagues[19] compared 720 term neonates after CC within 15 seconds, by delayed CC of 30, 60, 90, 120, 150, 180 seconds, and when umbilical cord pulsations ceased (n = 90 in each group). With the increase in the timing of CC, neonatal hematocrit at 24 hours was gradually increased.[19]

Gravity and positioning of the infant immediately after birth

Gravity affects the amount of placental transfusion that an infant receives and is interrelated with time of CC.[20,21] Holding the infant above the level of the placenta (>10 cm) slows the placental transfusion, and lowering the infant accelerates it (**Fig. 3**).[20] Clamping the cord at 1 minute with the infant on the maternal abdomen may reduce the placental transfusion by 50%.

Mercer and Erickson-Owens[21] measured the RPBV after infants were placed skin to skin and showed that a 5-minute delay in CC allowed the infant who is skin to skin to receive significantly more placental transfusion than a 2-minute delay (**Fig. 4**).

In contrast, a recent study reported no difference in weight in infants weighed quickly at birth, then placed on the maternal abdomen or lowered, and then weighed again after a 2-minute delay in CC. Weight gain was only half of what was expected after delayed CC.[22] An interpretation of these results is that a full placental transfusion was not completed after 2 minutes in either position.

Cord pulsations

Two recent studies on midwifery practices in the Netherlands and Italy report that umbilical artery flow and pulsations continue longer than the previously thought 1 to 3 minutes after birth.[23,24] Boere and colleagues[16] used Doppler to measure the blood flow

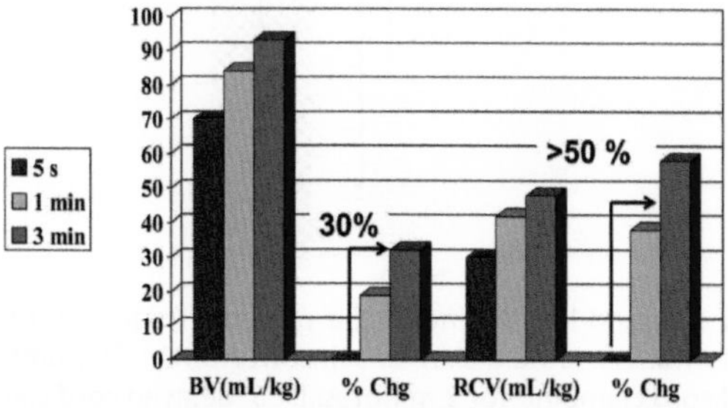
100
90
80
70
60
50
40
30
20
10
0
5 s
1 min
3 min
30%
>50 %
BV(mL/kg)
% Chg
RCV(mL/kg)
% Chg

Fig. 2. Percentage change (% Chg) in blood volume (BV) and red cell volume (RCV) caused by delayed CC. *From* Yao, Lind, et al, "Distribution of Blood between Infant and Placental after Birth," Lancet, Oct 25, 1969. Used with permission of Elsevier, Inc.

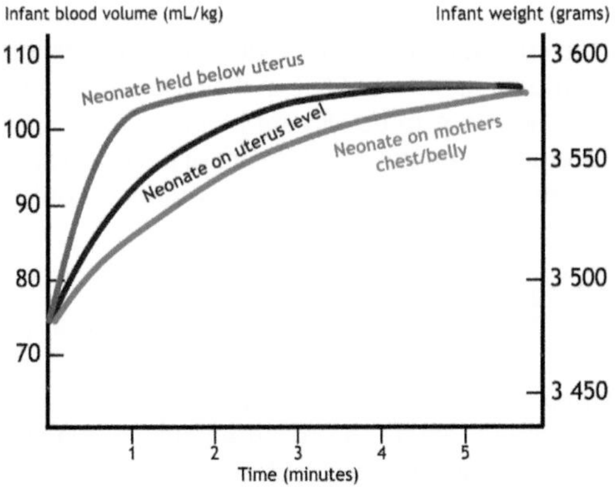
Infant blood volume (mL/kg)
Infant weight (grams)
110
100
90
80
70
3 600
3 550
3 500
3 450
Neonate held below uterus
Neonate on uterus level
Neonate on mothers chest/belly
1
2
3
4
5
Time (minutes)

Fig. 3. The speed and volume of placental transfusion in relation to time and relative position of neonate in relation to the placenta. Conceptual model.

and pulsations in the umbilical cord after birth and before CC. Umbilical artery flow was registered for a mean of 4.22 minutes after birth. When cord was clamped at 6 minutes (Dutch midwifery practice), 43% still had umbilical artery flow that was pulsatile, from the infant to the placenta, and similar to the infant's heartbeat.[16,23] The conclusion was that umbilical blood flow is likely unrelated to cessation of pulsations and that using pulsations as a time point for CC should be reconsidered.

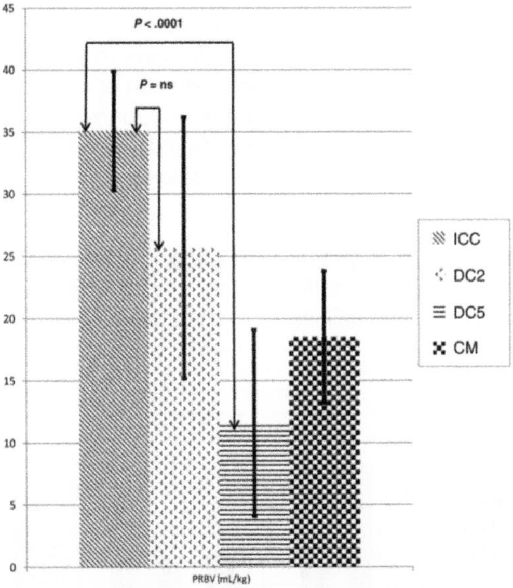
45
40
35
30
25
20
15
10
5
0
P < .0001
P = ns
ICC
DC2
DC5
CM
PRBV (mL/kg)

Fig. 4. The amount of blood left behind in the placenta (placental residual blood volume [PRBV]) when term infants are held skin to skin after birth. CM, umbilical cord milking 5 times; DC2, delayed cord clamping for 2 minutes; DC5, delayed cord clamping for 5 minutes; ICC, immediate CC. (*From* Mercer JS, Erickson-Owens DA. Rethinking placental transfusion and cord clamping issues. J Perinat Neonatal Nurs. Jul-Sep 2012;26(3):202-17; with permission.)

Di Tommaso and colleagues[24] reported that the median duration of palpated pulsation was 3.5 minutes (213 seconds). These 2 studies show that, for term infants, the ideal time of CC remains unknown but extends long after 1 minute. The end of palpable pulsations is likely not to be interpreted as cessation of placental transfusion.

What Cord Blood Contains

The residual placenta blood is body temperature and oxygenated with about 15 to 20 mL/kg of red blood cells, several million to a billion stem cells, and 10 to 15 mL/kg of plasma. The amount of iron provided by the placental transfusions is enough for a 3 to 8 months' supply for a term infant.[25] The large amount of stem cells represents an autologous transplant, which may reduce the infant's susceptibility to both neonatal and age-related diseases.[26]

Progesterone levels in term infants at birth are higher than the mothers' levels, and this high level may support the incorporation of the large volume of placental transfusion.[27] In addition, there are numerous cytokines, growth factors, and important messengers in cord blood that most likely support and drive the process of transition.[26–29] Recent research has shown associations between delayed CC and fewer oxidation reactions[30] as well as a decrease in cord blood lipids and an augmented antioxidant activity, which may moderate inflammatory-mediated effects induced during delivery.[31–33]

OBSTETRIC CONSIDERATIONS

Uterotonics and Uterine Contractions

Some investigators have raised concerns about giving uterotonics before CC. In a randomized controlled trial by Andersson and colleagues,[34] oxytocin was administered after 3 minutes and no negative effects were noticed. Vain and colleagues[35] recently reported that administration of intravenous oxytocin immediately after birth or after a 3-minute delay in CC did not alter the amount of placental transfusion received by term neonates born vigorous.

Cesarean Section

In planned/elective cesarean sections, 2 recent RCTs found increased hemoglobin level and hematocrit in the neonates after 60 seconds' delayed CC, without affecting maternal hemoglobin or blood losses.[36,37] In an observational study, Andersson and colleagues[38] found elective cesarean section combined with CC at 30 seconds resulted in higher iron stores at 4 months of age compared with early CC after vaginal birth. After a pilot trial, Chantry and colleagues[39] suggested CC can be delayed to 120 seconds during elective cesarean section without increased risk of excessive maternal blood loss. The authors conclude that it is safe and beneficial for neonates to clamp the umbilical cord after at 60 seconds in planned/elective cesarean sections.

CORD MILKING

Umbilical cord milking (UCM) at birth speeds up the process of providing a partial placental transfusion to a newborn and, although not physiologic, may provide a placental transfusion in infants that require immediate resuscitation.[40] McAdams and colleagues[41] reported a smaller blood volume with UCM compared with what is reported with a 3-minute delay (**Fig. 5**).

UCM is usually done by stripping the cord from placental end to the neonate over 2 seconds, releasing to allow refill and repeating 3 to 5 times. Studies on term infants show effects on short-term hematological outcomes from UCM comparable with

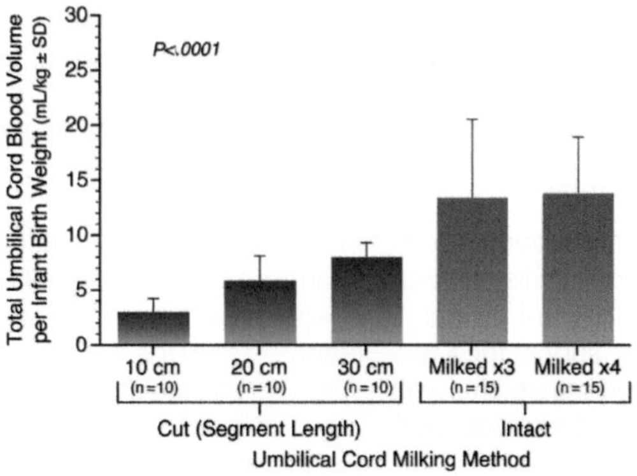
Total Umbilical Cord Blood Volume per Infant Birth Weight (mL/kg ± SD)
P<.0001
10 cm (n=10)
20 cm (n=10)
30 cm (n=10)
Milked x3 (n=15)
Milked x4 (n=15)
Cut (Segment Length)
Intact
Umbilical Cord Milking Method

Fig. 5. Total milked cord blood volume per newborn birth weight. Total umbilical cord milked blood volume in relation to infant birth weight is compared between milked cord segments cut at different lengths (10, 20, and 30 cm) and intact cords milked either 3 or 4 times. (*From* McAdams RM, Fay E, Delaney S. Whole blood volumes associated with milking intact and cut umbilical cords in term newborns. J Perinatol. 2018;38(3):245-250; with permission.)

delayed CC without any apparent harm.[42] In contrast, in the more susceptible population of preterm infants, 1 large RCT and registry studies find increased intraventricular hemorrhage after UCM compared with delayed CC.[43–45]

MAJOR BENEFITS OF DELAYED CORD CLAMPING FOR TERM INFANTS

The major effects of delayed CC/placental transfusion on term infants are outlined in **Fig. 6**. Briefly, the placental transfusion increases hemoglobin level and hematocrit

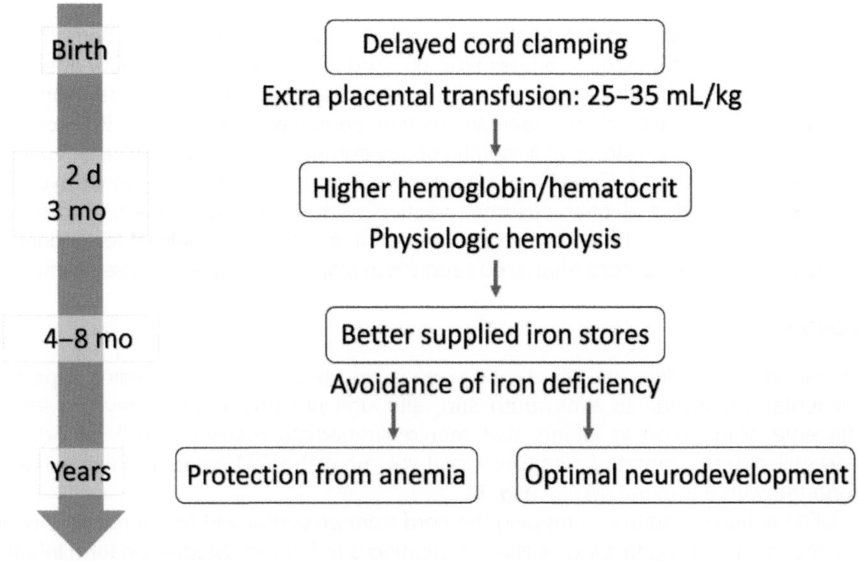
Birth
2 d
3 mo
4–8 mo
Years
Delayed cord clamping
Extra placental transfusion: 25–35 mL/kg
Higher hemoglobin/hematocrit
Physiologic hemolysis
Better supplied iron stores
Avoidance of iron deficiency
Protection from anemia
Optimal neurodevelopment

Fig. 6. The placental transfusion model.

within hours after delivery. Although physiologic hemolysis diminishes this effect on hemoglobin/hematocrit, iron stores are higher in infants with delayed CC.[2] A full placental transfusion increases iron stores for up to 8 months when CC is performed after 3 minutes.[46] This higher availability of iron helps to protect against anemia later in infancy.[3] Iron also provides substrate for an optimized neurodevelopment, including increased myelin content in the early developing brain up to 12 months of age and improved fine motor development and social behavior at 4 years of age.[5,6,47]

Ferritin and Iron Deficiency

Iron is mainly stored as ferritin in the body. Serum ferritin is considered an accurate indicator of body iron stores and is the most commonly used biomarker for identifying iron deficiency (ID).[46] In CC studies, ferritin level has been shown to be significantly higher at 3 to 8 months after birth, comparing CC before 1 minute with after 3 minutes.[2,3,10,48]

A higher ferritin level reduces the numbers of infants with ID, shown at 4 months in Sweden (from 6% to 0.6% of infants having ID), at 6 months in Mexico (from 7% to 1%), and at 8 months in Nepal (from 38% to 22%).[2,3,10,48]

Anemia

Anemia, or low hemoglobin content, leads to impaired oxygen delivery to the body's tissues, which in turn is associated with affected growth and cognitive development in children. Infant hemoglobin levels improved by 0.9 g/dL and anemia was significantly reduced at 8 months postpartum after introduction of a delayed-CC policy in a Peruvian hospital, resulting in an increase in CC timing from 57 seconds to 170 seconds.[49] In an RCT in Nepal, comparing early CC at less than 60 seconds with delayed CC after 180 seconds, anemia was reduced by 11% at 8 months, and by 9% at 12 months.[3]

Optimized Neurodevelopment

The late fetal period and postnatal period through the first 3 years of life are critical periods of rapid development for the brain.[47] Despite its high iron demand, the brain is not the highest-priority organ system for iron distribution because the red blood cells receive priority.[50] Neurodevelopmental studies in nonanemic term neonates as well as infants and toddlers show that ID causes neurodevelopmental abnormalities in brain circuits with high iron requirements. These abnormalities include reduced recognition memory, affect, and motor movements.[47]

Myelin

Iron also contributes to the maturation and functioning of the oligodendrocytes responsible for brain myelination. Myelination progresses rapidly during infancy and is essential for establishing brain connectivity and cognitive function.[47,51]

Mercer and colleagues[4,5] examined brain myelinization by MRI at 4 and 12 months of age in a study on 73 healthy term neonates randomized to either delayed CC (>5 minutes) or immediate CC (<20 seconds). At 4 and 12 months, infants with delayed CC had higher ferritin levels and greater myelin content in brain regions associated with motor, visual, and sensory processing/function. Developmental testing was not significantly different between the 2 groups.[5]

Development

Andersson and colleagues[52] also did not find any differences in neurodevelopment at 12 months of age after 3 minutes or immediate CC assessed by Ages and Stages Questionnaire (ASQ), second edition. However, they performed a longer-term follow-up at 4 years of age.[6] Delayed CC improved the ASQ personal-social and fine motor domains, and the Strengths and Difficulties Questionnaire prosocial subscale. Fewer children in the delayed-CC group had results below the cutoff in the Movement ABC bicycle-trail task. The effect of delayed CC seemed to be more evident in boys, who also showed significantly improved processing-speed quotient in the Wechsler Preschool and Primary Scale of Intelligence test.[6]

Rana used the ASQ third edition to assess development in 332 out of originally 540 infants randomized to either delayed (>3 minutes) or early CC (<60 seconds) and found delayed CC to be associated with an improvement of the overall neurodevelopment, with the most pronounced effects in the communication and personal-social domains.[7]

A summary of the research on delayed CC in term infants is shown in **Fig. 6**.

ARE THERE RISKS ASSOCIATED WITH PLACENTAL TRANSFUSION?

The theoretic risks associated with placental transfusion are a potential increase in hyperbilirubinemia, symptomatic polycythemia, hypothermia, and delayed resuscitation. None of these risks have been shown to be substantial in current RCTs and observational studies (**Table 1**).

There is a widespread misconception that placental transfusion increases an infant's risk for hyperbilirubinemia, repeatedly reiterated in official guidelines,[53,54] mainly referencing a 2013 Cochrane Review, the results of which may be questioned (discussed later).[2]

Systematic Reviews

Two systematic reviews have evaluated jaundice, hyperbilirubinemia, and use of phototherapy in term infants with regard to CC.[2,55] Hutton and Hassan[55] could not find a significant difference between early and late CC. A pooled analysis of data from 8 trials (1009 infants) did not show an increased risk of developing neonatal jaundice associated with late CC.

In 2013, the latest Cochrane Systematic Review reported a significant increase of 1.7% for jaundice requiring phototherapy but no significant difference in clinical jaundice. Neither term is defined in the report. Seven trials with data for 2324 infants.[2]

Recent Studies on Cord Clamping

A summary of findings from recent studies regarding possible risks associated with delayed CC is presented in **Table 1**.[12,19,56–65] No study reported any differences in hypothermia or respiratory distress between delayed and early CC groups.

Mercer and colleagues[12] reported more infants in the delayed-CC group needing phototherapy by intention-to-treat analysis, whereas analysis by actual treatment revealed that there were 2 infants in each group who received phototherapy during hospital stay without differences in peak total serum bilirubin levels or symptomatic polycythemia between the groups.[12]

Rincón and colleagues[60] observed an increase in the number of cases of blood hematocrit greater than 65% in the group with delayed CC after 3 minutes, but no symptomatic polycythemia was reported.

In the light of recent studies, our conclusion is that the risk of jaundice, hyperbilirubinemia, and need of phototherapy is much exaggerated, and rests on invalid conclusions mainly from an unpublished study performed more than 20 years ago. It has become a habit to refer to this risk in recent guidelines, but the authors implore future writers of guidelines to evaluate the evidence before repeating this warning. As for polycythemia, it may be unavoidable to detect an increased occurrence of this as

Table 1
Findings on possible risks of delayed cord clamping in the most recent meta-analyses and studies published after those

	Hyperbilirubinemia	Phototherapy	Hematocrit>65%	Symptomatic Polycythemia
Systematic Review/Meta-analyses				
Hutton & Hassan,[55] 2007	0	0	+	0
McDonald et al,[2] 2013	—	+	0	—
Randomized Trials				
Salari et al,[56] 2014 (n = 56, 180 s vs <10 s)	—	—	0	—
Nesheli et al,[57] 2014 (n = 60, 50–60 s vs ICC)	0	—	0	—
Mercer et al,[12] 2016 (n = 73, ≥5 min vs <20 s)	0	+	+	0
Chen et al,[19] 2018 (n = 720, within 15 s, by 30, 60, 90, 120, 150, or 180 s, or pulsation ceased)	0	0	—	—
Rana et al,[7] 2019 (n = 524, >60 s vs 180 s)	0	0	—	—
Mohammad et al,[59] 2021 (n = 128, 90 s vs <30 s)	0	—	—	—
Nonrandomized Studies				
Rincón et al,[60] 2014 (n = 80, <1 min; n = 31, 1–2 min; and n = 131, 2–3 min)	0	0	+	—
Ertekin et al,[61] 2016 (n = 150, at 90–120 s vs <30 s)	0	0	—	—
Yang et al,[62] 2019 (n = 424, >60 s vs early CC)	+[a], 0[b]	0	—	—

(*continued on next page*)

Table 1
(*continued*)

	Hyperbilirubinemia	Phototherapy	Hematocrit>65%	Symptomatic Polycythemia
Qian et al,[63] 2020 (n = 949, 30–120 s: 3 subgroups [30–60 s, 61–90 s, 91–120 s] vs n = 1005, <15 s)	0	—	+[c], 0[d]	—
Shinohara & Kataoka,[64] 2020 (n = 1211, DCC unspecified)	0	0	—	—
Carvalho et al,[65] 2019 (n = 117, <1 min; n = 228, between 1 and 3 min; and n = 53, >3 min)	0	0	0	—

Abbreviations: DCC, delayed CC; ICC, immediate CC.
[a] Serum.
[b] Transcutaneous.
[c] First day.
[d] Second and third day.

defined, because the placental transfusion increases hemoglobin content and hematocrit in the blood of neonates after birth. To date, no "symptomatic" polycythemia or hyperviscosity syndrome has been reported in the literature to our knowledge.

Conditions Associated with Risk

Small for gestational age and large for gestational age

Although polycythemia is more prevalent in small-for-gestational-age (SGA) as well as large-for-gestational-age (LGA) neonates, in the latter group especially with diabetic mothers,[66] current studies on delayed CC do not report concern for symptomatic polycythemia. In a South African cohort of 104 term newborns with a subnormal distribution of birth weight (39% had a birth weight <2500 g), neither hyperbilirubinemia nor hyperviscosity was observed.[67] In an RCT, Chopra and colleagues[68] reported that delayed CC improved iron stores in SGA infants greater than or equal to 35 weeks at 3 months of age without increasing the risk of symptomatic polycythemia at birth, the need for partial exchange transfusions or morbidities associated with polycythemia. A prospective randomized study on 51 term LGA infants, with 13 (25%) having a mother with diabetes mellitus, found similar rates of polycythemia and levels of bilirubin.[69]

Alloimmunization

An increased rate of hemolysis, as is present in blood group incompatibility (alloimmunization) between the mother and fetus, is associated with higher prevalence of hyperbilirubinemia and jaundice. A few studies have examined the effects of delayed CC in patients with alloimmunization. Garabedian and colleagues[70] studied 72 neonates with fetal anemia caused by Rh incompatibility and reported decreased exchange transfusion needs, improved hemoglobin level at birth, and longer delay between birth and first transfusion, with no severe hyperbilirubinemia after delayed CC. In a retrospective study on 336 cesarean-delivered term and late preterm neonates with ABO alloimmunization, Ghirardello and colleagues[71] reported that delayed and immediate CC had similar bilirubin levels at newborn screening, but immediate CC received a mean of 28 hours of phototherapy compared with 19 hours in the delayed-CC group, whereas delayed CC was associated with more phototherapy and longer time to discharge. Sahoo and colleagues[72] studied 70 Rh-alloimmunized infants after delayed or early CC in an RCT. Hematocrit was higher after 2 hours in the delayed-CC group, whereas there were no differences in the incidence of exchange transfusion or phototherapy.

Human immunodeficiency virus
The risk of virus transmission when the mother is infected with human immunodeficiency virus (HIV) has been studied on 64 mothers and their infants. Delayed CC 2 minutes after birth was not associated with any virus transmission and reduced the risk of neonatal anemia without any differences in polycythemia or need of phototherapy.[73]

INTACT CORD RESUSCITATION

As studies have shown improved outcomes on preterm as well as vigorous term infants after delayed CC, the concept of performing resuscitation with an intact cord has gained scientific interest. The rational is simple and is shown in **Fig. 7**. In addition to the placental transfusion, there is a possibility for the neonate to exchange carbon dioxide and oxygen while the placenta is still attached to the uterus.[17]

Midwives have used this approach for centuries and are inclined to practice intact cord resuscitation (ICR) at birth centers and planned home births.[74] Experience-derived knowledge is that neonates continue to receive placental support during the immediate transition, including when resuscitation is needed.[75]

Since 2013, animal studies have shown loss of preload and decrease in cardiac output producing bradycardia and disturbances in blood flow to the cerebral, visceral, and pulmonary circulation if CC is performed before ventilation.[76–78] Recently, a prolonged CC (10 minutes) in lambs after hypoxia-induced asystole was shown to significantly reduce postasphyxial rebound hypertension while normalizing cerebral blood flow and cerebral oxygenation.[15]

The concept of ICR to reduce further injury in term infants has been explored in a few pilot and/or feasibility trials. Katheria and colleagues[79] compared pregnancies at risk for resuscitation (n = 30 per group) in an RCT comparing 1 minute and 5 minutes of CC. The need for resuscitation was 63% in the 1-minute group and 43% in the 5-minute group. The 5-minute group had greater cerebral oxygenation and blood pressure at 12 hours of life.[79]

In a before-and-after design (n = 20 in each group), effects of ICR in neonates with congenital diaphragmatic hernia was studied. ICR resulted in higher pH and significantly lower plasma lactate concentration. Mean blood pressure was significantly higher 1, 6, and 12 hours after birth in the ICR group.[80] In another study on ICR and congenital diaphragmatic hernia, hemoglobin level and mean blood pressure at 1 hour of life were significantly higher in trial participants (n = 19, CC at 3 minutes) than historical controls.[81]

In an Australian feasibility trial, 44 vigorous infants (≥32 weeks) were enrolled and received greater than or equal to 2 minutes of delayed CC. It was feasible to provide

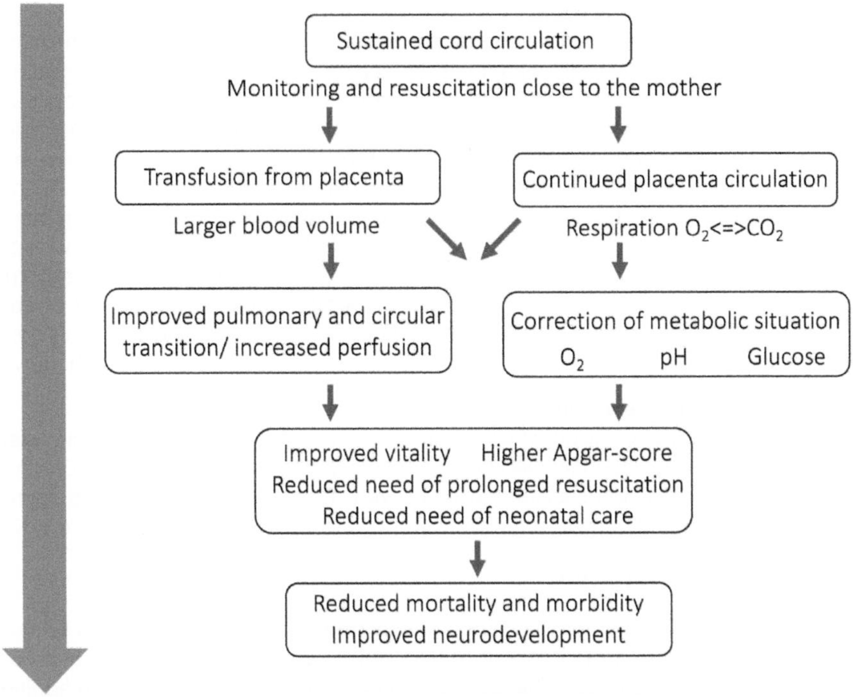

Sustained cord circulation
Monitoring and resuscitation close to the mother
Transfusion from placenta
Continued placenta circulation
Larger blood volume
Respiration O2<=>CO2
Improved pulmonary and circular transition/ increased perfusion
Correction of metabolic situation
O2 pH Glucose
Improved vitality Higher Apgar-score
Reduced need of prolonged resuscitation
Reduced need of neonatal care
Reduced mortality and morbidity
Improved neurodevelopment

Fig. 7. Effects of intact cord resuscitation with sustained cord circulation.

resuscitation to term and near-term infants during delayed CC, after both vaginal and cesarean births.[82]

The largest RCT to date on ICR, Nepcord III, was performed on neonates born vaginally at 35 weeks' gestational age or more randomized before delivery to ICR for 3 minutes (n = 134) or immediate CC (n = 97) and resuscitation.[83] Oxygen saturation and Apgar score were significantly higher in the ICR group at 1, 5, and 10 minutes. Newborn infants in the ICR group started to breathe and established regular breathing earlier than in the early-CC group.[83]

These studies provide new and important information on the effects of resuscitation with an intact cord. Newborns had improved oxygenation and higher Apgar score, and negative consequences were not recorded, similar to findings in preterm infants.[84] The model of ICR is very simple, cost neutral, and likely easily implemented, although with the possibility of almost surprisingly high impact on neonatal outcome.[85]

Nuchal Cord, Shoulder Dystocia, and the Cardiac Asystole Theory

During labor, and especially the second stage, the umbilical venous flow may be impeded by compression either because of a nuchal cord or pressure on the infant's body (occult cord), especially those infants at risk for shoulder dystocia. This condition causes blood to be sequestered in the placenta and can lead to severe hypovolemia at birth if the cord is clamped and cut immediately. The cardiac asystole theory suggests that, when this occurs, the pressure on the fetus in the birth canal functions like an antishock garment and helps to maintain central perfusion, keeping a normal pulse and blood pressure even when the blood volume is low.[86,87] At birth, the sudden release of pressure acts like a fast removal of the antishock garment, and the central blood volume flows rapidly into the peripheral circulation. This sudden and severe lack of central perfusion can result in hypovolemic shock and even asystole.[87–90]

Nuchal cord

Cutting a tight nuchal cord before birth can result in reduction in blood volume (60 mL of blood), resulting in hypovolemia and neonatal anemia.[91,92]

To restore blood volume after a nuchal cord, the Somersault maneuver is recommended (**Fig. 8**).[91] It involves somersaulting the body so that the infant's feet end up toward the mother's feet. The cord can then be unwrapped from the neck to preserve the integrity of the cord to allow for care at the perineum to avert hypovolemia from the blood sequestered in the placenta.[91,93]

Shoulder dystocia

Shoulder dystocia also places an infant at risk for hypovolemia, which may account for the poor condition of these infants at birth: worse than would be anticipated from shoulder dystocia alone.[94] Several cases, with and without nuchal cord, are found in the literature. Cases report head-to-shoulder birth times of 3 to 7 minutes, no prior evidence of fetal distress, asystole immediately after birth, poor Apgar scores, brain damage, and death. Iffy and Varadi[95] reported on 9 cases of shoulder dystocia with a nuchal cord cut before the birth, with 76% developing cerebral palsy. Five recently reported cases confirm these findings. Menticoglou and Schneider[89] present 2 fatal cases of asystole after shoulder dystocia. Heartbeats returned only after volume was administered, but the infants had profound brain damage and the babies did not survive. Cesari and colleagues[90] present a fatal case (after 35 minutes of resuscitation) where labor was uneventful, fetal heart rate tracing was normal until delivery, and resolution of the shoulder dystocia took less than 5 minutes. Two other cases were recently published by Ancora and colleagues,[88] of infants asystolic after delivery,

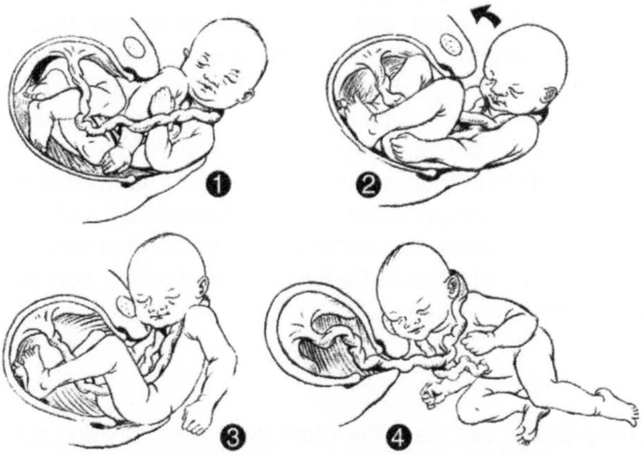

Somersault maneuver. The summersault maneuver involves holding the infant's head flexed and guiding it upward or sideways toward the pubic bone or thigh, so the baby does a "somersault," ending with the infant's feet toward the mother's knees and the head still at the perineum.

1. Once the nuchal cord is discovered, the anterior and posterior shoulders are slowly delivered under control without manipulating the cord.
2. As the shoulders are delivered, the head is flexed so that the face of the baby is pushed toward the maternal thigh
3. The baby's head is kept next to the perineum while the body is delivered and "somersaults" out.
4. The umbilical cord is then unwrapped, and the usual management ensues.

Fig. 8. Somersault maneuver. (*From* Mercer JS, Skovgaard RL, Peareara-Eaves J, Bowman TA. Nuchal cord management and nurse-midwifery practice. J Midwifery Womens Health. Sep-Oct 2005;50(5):373-9; with permission.)

with near-normal cord pH but very low pH on blood gas analysis obtained within 1 hour of life. The practice of immediate CC in such infants is harmful because it puts the newborn at risk for hypovolemic sequelae and death.[87]

Stem Cells

Cord blood is particularly rich in hematopoietic as well as nonhematopoietic stem cells, such as mesenchymal, unrestricted somatic, multilineage progenitor, embryoniclike, and oligodendrocyte progenitor cells.[28] Stem cells secrete neurotropic factors, growth factors, and cytokines, prevent cell death, decrease microglial activation, engraft and differentiate, and promote endogenous stem cell self-renewal.[96] They are part of the body's innate healing system.[26] Damaged tissue releases cytokines, which signal stem cells to travel to the damaged area and begin the healing process. Animal studies have shown that human umbilical cord blood stem cells help to heal almost any inflicted damage no matter how they are administered.

When infants receive the placental blood at the time of birth, they receive stem cells that are in the perfect medium along with the many cytokines, proangiogenic and anti-apoptotic messengers, and growth-stimulating factors. Tolosa and colleaues[97] argue that "artificial loss of stem cells at birth could ... predispose infants to diseases such as chronic lung disease, asthma, diabetes, cerebral palsy, infection, and neoplasm." When stem cells are given at later times, finding the appropriate medium is a major obstacle confronting stem cell therapies, especially when attempting proliferation of stem cells and translation of successful animal studies to humans.[98]

Cord Blood Banking

Cord blood banking involves collecting and storing umbilical cord blood after birth either in public banks or private banks. Stem cell therapy derived from cord blood can benefit individuals with selective genetic conditions, blood disorders, and cancers. However, as more studies show significant benefits to infants from placental transfusion and professional statements recommend delayed CC, ethical issues around cord blood banking become more prescient. The initial autologous autotransfusion that occurs with placental transfusion preserves all components of the residual placental and cord blood for the infant. Clinical trials examining administration of autologous stem cells to children for such conditions as autism, type 1 diabetes, hypoxic-ischemic encephalopathy, and cerebral palsy have not shown the expected improvements.[99,100]

The American College of Obstetricians and Gynecologists states that routine use of private cord blood banking is not supported by available evidence and should not alter routine practice of delayed umbilical CC, with the rare exception of medical indications for directed donation.[101] Parents should be fully informed before consenting to cord blood banking or donation.[102]

PRACTICE

At a normal birth, the provider can place the infant skin to skin, dry and cover the infant with a warm blanket, and leave the umbilical cord intact until the placenta is ready to deliver. Because blood flow continues after pulsations are palpable,[16] it is better to wait until the cord becomes pale, white, and flat and looks obviously emptied. This stage may or may not happen in 3 minutes and, if not, waiting longer is advised. Avoid tension on the cord because this is thought to cause the vessels to spasm and obstruct blood flow.

One caveat is that only infants with good tone should go immediately onto the maternal abdomen. When an infant has poor tone or is slow to start, the infant can be placed on a clean pad at the perineum if the bed is intact, held below the level of the placenta or placed on a cart or trolley placed close to the mother. Preliminary studies suggest that resuscitation can proceed but at the perineum (with an intact cord), rather than on the warmer.[79,83,103] Once the infant is breathing and tone is regained, the infant can be placed skin to skin.[104] It should not be assumed that, because the infant is now breathing, the blood volume has returned to normal: leave the cord intact a longer time for these infants. This method of resuscitation has been practiced for many years in out-of-hospital settings.[74,105,106]

As mentioned previously, if a baby has a nuchal cord or shoulder dystocia and looks floppy and pale and is not breathing, do not cut the cord but instead allow the baby to reperfuse with any resuscitation methods as needed. In the recently published American Heart Association Guidelines for Cardiopulmonary Resuscitation and Emergency Cardiovascular Care, it is recommended that it may be reasonable to delay CC for longer than 30 seconds in term infants who do not require resuscitation at birth.[107] The authors find this recommendation surprisingly unaware of the body of evidence on long-term positive effects of delayed CC, predominantly based on a CC after 180 seconds. For term infants in need of resuscitation, the statement has not changed from the 2015 recommendations.[108]

Cord Gas Collection

Cord gases provide a method to measure the metabolic status of the neonate at birth. It is suggested that the sample be drawn from a double-clamped segment of the umbilical cord and implies immediate CC.[109] The practice of placental transfusion and the collection of umbilical cord blood gases are not necessarily mutually exclusive. Nudelman and colleagues[110] performed a systematic review on 5 studies where blood gases were acquired after delayed CC up to 120 seconds. This delay had either no or only a small and not clinically significant effect on cord blood gas values. In Sweden, blood gases are drawn routinely from the intact, pulsating cord (**Fig. 9**). Andersson and colleagues[34] report this practice in an RCT, showing a preserved placental transfusion and comparable blood gas values.

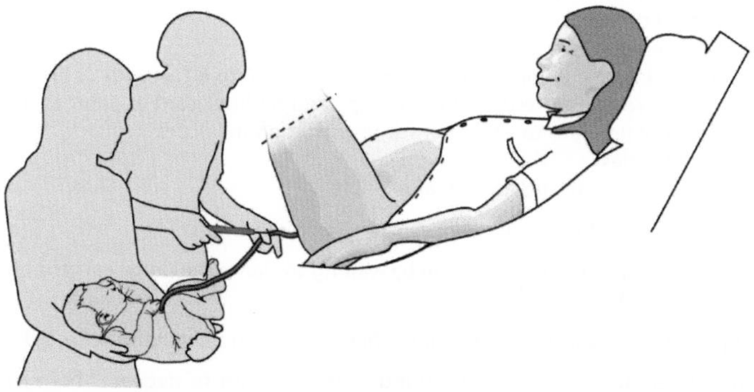

Fig. 9. Blood gas sampling from an unclamped umbilical cord. (*From* Andersson O, Hellstrom-Westas L, Andersson D, Clausen J, Domellof M. Effects of delayed compared with early umbilical cord clamping on maternal postpartum hemorrhage and cord blood gas sampling: a randomized trial. Acta Obstet Gynecol Scand. May 2013;92(5):567-74; with permission.)

CURRENT AND FUTURE RESEARCH ON PLACENTAL TRANSFUSION

Term infants gain ~80 to 100 mL of blood by delayed CC after at least 3 minutes when held at the level of the perineum or placed on the mother's abdomen.[11,13] However, the normal mechanisms of birth, including how umbilical cord circulation is regulated and ended after delivery, are not fully known or understood.

Trials on ICR in term infants are important, to ensure safety, as well as to establish possible long-term effects. Because term infants needing resuscitation are often not identifiable before birth, research involves enrolling large numbers of women before or during labor is an expensive, difficult, and ethically challenging task. A full-scale study in Sweden is expected to include at least 8000 deliveries to yield 600 neonates in need of resuscitation (NCT04070560). Alternatives, such as obtaining a waiver for randomization before enrollment, would make these trials more cost-effective to run. However, waivers for randomization before enrollment are difficult to obtain from institutional research boards because ethics are questioned by some for this method.[111] One trial on cord milking times 4 compared with immediate CC for infants needing resuscitation has been successful in obtaining waivers (NCT03631940).

For the study of rare events such as resuscitation of term infants, case, cohort, and epidemiologic studies, and quality improvement projects are essential and need consideration and the best level of evidence. Preplanning and careful coordination of staff are essential for success.[103,112] A few studies have evaluated parents and staff perceptions of ICR, whereas more research in different contexts and on broader outcomes is needed.[113–115]

For future studies, the authors urge researchers to use bilirubin levels rather than the subjective designation of jaundice or use of phototherapy. Use of a risk tool such as the Bhutani Nomogram for designation of hyperbilirubinemia allows a more objective quantification of levels of risk in comparing 2 groups of infants over time.[116,117] Because intention-to-treat analyses are designed to show the compliance with the protocol, we recommend that results also be analyzed by sensitivity analyses to allow the reader to see the actual effect of delayed CC on hyperbilirubinemia.

Best practices

What is the current practice?

Umbilical CC in term infants

Best practice/guideline/care path objectives

- Vaginal deliveries
  - In vigorous infants, clamp the umbilical cord after 30 to 60 seconds or later
  - In neonates requiring resuscitation, clamp the umbilical cord as soon as possible and transport the neonate to a warmer for resuscitation measures
- Cesarean deliveries
  - Clamp the umbilical cord as soon as possible

What changes in current practice are likely to improve outcomes?

- Allowing for a full placental transfusion by waiting to clamp the umbilical cord until it turns pale (>180 seconds)
- Initiating ventilation during resuscitation while there is an intact umbilical cord circulation
- Providing placental transfusion and smooth transition also to neonates born by cesarean section

Major recommendations

- Vaginal deliveries

- In vigorous infants, clamp the umbilical cord after the umbilical cord turns pale (at least 180 seconds)
- In neonates requiring resuscitation, perform resuscitation measures with an intact umbilical cord (in a research setting)

- Cesarean deliveries
  - Clamp the umbilical cord after 60 seconds or perform resuscitation measures with an intact umbilical cord (in a research setting)

Summary statement

Allowing for an intact cord circulation and full placental transfusion provides a facilitated transition, reduces ID early in infancy, and is associated with improved myelinization and neurodevelopment up to 4 years of age.

Data from Mercer JS, Erickson-Owens DA, Deoni SCL, et al. The Effects of Delayed Cord Clamping on 12-Month Brain Myelin Content and Neurodevelopment: A Randomized Controlled Trial. Am J Perinatol. Jul 21 2020;(EFirst)https://doi.org/10.1055/s-0040-1714258; Andersson O, Lindquist B, Lindgren M, Stjernqvist K, Domellof M, Hellstrom-Westas L. Effect of Delayed Cord Clamping on Neurodevelopment at 4 Years of Age: A Randomized Clinical Trial. JAMA Pediatr. Jul 2015;169(7):631-8. https://doi.org/10.1001/jamapediatrics.2015.0358; Katheria AC, Lakshminrusimha S, Rabe H, McAdams R, Mercer JS. Placental transfusion: a review. J Perinatol. Feb 2017;37(2):105-111. https://doi.org/10.1038/jp.2016.151.

SUMMARY

Placental transfusion is an essential part of the birthing process. The enhanced blood volume provided by an intact cord circulation is involved in interactions with all organ systems to help postdelivery adaption and support the complexity of internal stability during transition.[118] Considering the many interactions in the infant's attempt to regain and maintain homeostasis during transition and placing an emphasis on the effects of an intact cord circulation may help clinicians make further advancements in the prevention and treatment of conditions such as hypoxic-ischemic encephalopathy, bronchopulmonary dysplasia, and neurodevelopmental injury for infants of all gestational ages.

CLINICS CARE POINTS

- Keep the umbilical cord intact for at least 3 minutes or until the cord is flat and white.
- Placental transfusion allows for transfer of the infant's blood volume from the placenta to the infant's body, lungs, and other vital organs.
- Uterotonics may be used at the provider's discretion before, during, or after cord clamping.
- Avoid cutting a nuchal cord before birth - allow infants with nuchal cord and/or shoulder dystocia time to reperfuse via an intact cord after birth.
- Keep infants with poor tone at the level of the perineum.
- Learn how to collect cord blood gases from an intact cord when necessary.
- Resuscitation with an intact cord offers an infant continued placental circulation and oxygenation, improved transition, higher Apgar scores and oxygen saturation at 10 minutes of life but requires a conscious paradigm shift.
- Providing a placental transfusion is an interdisciplinary issue: therefore midwifery, obstetrics, neonatology/pediatrics, and nursing need to collaborate on education and quality improvements to increase utilization of optimal cord management.

DISCLOSURE

The authors have nothing to disclose.

REFERENCES

1. Downey CL, Bewley S. Historical perspectives on umbilical cord clamping and neonatal transition. J R Soc Med 2012;105(8):325–9.
2. McDonald SJ, Middleton P, Dowswell T, et al. Effect of timing of umbilical cord clamping of term infants on maternal and neonatal outcomes. Cochrane Database Syst Rev 2013;(7):CD004074.
3. Kc A, Rana N, Malqvist M, et al. Effects of delayed umbilical cord clamping vs early clamping on anemia in infants at 8 and 12 months: a randomized clinical trial. JAMA Pediatr 2017;171(3):264–70.
4. Mercer JS, Erickson-Owens DA, Deoni SCL, et al. Effects of delayed cord clamping on 4-month ferritin levels, brain myelin content, and neurodevelopment: a randomized controlled trial. J Pediatr 2018;203:266–72.e2.
5. Mercer JS, Erickson-Owens DA, Deoni SCL, et al. The effects of delayed cord clamping on 12-month brain myelin content and neurodevelopment: a randomized controlled trial. Am J Perinatol 2020. https://doi.org/10.1055/s-0040-1714258.
6. Andersson O, Lindquist B, Lindgren M, et al. Effect of delayed cord clamping on neurodevelopment at 4 years of age: a randomized clinical trial. JAMA Pediatr 2015;169(7):631–8.
7. Rana N, Kc A, Malqvist M, et al. Effect of delayed cord clamping of term babies on neurodevelopment at 12 months: a randomized controlled trial. Neonatólogy 2019;115(1):36–42.
8. Linderkamp O. Placental transfusion: determinants and effects. Clin Perinatol 1982;9(3):559–92.
9. Katheria AC, Lakshminrusimha S, Rabe H, et al. Placental transfusion: a review. J Perinatol 2017;37(2):105–11.
10. Andersson O, Hellstrom-Westas L, Andersson D, et al. Effect of delayed versus early umbilical cord clamping on neonatal outcomes and iron status at 4 months: a randomised controlled trial. BMJ 2011;343:d7157.
11. Yao AC, Moinian M, Lind J. Distribution of blood between infant and placenta after birth. Lancet 1969;2(7626):871–3.
12. Mercer JS, Erickson-Owens DA, Collins J, et al. Effects of delayed cord clamping on residual placental blood volume, hemoglobin and bilirubin levels in term infants: a randomized controlled trial. Original Article. J Perinatol 2016. https://doi.org/10.1038/jp.2016.222.
13. Farrar D, Airey R, Law GR, et al. Measuring placental transfusion for term births: weighing babies with cord intact. BJOG 2011;118(1):70–5.
14. Štembera ZK, Hodr J, Janda J. Umbilical blood flow in healthy newborn infants during the first minutes after birth. Am J Obstet Gynecol 1965;91(4):568–74.
15. Polglase GR, Schmölzer GM, Roberts CT, et al. Cardiopulmonary resuscitation of asystolic newborn lambs prior to umbilical cord clamping; the timing of cord clamping matters! Front Physiol 2020;11. https://doi.org/10.3389/fphys.2020.00902.
16. Boere I, Roest AA, Wallace E, et al. Umbilical blood flow patterns directly after birth before delayed cord clamping. Arch Dis Child Fetal Neonatal Ed 2015;100(2):F121–5.

17. Marquis L, Ackerman BD. Placental respiration in the immediate neonatal period. Am J Obstet Gynecol 1973;117(3):358–63.
18. Yao AC, Hirvensalo M, Lind J. Placental transfusion-rate and uterine contraction. Lancet 1968;1(7539):380–3.
19. Chen X, Li X, Chang Y, et al. Effect and safety of timing of cord clamping on neonatal hematocrit values and clinical outcomes in term infants: a randomized controlled trial. J Perinatol 2018;38(3):251–7.
20. Yao AC, Lind J. Effect of gravity on placental transfusion. Lancet 1969;2(7619): 505–8.
21. Mercer JS, Erickson-Owens DA. Rethinking placental transfusion and cord clamping issues. J Perinat Neonatal Nurs 2012;26(3):202–17 [quiz: 218–9].
22. Vain NE, Satragno DS, Gorenstein AN, et al. Effect of gravity on volume of placental transfusion: a multicentre, randomised, non-inferiority trial. Lancet 2014;384(9939):235–40.
23. Boere I, Smit M, Roest AAW, et al. Current practice of cord clamping in The Netherlands: a questionnaire study. Neonatology 2015;107(1):50–5.
24. Di Tommaso M, Carotenuto B, Seravalli V, et al. Evaluation of umbilical cord pulsatility after vaginal delivery in singleton pregnancies at term. Eur J Obstet Gynecol Reprod Biol 2019;236:94–7.
25. Dewey KG, Chaparro CM. Session 4: mineral metabolism and body composition Iron status of breast-fed infants. Proc Nutr Soc 2007;66(3):412–22.
26. Lawton C, Acosta S, Watson N, et al. Enhancing endogenous stem cells in the newborn via delayed umbilical cord clamping. Neural Regen Res 2015;10(9): 1359–62.
27. Sippell WG, Becker H, Versmold HT, et al. Longitudinal studies of plasma aldosterone, corticosterone, deoxycorticosterone, progesterone, 17-hydroxyprogesterone, cortisol, and cortisone determined simultaneously in mother and child at birth and during the early neonatal period. I. Spontaneous delivery. J Clin Endocrinol Metab 1978;46(6):971–85.
28. Chaudhury S, Saqibuddin J, Birkett R, et al. Variations in umbilical cord hematopoietic and mesenchymal stem cells with bronchopulmonary dysplasia. Front Pediatr 2019;7. https://doi.org/10.3389/fped.2019.00475.
29. González-Orozco JC, Camacho-Arroyo I. Progesterone actions during central nervous system development. Front Neurosci 2019;13. https://doi.org/10.3389/fnins.2019.00503.
30. Vatansever B, Demirel G, Ciler Eren E, et al. Is early cord clamping, delayed cord clamping or cord milking best? J Matern Fetal Neonatal Med 2018;31(7): 877–80.
31. Moustafa AN, Ibrahim MH, Mousa SO, et al. Association between oxidative stress and cord serum lipids in relation to delayed cord clamping in term neonates. Lipids Health Dis 2017;16(1). https://doi.org/10.1186/s12944-017-0599-y.
32. Diaz-Castro J, Florido J, Kajarabille N, et al. The timing of cord clamping and oxidative stress in term newborns. Pediatrics 2014;134(2):257–64.
33. Florido J, De Paco-Matallana C, Quezada MS, et al. Umbilical cord serum lipids between early and late clamping in full-term newborns. A systematic assignment treatment group. J Matern Fetal Neonatal Med 2015;28(2):186–9.
34. Andersson O, Hellstrom-Westas L, Andersson D, et al. Effects of delayed compared with early umbilical cord clamping on maternal postpartum hemorrhage and cord blood gas sampling: a randomized trial. Acta Obstet Gynecol Scand 2013;92(5):567–74.

35. Vain NE, Satragno DS, Gordillo JE, et al. Postpartum use of oxytocin and volume of placental transfusion: a randomised controlled trial. Arch Dis Child Fetal Neonatal Ed 2020;105(1):14–7.
36. Cavallin F, Galeazzo B, Loretelli V, et al. Delayed cord clamping versus early cord clamping in elective cesarean section: a randomized controlled trial. Neonatology 2019;116(3):252–9.
37. Purisch SE, Ananth CV, Arditi B, et al. Effect of delayed vs immediate umbilical cord clamping on maternal blood loss in term cesarean delivery. JAMA 2019; 322(19):1869.
38. Andersson O, Hellstrom-Westas L, Domellof M. Elective caesarean: does delay in cord clamping for 30 s ensure sufficient iron stores at 4 months of age? A historical cohort control study. BMJ Open 2016;6(11):e012995.
39. Chantry CJ, Blanton A, Taché V, et al. Delayed cord clamping during elective cesarean deliveries: results of a pilot safety trial. Matern Health Neonatol Perinatol 2018;4(1). https://doi.org/10.1186/s40748-018-0083-3.
40. Ortiz-Esquinas I, Rodríguez-Almagro J, Gómez-Salgado J, et al. Effects of cord milking in late preterm infants and full-term infants: a systematic review and meta-analysis. Birth 2020;47(3):259–69.
41. McAdams RM, Fay E, Delaney S. Whole blood volumes associated with milking intact and cut umbilical cords in term newborns. J Perinatol 2018;38(3):245–50.
42. Jeevan A, Ananthan A, Bhuwan M, et al. Umbilical cord milking versus delayed cord clamping in term and late-preterm infants: a systematic review and meta-analysis. J Matern Fetal Neonatal Med 2021;1–11. https://doi.org/10.1080/14767058.2021.1884676.
43. Katheria A, Reister F, Essers J, et al. Association of umbilical cord milking vs delayed umbilical cord clamping with death or severe intraventricular hemorrhage among preterm infants. JAMA 2019;322(19):1877–86.
44. Balasubramanian H, Ananthan A, Jain V, et al. Umbilical cord milking in preterm infants: a systematic review and meta-analysis. Arch Dis Child Fetal Neonatal Ed 2020;105(6):572–80.
45. El-Naggar W, Afifi J, Dorling J, et al. A comparison of strategies for managing the umbilical cord at birth in preterm infants. J Pediatr 2020;225:58–64.e4.
46. Domellof M, Braegger C, Campoy C, et al. Iron requirements of infants and toddlers. J Pediatr Gastroenterol Nutr 2014;58(1):119–29.
47. Georgieff MK. Iron assessment to protect the developing brain. Am J Clin Nutr 2017;106(Supplement 6):1588S–93S.
48. Chaparro CM, Neufeld LM, Tena Alavez G, et al. Effect of timing of umbilical cord clamping on iron status in Mexican infants: a randomised controlled trial. Lancet 2006;367(9527):1997–2004.
49. Gyorkos TW, Maheu-Giroux M, Blouin B, et al. A hospital policy change toward delayed cord clamping is effective in improving hemoglobin levels and anemia status of 8-month-old Peruvian infants. J Trop Pediatr Dec 2012;58(6):435–40.
50. Zamora TG, Guiang SF, Widness JA, et al. Iron is prioritized to red blood cells over the brain in phlebotomized anemic newborn lambs. Pediatr Res 2016; 79(6):922–8.
51. Todorich B, Pasquini JM, Garcia CI, et al. Oligodendrocytes and myelination: the role of iron. Glia 2009;57(5):467–78.
52. Andersson O, Domellof M, Andersson D, et al. Effect of delayed vs early umbilical cord clamping on iron status and neurodevelopment at age 12 months: a randomized clinical trial. JAMA Pediatr 2014;168(6):547–54.

53. Delgado Nunes V, Gholitabar M, Sims JM, et al. Intrapartum care of healthy women and their babies: summary of updated NICE guidance. BMJ 2014; 349:g6886.
54. Delayed umbilical cord clamping after birth: ACOG committee opinion, number 814. Obstet Gynecol 2020;136(6):e100–6.
55. Hutton EK, Hassan ES. Late vs early clamping of the umbilical cord in full-term neonates: systematic review and meta-analysis of controlled trials. JAMA 2007; 297(11):1241–52.
56. Salari Z, Rezapour M, Khalili N. Late umbilical cord clamping, neonatal hematocrit and Apgar scores: a randomized controlled trial. J Neonatal Perinatal Med 2014;7(4):287–91.
57. Nesheli HM, Esmailzadeh S, Haghshenas M, et al. Effect of late vs early clamping of the umbilical cord (on haemoglobin level) in full-term neonates. J Pak Med Assoc 2014;64(11):1303–5.
58. Rana N, Ranneberg LJ, Malqvist M, et al. Delayed cord clamping was not associated with an increased risk of hyperbilirubinaemia on the day of birth or jaundice in the first 4 weeks. Acta Paediatr 2020;109(1):71–7.
59. Mohammad K, Tailakh S, Fram K, et al. Effects of early umbilical cord clamping versus delayed clamping on maternal and neonatal outcomes: a Jordanian study. J Matern Fetal Neonatal Med 2021;34(2):231–7.
60. Rincón D, Foguet A, Rojas M, et al. Tiempo de pinzamiento del cordón umbilical y complicaciones neonatales, un estudio prospectivo. An Pediatr (Barc) 2014; 81(3):142–8.
61. Ertekin AA, Nihan Ozdemir N, Sahinoglu Z, et al. Term babies with delayed cord clamping: an approach in preventing anemia. J Matern Fetal Neonatal Med 2016;29(17):2813–6.
62. Yang S, Duffy JY, Johnston R, et al. Association of a delayed cord-clamping protocol with hyperbilirubinemia in term neonates. Obstet Gynecol 2019;133(4): 754–61.
63. Qian Y, Lu Q, Shao H, et al. Timing of umbilical cord clamping and neonatal jaundice in singleton term pregnancy. Early Hum Dev 2020;142:104948.
64. Shinohara E, Kataoka Y. Prevalence and risk factors for hyperbilirubinemia among newborns from a low-risk birth setting using delayed cord clamping in Japan. Jpn J Nurs Sci 2020. https://doi.org/10.1111/jjns.12372.
65. Carvalho OMC, Augusto MCC, Medeiros MQ, et al. Late umbilical cord clamping does not increase rates of jaundice and the need for phototherapy in pregnancies at normal risk. J Matern Fetal Neonatal Med 2019;32(22):3824–9.
66. Kates EH, Kates JS. Anemia and polycythemia in the newborn. Pediatr Rev 2007;28(1):33–4.
67. Tiemersma S, Heistein J, Ruijne R, et al. Delayed cord clamping in South African neonates with expected low birthweight: a randomised controlled trial. Trop Med Int Health 2015;20(2):177–83.
68. Chopra A, Thakur A, Garg P, et al. Early versus delayed cord clamping in small for gestational age infants and iron stores at 3 months of age - a randomized controlled trial. BMC Pediatr 2018;18(1):234.
69. Vural I, Ozdemir H, Teker G, et al. Delayed cord clamping in term large-for-gestational age infants: a prospective randomised study. J Paediatr Child Health 2019;55(5):555–60.
70. Garabedian C, Rakza T, Drumez E, et al. Benefits of delayed cord clamping in red blood cell alloimmunization. Pediatrics 2016;137(3):e20153236.

71. Ghirardello S, Crippa BL, Cortesi V, et al. Delayed cord clamping increased the need for phototherapy treatment in infants with AB0 alloimmunization born by cesarean section: a retrospective study. Front Pediatr 2018;6. https://doi.org/10.3389/fped.2018.00241.
72. Sahoo T, Thukral A, Sankar MJ, et al. Delayed cord clamping in Rh-alloimmunised infants: a randomised controlled trial. Eur J Pediatr 2020;179(6):881–9.
73. Pogliani L, Erba P, Nannini P, et al. Effects and safety of delayed versus early umbilical cord clamping in newborns of HIV-infected mothers. J Matern Fetal Neonatal Med 2019;32(4):646–9.
74. Fulton C, Stoll K, Thordarson D. Bedside resuscitation of newborns with an intact umbilical cord: experiences of midwives from British Columbia. Midwifery 2016;34:42–6.
75. Mercer JS, Nelson CC, Skovgaard RL. Umbilical cord clamping: beliefs and practices of American nurse-midwives. J Midwifery Womens Health 2000;45(1):58–66.
76. Bhatt S, Alison BJ, Wallace EM, et al. Delaying cord clamping until ventilation onset improves cardiovascular function at birth in preterm lambs. J Physiol 2013;591(8):2113–26.
77. Polglase GR, Dawson JA, Kluckow M, et al. Ventilation onset prior to umbilical cord clamping (physiological-based cord clamping) improves systemic and cerebral oxygenation in preterm lambs. PLoS One 2015;10(2):e0117504.
78. Hooper SB, Kitchen MJ, Polglase GR, et al. The physiology of neonatal resuscitation. Curr Opin Pediatr 2018;30(2):187–91.
79. Katheria AC, Brown MK, Faksh A, et al. Delayed cord clamping in newborns born at term at risk for resuscitation: a feasibility randomized clinical trial. J Pediatr 2017;187:313–7.e1.
80. Lefebvre C, Rakza T, Weslinck N, et al. Feasibility and safety of intact cord resuscitation in newborn infants with congenital diaphragmatic hernia (CDH). Resuscitation 2017;120:20–5.
81. Foglia EE, Ades A, Hedrick HL, et al. Initiating resuscitation before umbilical cord clamping in infants with congenital diaphragmatic hernia: a pilot feasibility trial. Arch Dis Child Fetal Neonatal Ed 2020;105(3):322–6.
82. Blank DA, Badurdeen S, Omar FKC, et al. Baby-directed umbilical cord clamping: a feasibility study. Resuscitation 2018;131:1–7.
83. Andersson O, Rana N, Ewald U, et al. Intact cord resuscitation versus early cord clamping in the treatment of depressed newborn infants during the first 10 minutes of birth (Nepcord III) - a randomized clinical trial. Matern Health Neonatol Perinatol 2019;5(1):15.
84. Knol R, Brouwer E, Van Den Akker T, et al. Physiological-based cord clamping in very preterm infants — randomised controlled trial on effectiveness of stabilisation. Resuscitation 2020;147:26–33.
85. Chou D, Daelmans B, Jolivet RR, et al. Ending preventable maternal and newborn mortality and stillbirths. BMJ 2015;351:h4255.
86. Miller S, Turan JM, Ojengbede A, et al. The pilot study of the non-pneumatic anti-shock garment (NASG) in women with severe obstetric hemorrhage: combined results from Egypt and Nigeria. Int J Gynaecol Obstet 2006;94(Suppl 2):S154–6.
87. Mercer J, Erickson-Owens D, Skovgaard R. Cardiac asystole at birth: is hypovolemic shock the cause? Med Hypotheses 2009;72(4):458–63.
88. Ancora G, Meloni C, Soffritti S, et al. Intrapartum asphyxiated newborns without fetal heart rate and cord blood gases abnormalities: two case reports of

shoulder dystocia to reflect upon. Front Pediatr 2020;8. https://doi.org/10.3389/fped.2020.570332.
89. Menticoglou S, Schneider C. Resuscitating the baby after shoulder dystocia. Case Rep Obstet Gynecol 2016;2016:1–3.
90. Cesari E, Ghirardello S, Brembilla G, et al. Clinical features of a fatal shoulder dystocia: the hypovolemic shock hypothesis. Med Hypotheses 2018;118:139–41.
91. Mercer JS, Skovgaard RL, Peareara-Eaves J, et al. Nuchal cord management and nurse-midwifery practice. J Midwifery Womens Health 2005;50(5):373–9.
92. Iffy L, Varadi V, Papp E. Untoward neonatal sequelae deriving from cutting of the umbilical cord before delivery. Med Law 2001;20(4):627–34.
93. Vanhaesebrouck P, Vanneste K, de Praeter C, et al. Tight nuchal cord and neonatal hypovolaemic shock. Arch Dis Child 1987;62(12):1276–7.
94. Hope P, Breslin S, Lamont L, et al. Fatal shoulder dystocia: a review of 56 cases reported to the confidential enquiry into stillbirths and deaths in infancy. Br J Obstet Gynaecol 1998;105(12):1256–61.
95. Iffy L, Varadi V. Cerebral palsy following cutting of the nuchal cord before delivery. Med Law 1994;13(3–4):323–30.
96. Liao Y, Cotten M, Tan S, et al. Rescuing the neonatal brain from hypoxic injury with autologous cord blood. Bone Marrow Transplant 2013;48(7):890–900.
97. Tolosa JN, Park D-H, Eve DJ, et al. Mankind's first natural stem cell transplant. J Cell Mol Med 2010;14(3):488–95.
98. Baker EK, Jacobs SE, Lim R, et al. Cell therapy for the preterm infant: promise and practicalities. Arch Dis Child Fetal Neonatal Ed 2020;105(5):563–8.
99. Peberdy L, Young J, Kearney L. Health care professionals' knowledge, attitudes and practices relating to umbilical cord blood banking and donation: an integrative review. BMC Pregnancy Childbirth 2016;16(1). https://doi.org/10.1186/s12884-016-0863-6.
100. Dawson G, Sun JM, Baker J, et al. A phase II randomized clinical trial of the safety and efficacy of intravenous umbilical cord blood infusion for treatment of children with autism spectrum disorder. J Pediatr 2020;222:164–73.e5.
101. ACOG committee opinion No. 771: umbilical cord blood banking. Obstet Gynecol 2019;133(3):e249–53.
102. Brown N, Williams R. Cord blood banking – bio-objects on the borderlands between community and immunity. Life Sci Soc Policy 2015;11(1). https://doi.org/10.1186/s40504-015-0029-8.
103. Saether E, Gulpen FR, Jensen C, et al. Neonatal transitional support with intact umbilical cord in assisted vaginal deliveries: a quality-improvement cohort study. BMC Pregnancy Childbirth 2020;20(1):496.
104. Katheria AC, Brown MK, Rich W, et al. Providing a placental transfusion in newborns who need resuscitation. Front Pediatr 2017;5:1.
105. Mercer JS, Skovgaard RL. Neonatal transitional physiology: a new paradigm. J Perinat Neonatal Nurs 2002;15(4):56–75.
106. Leslie MS, Erickson-Owens D, Park J. Umbilical cord practices of members of the American College of nurse-midwives. J Midwifery Womens Health 2020;65(4):520–8.
107. Aziz K, Lee HC, Escobedo MB, et al. Part 5: neonatal resuscitation: 2020 American Heart Association guidelines for cardiopulmonary resuscitation and emergency cardiovascular care. Circulation 2020;142(16_suppl_2). https://doi.org/10.1161/cir.0000000000000902.

108. Perlman JM, Wyllie J, Kattwinkel J, et al. Part 7: neonatal resuscitation: 2015 international consensus on cardiopulmonary resuscitation and emergency cardiovascular care science with treatment recommendations. Circulation 2015; 132(16 suppl 1):S204–41.
109. Armstrong L, Stenson BJ. Use of umbilical cord blood gas analysis in the assessment of the newborn. Arch Dis Child Fetal Neonatal Ed 2007;92(6): F430–4.
110. Nudelman MJR, Belogolovsky E, Jegatheesan P, et al. Effect of delayed cord clamping on umbilical blood gas values in term newborns. Obstet Gynecol 2020;135(3):576–82.
111. Katheria AC, Allman P, Szychowski JM, et al. Perinatal outcomes of subjects enrolled in a multicenter trial with a waiver of antenatal consent. Am J Perinatol 2020. https://doi.org/10.1055/s-0040-1719184.
112. Anton O, Jordan H, Rabe H. Strategies for implementing placental transfusion at birth: a systematic review. Birth 2019;46(3):411–27.
113. Sawyer A, Ayers S, Bertullies S, et al. Providing immediate neonatal care and resuscitation at birth beside the mother: parents' views, a qualitative study. BMJ Open 2015;5(9):e008495.
114. Katheria AC, Sorkhi SR, Hassen K, et al. Acceptability of bedside resuscitation with intact umbilical cord to clinicians and patients' families in the United States. Front Pediatr 2018;6:100.
115. Thomas M, Yoxall C, Weeks A, et al. Providing newborn resuscitation at the mother's bedside: assessing the safety, usability and acceptability of a mobile trolley. BMC Pediatr 2014;14(1):135.
116. Bhutani VK, Gourley GR, Adler S, et al. Noninvasive measurement of total serum bilirubin in a multiracial predischarge newborn population to assess the risk of severe hyperbilirubinemia. Pediatrics 2000;106(2):e17.
117. American Academy of Pediatrics Subcommittee on H. Management of hyperbilirubinemia in the newborn infant 35 or more weeks of gestation. Pediatrics 2004;114(1):297–316.
118. Billman GE. Homeostasis: the underappreciated and far too often ignored central organizing principle of physiology. Front Physiol 2020;11. https://doi.org/10.3389/fphys.2020.00200.

The Term Newborn

Early-Onset Sepsis

Karen M. Puopolo, MD, PhD[a,b,*],
Sagori Mukhopadhay, MD, MMSc[a,b], Adam Frymoyer, MD[c],
William E. Benitz, MD[c]

KEYWORDS

• Newborn • Early-onset sepsis • Antibiotics • Risk assessment

KEY POINTS

- Although early-onset sepsis (EOS) has become a rare disease, its risk remains among the most common reasons for medical interventions in term newborns, leading to diagnostic evaluations and empirical antibiotic treatment of far more infants than are actually infected.
- Despite substantial reduction of its incidence by intrapartum maternal prophylaxis, group B *Streptococcus* remains the organism most commonly isolated from term infants with EOS.
- When compared with historical categorical approaches, strategies for individualized risk assessment can markedly reduce testing and treatment of well-appearing term infants.
- Ampicillin and gentamicin remain the first-line choice for empirical treatment of EOS.
- Results of properly collected bacterial cultures allow neonatal care providers to discontinue antibiotic treatment when cultures are sterile and narrow the antibiotic regimen when infection is confirmed, reducing selection pressure for antibiotic-resistant pathogens.

INTRODUCTION

In 2017, bacterial sepsis was the fifth most common cause of death in the neonatal period in the United States, resulting in 576 deaths.[1] Neonatal early-onset sepsis (EOS) is typically defined for term infants (born ≥37 weeks' gestations) as invasive bacterial infection detected within 0 to 2 days (<72 hours) after birth,[2,3] although cases may present up to 6 days after birth.[4] Since 2005, the overall EOS incidence among preterm and term infants has remained stable at 0.7 to 0.8 cases per 1000 live births

[a] Division of Neonatology, Department of Pediatrics, Children's Hospital of Philadelphia Newborn Care at Pennsylvania Hospital, 800 Spruce Street, Philadelphia, PA 19107, USA; [b] Department of Pediatrics, University of Pennsylvania Perelman School of Medicine, Philadelphia, PA, USA; [c] Department of Pediatrics-Neonatology, Stanford University, 453 Quarry Road, MC: 5660, Palo Alto, CA 94304, USA
* Corresponding author. Children's Hospital of Philadelphia Newborn Care, Pennsylvania Hospital, 800 Spruce Street, Philadelphia, PA 19107.
E-mail address: puopolok@chop.edu

Clin Perinatol 48 (2021) 471–484
https://doi.org/10.1016/j.clp.2021.05.003

(LB).[2,3] Identifying and managing infants at risk for EOS is part of routine care provided by neonatal clinicians, and most centers use standardized screening approaches to facilitate consistent care.[5] Similarly, infants undergoing sepsis evaluations comprise a substantial proportion of neonatal intensive care unit (NICU) admissions.[6–8] Many of these admissions are well-appearing term infants, in whom the risks of evaluating for sepsis, including mother-infant separation and exposure to antibiotics, must be balanced with the risk from unidentified infection.[7,9] The challenge of minimizing unnecessary medicalization of term newborns while maintaining safety is well recognized,[10] and different approaches to improving this balance have been reported.[11–14] In this article, we describe the current epidemiology and outline the recommended approaches to the timely identification and management of EOS among term infants.[15]

EPIDEMIOLOGY AND MICROBIOLOGY OF EARLY-ONSET SEPSIS AMONG TERM INFANTS

The incidence of EOS among term infants is approximately 0.5 cases per 1000 LB.[2] The 2 most common pathogens causing EOS are group B *Streptococcus* (GBS) followed by *Escherichia coli*.[3,16] In contrast, *E coli* is the most commonly isolated organism among very-low-birth-weight preterm infants.[3,16] Other pathogens isolated in EOS cases, across gestational ages and specifically among term infants, are shown in **Table 1**.

National estimates for incidence of GBS EOS among term infants decreased from 0.30 to 0.17 per 1000 LB (2006–2015), whereas those for *E coli* remained stable at ~0.08 per 1000 LB (2005–2014).[3,4] In a cohort study (2015–2017) across 18 academic sites that enrich for high-risk deliveries, EOS incidence rates were comparable to the national estimates, including all-cause EOS (0.56 per 1000 LB), GBS EOS (0.29 per 1000 LB), and *E coli* EOS (0.10 per 1000 LB).[16] Among infants born at 37 weeks' gestation or more in the United States, the rate of all-cause EOS is ~1.1 per 1000 LB in black infants and ~0.4 per 1000 LB in nonblack infants.[3] Case fatality rates are low in term infants. In a population surveillance study from 2005 to 2008, the risk-adjusted case fatality rate for a national estimate of 1740 term infants with EOS per year was 2%, ranging from 0% for cases caused by GBS to 9% for those caused by *E coli*.[2] A more recent (2015–2017) multicenter report found no fatalities reported among 104 term infants with EOS.[16]

EOS is vertically transmitted from mother to child either transplacentally (rarely) or more commonly, during labor and delivery with colonization of the fetus/newborn with maternal gastrointestinal and genitourinary microorganisms that subsequently cause invasive infection in the newborn.[18] Because the microbiology of EOS reflects colonization from maternal sources soon before or at delivery, prevention measures involve identification of at-risk mothers and subsequent intrapartum antibiotic administration to either alter pathogenic maternal-fetal colonization or as early treatment to the fetus via the mother. In the United States, preventative methods include universal GBS screening of pregnant women at 36 to 37 weeks' gestation and administration of intrapartum antibiotic prophylaxis (IAP) to women who are GBS colonized or to women with signs and symptoms of intra-amniotic infection.[19,20] Reduction in the estimated number of GBS EOS cases in the United States from 2600 in 1997 to 930 in 2018[21] has been attributed to these national policies of intrapartum care. National surveillance for ongoing GBS EOS from 2006 to 2015 found that among 1277 GBS EOS cases, 48% occurred in women who did not meet criteria to receive GBS IAP, 22% among women who met criteria but were not started on IAP, and 30% among women who

Table 1
Organisms causing early-onset sepsis

Organism	Ref. A n = 1484	Ref. B n = 1178	Ref. C n = 235
Gram-positive, n (% total)			
Group B *Streptococcus*	532 (35.8)	473 (40.2)	70 (29.8)
Streptococcus viridans	280 (18.9)	-	7 (3.0)
Enterococcus	46 (3.1)	63 (5.3)	13 (5.5)
Group D *Streptococcus/Streptococcus bovis*	21 (1.4)	-	6 (2.6)
Listeria spp.	19 (1.3)	4 (0.3)	2 (0.9)
Streptococcus pneumoniae	14 (0.9)	11 (0.9)	3 (1.3)
Staphylococcus aureus	52 (3.5)	23 (2.0)	3 (1.3)
Group A *Streptococcus*	-	1 (0.1)	9 (3.8)
CONS	-	18 (1.5)	2 (0.9)
Other gram-positive cocci	-	208 (17.7)	5 (2.1)
Gram-negative			
E coli	368 (24.8)	145 (12.3)	83 (35.3)
Hemophilus influenzae	67 (4.5)	23 (2.0)	9 (3.8)
Klebsiella spp.	14 (0.9)	7 (0.6)	7 (3.0)
Citrobacter spp.	-	3 (0.3)	1 (0.4)
Enterobacter spp.	-	4 (0.3)	1 (0.4)
Pseudomonas spp.	-	2 (0.2)	1 (0.4)
Other gram-negative rods	-	43 (3.7)	5 (2.1)
Other			
Candida spp.	-	1 (0.1)	4 (1.7)
Other/unknown*	71 (4.8)	149 (12.6)	4 (1.7)

Individual organisms and categories listed if identified in more than 1 study. Reference A includes infants born at 23 weeks' gestation or more, from CDC multistate active surveillance, 2005 to 2014.[3] Reference B includes infants born at 37 to 42 weeks' gestation, at Pediatrix-managed facilities, 2011 to 2016.[17] Reference C includes infants born at 22 weeks' gestation or more at 18 centers participant in the NICHD Neonatal Research Network, 2015 to 2018.[16]

*Other/unknown category refers to (1) any species for which less than 10 isolates were identified (reference A), (2) isolates not identified by name in the data base (reference B), or (3) polymicrobial infections (reference C).

Abbreviations: CDC, Centers for Disease Control and Prevention; CONS, coagulase-negative *Staphylococci;* Ref., reference; NICHD, *Eunice Kennedy Shriver* National Institute of Child Health and Human Development.

received inadequate duration or content of IAP.[4] Thus, despite the success of prevention methods, not all cases are captured with current screening strategies or are preventable.

The content of intrapartum antibiotics is informed by antibiotic susceptibility of the most common EOS isolates. All GBS bacteria remain sensitive to penicillin and ampicillin, but increasing prevalence of resistance to clindamycin (21-47% of isolates) and erythromycin (49-58% of isolates) has been reported and is relevant for intrapartum management.[4,21] *E coli* strains causing EOS, in contrast, are more likely to be resistant to the common first-line antibiotics (ampicillin and gentamicin), particularly among preterm infants and after prolonged exposure to maternal intrapartum antibiotics.[3,22] Among 255 cases of *E coli* in infants of all gestations in a national surveillance from 2007 to 2014, 66% were resistant to ampicillin and 10% to gentamicin.[3] In a recent report of susceptibility patterns of 218 *E coli* isolates from EOS cases in 170 NICUs across the United States, 68% were resistant to ampicillin and 10% were resistant to both ampicillin and gentamicin.[23] These patterns were also present among more mature infants: among the 129 cases in infants with birth weight greater than 1500 g, 67% were resistant to ampicillin and 8% were resistant to both ampicillin and gentamicin. These susceptibilities are likely to evolve in the future and highlight the importance of ongoing surveillance, and the efforts to optimized selection pressure from antibiotic use both among mothers and in neonates.

RISK FACTORS AND CLINICAL PRESENTATION OF EARLY-ONSET SEPSIS

Mother to child transmission of colonizing microorganisms is described as part of normal vaginal delivery.[24] However, EOS cases are associated with pathogenic colonization and infection, which may be reflected in a constellation of clinical factors that represent either the opportunity for such colonization, such as prolonged membrane rupture, or a manifestation of infection, such as maternal fever. These clinical factors occur significantly more often in EOS deliveries than in uninfected deliveries. Historically, before adoption of GBS screening and IAP policies, many risk factors were noted in GBS cases.[10] However, risk factors that perform well (ie, occur infrequently in deliveries of uninfected infants and capture most cases of EOS), including maternal intrapartum fever, maternal diagnosis of intra-amniotic infection, and prolonged duration of rupture of membranes, are also described in the post-GBS IAP period and for other pathogens such as *E coli*.[16,25,26]

Clinical examination findings are important in discriminating EOS cases. Asymptomatic status in the period after delivery reduces the odds of EOS.[12,25] In a study of 235 EOS cases, 93% of infants (including 85% and 94% of term infants with GBS and *E coli* infection, respectively) had documented signs of infection within the first 3 days after birth.[16] These signs most frequently included tachypnea (>60 breaths/min sustained over 30 minutes), increased work of breathing, and tachycardia (>160 beats/min), followed by acidosis and hypotension. A study of 81 term EOS cases delivered to women with a diagnosis of chorioamnionitis, most of whom were treated with empirical antibiotics within 6 hours of birth, reported that a higher proportion of infants (22%) with EOS remained asymptomatic during the first 72 hours.[27]

RISK ASSESSMENT

Risk assessment in medicine, although aimed at risk mitigation, requires a certain degree of risk acceptance. Screening protocols that target patients before manifest disease must consider harms from screening versus gains from early detection. As disease incidence decreases, the risk or benefit of screening will change. The numbers needed to treat or harm can be calculated, but the choice of an acceptable risk threshold is subjective.

EOS risk assessment can involve consideration of perinatal risk factors, clinical examination, and laboratory test results. These factors do not contribute equally to decision making: critical illness often supersedes other factors, at least for immediate management. Similarly, isolation of a pathogen from a blood culture usually supersedes normal host immune markers and reassuring clinical examination. In the following, we focus on the decision to initiate antibiotics in well-appearing newborns, which is most challenging because of the relatively low probability of true disease.

We describe 3 different approaches that share some common features: each approach consists of a set of steps that incorporate information from history and/or examination into a standardized workflow to assist the clinician in consistently identifying at-risk infants. The approaches differ in how the risk factors are incorporated, in actionable risk thresholds, and in recommended clinical actions.

Categorical Approach

In the categorical approach, risk factors are arranged sequentially, often in an order that allows an "if this, then that" pathway for management. Easily visualized as flowcharts, such approaches have been advocated since the first GBS prevention guidelines were published in 1993 and have evolved in subsequent recommendations.[15,20,28,29] Factors frequently considered include gestational age, duration of membrane rupture, suspected maternal chorioamnionitis, maternal GBS status and adequacy of IAP, and infant clinical status. The risk factors are considered in a dichotomous manner in which the answers are yes or no, requiring creation of cutoffs for continuous variables (such as gestational age <35 or <37 weeks and duration of membrane rupture ≥18 hours.) Advantages of the categorical approach include the familiarity of such approaches in medicine and the ease of use. The disadvantages are loss of information in the dichotomization of variables and a simplified presentation of risk factor relationships that may be, in reality, complex. A primary concern with these approaches includes the overidentification of at-risk infants due to the prevalence of commonly included risk factors compared with the incidence of EOS, with associated consequences of mother-infant separation and resource utilization.[7,9,30]

Multivariate Risk Estimation

Variables associated with increased risk of EOS may not occur one at a time, and when occurring together may have complex interactions. For a newborn with multiple factors, the risk of EOS is different from that estimated by consideration of each perinatal variable separately. The Kaiser Permanente neonatal EOS calculator (https://neonatalsepsiscalculator.kaiserpermanente.org) is a combination of 2 multivariable prediction models that incorporate perinatal risk factors including maternal intrapartum antibiotic administration, as well as the infant's evolving clinical condition, to calculate the risk estimate for an individual infant. The perinatal model uses the known incidence of EOS in the term population and incorporates 5 factors known to affect risk of infection (gestational age, duration of membrane rupture, highest maternal temperature during labor, type and timing of administration of maternal antibiotics during labor, and maternal GBS status) to provide the probability of EOS at the time of birth for that infant.[12,31,32] The user can then categorize the evolving clinical examination over the next 12 to 24 hours into well-appearing, equivocal, or clinical illness, based on prespecified definitions, and incorporate the risk model for clinical condition to obtain a final probability of infection. The calculator models do not use laboratory test findings. The probability of EOS is expressed as the predicted number of EOS cases per 1000 LB. The recommendations on the current sepsis risk calculator Web site are to obtain blood culture and use close clinical observation if the final risk estimate is greater than 1 per 1000 LB and to administer empirical antibiotic treatment if the final risk estimate is greater than 3 per 1000 LB.[32] The probability of EOS calculated by the models is based on a robust study of cases and controls, whereas the recommendations for actions at particular thresholds were established by expert consensus and were subsequently prospectively validated in a large implementation study.[30,32,33] In this study, comparison of the categorical approach with the calculator was found to reduce EOS evaluations from 14% to 5% and antibiotic use in the first 24 hours after birth from 5% to 3%.[33] The study compared more than 90,000 infants managed with a categorical approach with more than 50,000 infants managed with the calculator and found similar rates of EOS and severe clinical illness from EOS. This study also demonstrated that after birth hospital discharge, the rate of readmission with culture-confirmed EOS in the week after birth was very low (approximately 5 cases per 100,000 LB) and not different when using categorical or calculator approaches. A meta-analysis of 13 studies found that adoption of the sepsis risk calculator was associated with significant reduction in empirical antibiotic use, with no difference in proportion of missed cases (defined as newborns with EOS not initiated on antibiotic therapy within 24 hours after birth).[34] Thus in the setting of similar safety profiles, the multivariate risk model was significantly more efficient, cost effective, and reduced unnecessary antibiotic exposure for infants.[35]

Serial Clinical Observation

A third strategy for ascertainment of newborn infants who have EOS relies on serial clinical observation of newborn infants to achieve timely recognition of those who are or who become ill with EOS. This approach is justified by studies demonstrating that term newborn infants who do not exhibit clinical signs of illness rarely have EOS.[12,13,36,37] Even among the high-risk group of infants exposed to maternal chorioamnionitis, the EOS rate is approximately 3 per 1000 LB or less among those who appear well at birth.[38–40] Strategies based on serial clinical observation, without use of empirical antibiotics based on maternal risk factors, have been recommended for very specific scenarios in the United Kingdom[41] but more generally adopted in the Friuli-Venezia Giulia[37] and Emilia-Romagna regions of Italy,[42] and have been endorsed as an option for EOS risk assessment in the United States.[15,20]

The specific details of observation-based strategies vary among different implementations, but all share common features,[43] which overlap with components of the sepsis risk calculator.[32] Most importantly, all incorporate structured programs of serial examinations of newborn infants over the first 12 to 48 hours after birth, most frequently over the first 6 to 8 hours and less so thereafter. Implementation at Stanford University birth hospitals in the United States now includes serial examinations of all newborn infants $\geq$35 weeks' gestation,[44] whereas other approaches focus only on those exposed to chorioamnionitis or with risk factors and inadequate intrapartum prophylaxis.[37,41,42] Components of the assessments differ (and are not as specific as those that inform the sepsis risk calculator), but typically include skin color and perfusion, signs of respiratory distress, temperature instability, and general well-being (lethargy, irritability, seizures).[43] Criteria for diagnostic evaluation and/or treatment based on examination findings vary by center.

Reports of observation-based strategies address safety and effectiveness. Well-appearing term infants were compared in 1-year epochs before (7628 infants) and after (7611 infants) transition from a categorical risk strategy with serial observation in Friuli-Venezia Giulia. Rates of laboratory testing decreased from 6.3% to 0.5% and antibiotic treatment from 1.2% to 0.5%.[37] Retrospective analysis of 1000 well-appearing at-risk infants born at 35 weeks' gestation or more at a single center in Emilia-Romagna showed reduction of laboratory testing from 11.6% to 1.6% and antibiotic treatment from 2.8% to 0.6% after adoption of an observation-based strategy.[13] In a subsequent analysis of EOS in the birth cohort of this region after adoption of observation-based strategies (48 cases among 265,508 LB $\geq$35 weeks' gestation during 2010–2016), no case infant had an adverse outcome resulting from this strategy. However, 75% of centers also obtained blood cultures and white blood counts at birth in neonates exposed to intrapartum fever.[45] Notably, 15 infants with EOS had been deemed "not at-risk" and were identified when they exhibited signs of illness, emphasizing the value of serial clinical observation in the identification of infected newborns without specific perinatal risk factors. A single-center experience reported from

California is consistent with these observations.[14,40,44] Among infants born to women with clinical chorioamnionitis, adoption of an observation-based protocol reduced antibiotic exposure from 100% (in compliance with Centers for Disease Control and Prevention [CDC] recommendations at the time of the study[29]) to 21.0%[14] and subsequently to 10.3%.[40] In the entire cohort of 20,394 infants 35 weeks' gestation or more born after adoption of the observation-based protocol, antibiotic exposure declined by 63%. All 7 infants with EOS born during the observation-based protocol period were identified based on development of clinical signs of illness, and no adverse outcomes were attributed to the observation-based strategy.[44] In this cohort, treatment based on clinical signs of illness still resulted in antibiotic administration to 120 infants for each case of EOS, indicating a persistent need for tools that can help identify infants who do not have EOS despite not appearing well.

LABORATORY STUDIES

Blood Culture

EOS is traditionally diagnosed by isolation of pathogenic organisms from normally sterile sites, primarily blood and cerebrospinal fluid (CSF). In the first 72 hours after birth, the yield of urine cultures is very low, and these are not indicated. Cultures of surface swabs (ear, skin, umbilical stump) or gastric aspirate specimens are not informative. If adequate volumes of blood (≥1 mL) are obtained, current blood culture techniques incorporating enriched medium with antibiotic neutralization resins in continuous-reading detection systems reliably detect bacteremia at levels of 1 to 10 colony-forming units per milliliter of blood.[46] Ultralow-level bacteremia below this detection limit is rare in bacteremic newborns, in whom the density of bacteremia exceeds 10 colony-forming unit/mL in 90% of cases.[47] Inoculation of 2 culture bottles may help distinguish contaminant species from true infections, but most clinicians do not obtain paired specimens from separate sites for EOS evaluation. Anaerobic cultures optimize recovery of strictly anaerobic pathogens, which may account for approximately 15% of EOS cases in very-low-birth-weight infants,[48] but uncertainty about the role of anaerobic infections in term infants has hindered adoption of routine anaerobic culture in this population. Growth of an organism is reported by the laboratory after 36 hours or less of incubation in 95% of cultures that test positive,[49,50] justifying decisions to discontinue empirical therapy at that time. Continuing antibiotics beyond 36 hours to avoid interruption of treatment in infants with (yet unreported) bacteremia is estimated to require treatment of nearly 3600 infants who ultimately have definitively sterile cultures.[50]

Although a positive result of blood culture is a consensus criterion for diagnosis of EOS, both false-positive and false-negative results may occur. False-positive results most commonly result from isolation of nonpathogenic organisms introduced during specimen collection. Isolation of pathogens such as GBS or *E coli* from infants who remain well and have sterile follow-up cultures before antibiotic treatment suggest that asymptomatic, transient bacteremia may not be uncommon.[33] Sterile results are unlikely in infants who are bacteremic with an organism the cultures are designed to detect if cultures are properly obtained. However, some infants with serious bacterial infections such as pneumonia are not bacteremic and have sterile blood cultures; the content and duration of antibiotic treatment in such cases is left to clinical judgment.

Cerebrospinal Fluid Culture

As the incidence of EOS has decreased over the last 2 decades, so has the proportion of infants with EOS who have meningitis, making criteria for obtaining cultures of CSF more difficult to define and more controversial. Although selective use of lumbar puncture may have led to underascertainment of meningitis cases, only 4% of infants of all gestational ages with EOS in a 2005 to 2014 CDC surveillance cohort[3] and 3% of those in a 2015 to 2017 NICHD Neonatal Research Network cohort[16] were diagnosed with meningitis. The rationale for CSF culture as part of routine EOS evaluation is based on the observation that some proportion of neonates with culture-confirmed bacterial meningitis do not have positive result of blood cultures, but the incidence for all organisms among all newborns is very low (1–2 per 100,000 LB).[15] Among GBS EOS cases occurring in term infants, national surveillance from 2006 to 2015 found GBS isolated from CSF alone in approximately 2 cases per 1,000,000 LB.[4] In data from an earlier era, no cases of meningitis were identified among 284 asymptomatic infants who underwent lumbar puncture because of maternal risk factors.[51] The proportion of term infants who are treated for suspected EOS in contemporary studies and found to be bacteremic is at present less than 1%.[33,44] In most cases, therefore, and definitively among well-appearing term infants, lumbar puncture can be deferred until blood culture yields a pathogen. Lumbar puncture is indicated if other findings (eg, seizures) point specifically to central nervous system disease. Although deferring CSF culture may compromise opportunities for pathogen isolation, fluid analysis can still be useful to optimize content and duration of antibiotic treatment. In the rare circumstance of meningitis without bacteremia, CSF analysis by multiplex PCR panel may allow identification of a causative organism for up to several days after initiation of treatment.[52] Selection of at-risk infants for lumbar puncture based on elevation of serum C-reactive protein (CRP) levels is not supported by empirical data, which show poor performance of CRP in identification of cases of definite or probable meningitis among sick infants evaluated for sepsis.[53]

Nucleic Acid Amplification

Methodologies using nucleic acid amplification to rapidly identify and characterize bacterial DNA in blood or other tissue fluids are becoming available for clinical use. These methods can provide more rapid pathogen identification from positive results of blood cultures compared with traditional microbiology techniques. Such methods also may potentially be more sensitive than blood cultures and may yield results from infants with ultralow-density bacteremia or following antibiotic exposure.[54] These possibilities have not been confirmed in prospective trials addressing sensitivity and specificity compared with culture-based diagnostics.[55] False-positive results, in which bacterial DNA is detected in the absence of viable circulating organisms, are problematic for the diagnosis and treatment of EOS.[56] Additional experience with these methods will be necessary before they are adopted into routine practice.

White Blood Cell Count, C-Reactive Protein, Procalcitonin, and Other Tests

Ancillary diagnostic tests, including hematological counts, acute-phase reactants, and a variety of cytokines or chemokines, have been evaluated as potential indicators of neonatal sepsis.[54,57] Much of the literature on these biomarkers is compromised by failure to use age-appropriate reference ranges and/or by comparison of infants who are sick (but without EOS) with well controls. Virtually all suffer from very low sensitivity at or soon after the onset of infection and most are quite nonspecific in the immediate newborn period. As such, these laboratory tests have no utility in making decisions about initiating or withholding antibiotic therapy in infants at risk for EOS.

Various components of the complete blood cell count and differential have been used in the evaluation of infants at risk for EOS for many years. Multicenter studies evaluating the utility of white blood cell counts found that extreme values (total white cell count <5000/μL or <1000/μL, absolute neutrophil count <1000/μL or <2000/μL, immature:total neutrophil ratio >0.3 or >0.5) were associated with high positive likelihood ratios but very low sensitivity.[58,59] These results are consistent across numerous studies.[57] Because of the low incidence of EOS, even the best performing indices have low positive predictive value and high negative predictive value and provide very little diagnostic information. Therefore, hematological values are sufficient neither to support a decision to defer treatment in an infant who has clinical signs of illness nor to initiate treatment in one who does not. Serial normal blood cell counts have been associated with low probabilities of EOS, but do not add appreciably to culture results as guides to management.

Serial measurements of acute-phase reactants may correlate with sterile culture results. A recent post hoc analysis of data from the Neonatal Procalcitonin Intervention Study (NeoPIns) cohort found that serial CRP or procalcitonin (PCT) measurements over the first 36 hours after birth, with cutoff thresholds at 16 mg/L and 2.8 ng/L, respectively, had negative predictive values of 100% for distinguishing no sepsis from culture-confirmed infection.[60] The investigators concluded that serial normal levels of these markers at 36 hours of age provided sufficient reassurance to stop antibiotic therapy. It remains unclear why serial acute-phase reactants that correlate with sterile blood culture results are necessary, although those with concern for "culture-negative" sepsis may find such test results reassuring. These tests have very low positive predictive value for culture-confirmed bacteremia (<1% for CRP ≥10 mg/L at 18 hours of age among infants ≥35 weeks' gestation[61]; reliable data for PCT levels in term infants with confirmed sepsis are not available). There are no data to inform the utility of continuing antibiotics when test values do not correlate with properly obtained culture results. Elevated levels therefore do not justify continuation of antibiotic therapy in the face of sterile culture results.

EMPIRICAL AND DEFINITIVE TREATMENT

Empirical Treatment

Empirical treatment of suspected EOS is targeted to the 2 predominant pathogens, GBS and *E coli*. Given the susceptibility data reviewed earlier, the combination of ampicillin and gentamicin remains the currently preferred empirical treatment. This combination will also provide coverage for less common organisms causing EOS, including viridans streptococci, enterococci, *Listeria monocytogenes*, and many enteric gram-negative organisms. Use of third-generation cephalosporins, which will be effective for most resistant *E coli* strains but not for *Enterococcus* or *Listeria*, has been associated with increased mortality.[62] Extended-spectrum β-lactamase-producing organisms rarely cause EOS in term infants in the United States, so routine use of agents such as carbapenems is not indicated. However, given the data reviewed earlier regarding *E coli* with resistance to both ampicillin and gentamicin, the addition of a broader-spectrum antimicrobial should be reserved for term infants who are critically ill or responding poorly to treatment while cultures are pending or for whom preliminary culture results identify gram-negative bacilli.

Definitive Treatment

Definitive treatment of EOS depends on pathogen isolation in culture and determination of antibiotic susceptibilities and ideally consists of the narrowest-spectrum antibiotic appropriate to the clinical situation. Other considerations for definitive therapy include the presence or absence of meningitis, as well as any evidence of renal or hepatic dysfunction. GBS sepsis or meningitis can be treated with ampicillin or penicillin; dosing recommendations are included in updated GBS guidance.[20] For sepsis caused by ampicillin-sensitive *E coli*, ampicillin is sufficient; susceptibility data should guide the choice for ampicillin-resistant isolates. If gram-negative meningitis is suspected or confirmed, a cephalosporin or carbapenem, providing superior central nervous system penetration, is preferred. Consultation with infectious disease experts is recommended for cases of early-onset meningitis, as well as for optimal management of less common microbial causes of EOS.

SUMMARY

The changing epidemiology of EOS among term infants has required reappraisal of approaches to management of newborn infants at potential risk. As this is now a rare disease, new strategies for reduction in diagnostic testing and empirical treatment have been developed. Adoption and refinement of these strategies should be a priority for all facilities where babies are born.

CLINICS CARE POINTS

- EOS occurs in approximately 1 in 2000 term newborns
- The most common organisms isolated in EOS cases among term infants are GBS and *E. coli*
- Term newborns can be evaluated for EOS using categorical algorithms, multivariate risk models or approaches based primarily on serial clinical examination.
- Ampicillin and gentamicin remain the most appropriate empiric antibiotic combination for term infants at risk for EOS. Addition of broader-spectrum antibiotics may be considered for term infants at highest risk, particularly those with critical illness.

DISCLOSURE

Dr Mukhopadhyay is supported by grant K23-HD088753 from the *Eunice Kennedy Shriver* National Institute of Child Health and Human Development.

Best Practices

What is the current practice for identifying and managing term infants at risk for early onset neonatal sepsis?

Best practices and guidelines

- Current obstetric practices for prevention of early-onset neonatal sepsis are effective and should be continued.
- Recognition of the current low incidence of early-onset sepsis in term infants, including those with risk factors such as exposure to chorioamnionitis, has required reassessment of strategies for ascertainment and management of serious bacterial infections in term infants.
- Guidelines for management of infants at risk for early-onset neonatal sepsis have been provided by the American Academy of Pediatrics[15,20] and endorsed by the Centers for Disease Control and Prevention.

Major recommendations

- Systematic strategies for reduction of unnecessary diagnostic testing, empirical antibiotic administration, and disruption of mother-infant bonding, while maintaining a high level of vigilance for neonatal sepsis, should be adopted by every birthing facility.
- No matter what approach is taken to the initial evaluation for ascertainment of infants with sepsis, ongoing careful observation of all infants is necessary over the first 24 to 48 hours to ensure recognition of infants who become ill from any cause within that time period.

- With some exceptions, ampicillin and gentamicin remain the preferred antibiotics for empirical treatment of infants who meet threshold criteria.
- Antibiotic therapy should be focused to use the narrowest-spectrum agent to which the culture isolate is susceptible, or discontinued after 36 hours if blood cultures are sterile (in the absence of evidence of a focal serious bacterial infection).

Summary statement

Reappraisal of current epidemiology of early-onset neonatal sepsis has engendered revision of guidelines for the management of neonates potentially at risk. These changes have been particularly substantial for term infants. Adoption of strategies for limiting diagnostic testing and antibiotic use in this population, as well as continued efforts to improve upon those strategies, is essential.

REFERENCES

1. Heron M. Deaths: leading causes for 2017. Natl Vital Stat Rep 2019;68:1–77.
2. Weston EJ, Pondo T, Lewis MM, et al. The burden of invasive early-onset neonatal sepsis in the United States, 2005-2008. Pediatr Infect Dis J 2011;30: 937–41.
3. Schrag SJ, Farley MM, Petit S, et al. Epidemiology of invasive early-onset neonatal sepsis, 2005 to 2014. Pediatrics 2016;138:e20162013.
4. Nanduri SA, Petit S, Smelser C, et al. Epidemiology of invasive early-onset and late-onset group B streptococcal disease in the United States, 2006 to 2015: multistate laboratory and population-based surveillance. JAMA Pediatr 2019; 173:224–33.
5. Mukhopadhyay S, Taylor JA, Von Kohorn I, et al. Variation in sepsis evaluation across a national network of nurseries. Pediatrics 2017;139:e20162845.
6. Haidari ES, Lee HC, Illuzzi JL, et al. Hospital variation in admissions to neonatal intensive care units by diagnosis severity and category. J Perinatol 2021;41(3): 468–77.
7. Mukhopadhyay S, Dukhovny D, Mao W, et al. 2010 perinatal GBS prevention guideline and resource utilization. Pediatrics 2014;133:196–203.
8. Zupancic JA, Richardson DK. Characterization of the triage process in neonatal intensive care. Pediatrics 1998;102:1432–6.
9. Mukhopadhyay S, Lieberman ES, Puopolo KM, et al. Effect of early-onset sepsis evaluations on in-hospital breastfeeding practices among asymptomatic term neonates. Hosp Pediatr 2015;5:203–10.
10. Benitz WE, Gould JB, Druzin ML. Risk factors for early-onset group B streptococcal sepsis: estimation of odds ratios by critical literature review. Pediatrics 1999;103:e77.
11. Puopolo KM, Escobar GJ. Early-onset sepsis: a predictive model based on maternal risk factors. Curr Opin Pediatr 2013;25:161–6.
12. Escobar GJ, Puopolo KM, Wi S, et al. Stratification of risk of early-onset sepsis in newborns ≥ 34 weeks' gestation. Pediatrics 2014;133:30–6.
13. Berardi A, Fornaciari S, Rossi C, et al. Safety of physical examination alone for managing well-appearing neonates ≥ 35 weeks' gestation at risk for early-onset sepsis. J Matern Fetal Neonatal Med 2015;28:1123–7.
14. Joshi NS, Gupta A, Allan JM, et al. Clinical monitoring of well-appearing infants born to mothers with chorioamnionitis. Pediatrics 2018;141:e20172056.
15. Puopolo K, Benitz WE, Zaoutis TE, et al. Management of neonates born ≥35 0/7 weeks gestation with suspected or proven early-onset bacterial sepsis. Pediatrics 2018;142:e20182894.

16. Stoll BJ, Puopolo KM, Hansen NI, et al. Early-onset neonatal sepsis 2015 to 2017, the rise of *Escherichia coli*, and the need for novel prevention strategies. JAMA Pediatr 2020;174:e200593.
17. Polcwiartek LB, Smith PB, Benjamin DK, et al. Early-onset sepsis in term infants admitted to neonatal intensive care units (2011-2016). J Perinatol 2020;41(1):157–63.
18. Benirschke K. Routes and types of infection in the fetus and the newborn. AMA J Dis Child 1960;99:714–21.
19. Committee on obstetric practice. Committee Opinion No. 712: intrapartum management of intraamniotic infection. Obstet Gynecol 2017;130:e95–101.
20. Puopolo KM, Lynfield R, Cummings JJ, et al. Management of infants at risk for group B streptococcal disease. Pediatrics 2019;144:e20191881.
21. Active bacterial Core surveillance (ABCs): Bact Facts Interactive Beta v8.2. In: Centers for Disease Control and Prevention. 2020. Available at: https://wwwn.cdc.gov/BactFacts/index.html. Accessed November 30, 2020.
22. Bizzarro MJ, Dembry LM, Baltimore RS, et al. Changing patterns in neonatal *Escherichia coli* sepsis and ampicillin resistance in the era of intrapartum antibiotic prophylaxis. Pediatrics 2008;121:689–96.
23. Flannery DD, Akinboyo IC, Mukhopadhyay S, et al. Antibiotic susceptibility of *Escherichia coli* among infants admitted to neonatal intensive care units across the US from 2009 to 2017. JAMA Pediatr 2021;175(2):168–75.
24. Dominguez-Bello MG, Costello EK, Contreras M, et al. Delivery mode shapes the acquisition and structure of the initial microbiota across multiple body habitats in newborns. Proc Natl Acad Sci U S A 2010;107:11971–5.
25. Escobar GJ, Li DK, Armstrong MA, et al. Neonatal sepsis workups in infants $\geq$ 2000 grams at birth: a population-based study. Pediatrics 2000;106:256–63.
26. Schrag SJ, Hadler JL, Arnold KE, et al. Risk factors for invasive, early-onset *Escherichia coli* infections in the era of widespread intrapartum antibiotic use. Pediatrics 2006;118:570–6.
27. Wortham JM, Hansen NI, Schrag SJ, et al. Chorioamnionitis and culture-confirmed, early-onset neonatal infections. Pediatrics 2016;137:e20152323.
28. Centers for Disease Control and Prevention. Prevention of perinatal group B streptococcal disease: a public health perspective. MMWR 1996;45:1–24.
29. Verani JR, McGee L, Schrag SJ. Prevention of perinatal group B streptococcal disease – revised guidelines from CDC, 2010. MMWR Recomm Rep 2010;59:1–36.
30. Dhudasia MB, Mukhopadhyay S, Puopolo KM. Implementation of the sepsis risk calculator at an academic birth hospital. Hosp Pediatr 2018;8:243–50.
31. Puopolo KM, Draper D, Wi S, et al. Estimating the probability of neonatal early-onset infection on the basis of maternal risk factors. Pediatrics 2011;128:e1155–63.
32. Kuzniewicz MW, Walsh EM, Li S, et al. Development and implementation of an early-onset sepsis calculator to guide antibiotic management in late preterm and term neonates. Jt Comm J Qual Patient Saf 2016;42:232–9.
33. Kuzniewicz MW, Puopolo KM, Fischer A, et al. A quantitative, risk-based approach to the management of neonatal early-onset sepsis. JAMA Pediatr 2017;171:365–71.
34. Achten NB, Klingenberg C, Benitz WE, et al. Association of use of the Neonatal Early-Onset Sepsis Calculator with reduction in antibiotic therapy and safety: a systematic review and meta-analysis. JAMA Pediatr 2019;173:1032–40.

35. Achten NB, Dorigo-Zetsma JW, van der Linden PD, et al. Sepsis calculator implementation reduces empiric antibiotics for suspected early-onset sepsis. Eur J Pediatr 2018;177:741–6.
36. Ottolini MC, Lundgren K, Mirkinson LJ, et al. Utility of complete blood count and blood culture screening to diagnose neonatal sepsis in the asymptomatic at risk newborn. Pediatr Infect Dis J 2003;22:430–4.
37. Cantoni L, Ronfani L, Da Riol R, et al. Physical examination instead of laboratory tests for most infants born to mothers colonized with group B *Streptococcus*: support for the Centers for Disease Control and Prevention's 2010 recommendations. J Pediatr 2013;163:568–73.
38. Shakib J, Buchi K, Smith E, et al. Management of newborns born to mothers with chorioamnionitis: is it time for a kinder, gentler approach? Acad Pediatr 2015;15: 340–4.
39. Money N, Newman J, Demissie S, et al. Anti-microbial stewardship: antibiotic use in well-appearing term neonates born to mothers with chorioamnionitis. J Perinatol 2017;37:1304–9.
40. Joshi NS, Gupta A, Allan JM, et al. Management of chorioamnionitis-exposed infants in the newborn nursery using a clinical examination-based approach. Hosp Pediatr 2019;9:227–33.
41. Hughes R, Brocklehurst P, Steer P, et al. Prevention of early-onset neonatal group B streptococcal disease. Green-top Guideline No. 36. BJOG 2017;124: e280–305.
42. Berardi A, Ficara M, Pietrella E, et al. Stewardship antimicrobica nel neonato e nel piccolo lattante [Antimicrobial stewardship in newborns and young infants: why and how to do it]. Medico e Bambino 2017;36:493–501.
43. Berardi A, Bedetti L, Spada C, et al. Serial clinical observation for management of newborns at risk of early-onset sepsis. Curr Opin Pediatr 2020;32:245–51.
44. Frymoyer A, Joshi NS, Allan JM, et al. Sustainability of a clinical examination-based approach for ascertainment of early-onset sepsis in late preterm and term neonates. J Pediatr 2020;225:263–8.
45. Berardi A, Spada C, Reggiani MLB, et al. Group B *Streptococcus* early-onset disease and observation of well-appearing newborns. PLoS One 2019;14:e0212784.
46. Cantey JB, Baird SD. Ending the culture of culture-negative sepsis in the neonatal ICU. Pediatrics 2017;140:e20170044.
47. Sabui T, Tudehope DI, Tilse M. Clinical significance of quantitative blood cultures in newborn infants. J Paediatr Child Health 1999;35:578–81.
48. Mukhopadhyay S, Puopolo KM. Clinical and microbiologic characteristics of early-onset sepsis among very low birth weight infants: opportunities for antibiotic stewardship. Pediatr Infect Dis J 2017;36:477–81.
49. Biondi EA, Mischler M, Jerardi KE, et al. Blood culture time to positivity in febrile infants with bacteremia. JAMA Pediatr 2014;168:844–9.
50. Kuzniewicz MW, Mukhopadhyay S, Li S, et al. Time to positivity of neonatal blood cultures for early-onset sepsis. Pediatr Infect Dis J 2020;39:634–40.
51. Fielkow S, Reuter S, Gotoff SP. Cerebrospinal fluid examination in symptom-free infants with risk factors for infection. J Pediatr 1991;119:971–3.
52. Arora HS, Asmar BI, Salimnia H, et al. Enhanced identification of group B *streptococcus* and *Escherichia coli* in young infants with meningitis using the Biofire Filmarray meningitis/Encephalitis panel. Pediatr Infect Dis J 2017;36:685–7.
53. Durrani NUR, Dutta S, Rochow N, et al. C-reactive protein as a predictor of meningitis in early onset neonatal sepsis: a single unit experience. J Perinat Med 2020;48:845–51.

54. Iroh Tam PY, Bendel CM. Diagnostics for neonatal sepsis: current approaches and future directions. Pediatr Res 2017;82:574–83.
55. Pammi M, Flores A, Versalovic J, et al. Molecular assays for the diagnosis of sepsis in neonates. Cochrane Database Syst Rev 2017;2:CD011926.
56. Liu CL, Ai HW, Wang WP, et al. Comparison of 16S rRNA gene PCR and blood culture for diagnosis of neonatal sepsis. Arch Pediatr 2014;21:162–9.
57. Benitz WE. Adjunct laboratory tests in the diagnosis of early-onset neonatal sepsis. Clin Perinatol 2010;37:421–38.
58. Hornik CP, Benjamin DK, Becker KC, et al. Use of the complete blood cell count in early-onset neonatal sepsis. Pediatr Infect Dis J 2012;31:799–802.
59. Newman TB, Puopolo KM, Wi S, et al. Interpreting complete blood counts soon after birth in newborns at risk for sepsis. Pediatrics 2010;126:903–9.
60. Stocker M, van Herk W, El Helou S, et al. C-reactive protein, procalcitonin, and white blood count to rule out neonatal early-onset sepsis within 36 hours: a secondary analysis of the Neonatal Procalcitonin Intervention Study. Clin Infect Dis 2020. https://doi.org/10.1093/cid/ciaa876.
61. Lacaze-Masmonteil T, Rosychuk RJ, Robinson JL. Value of a single C-reactive protein measurement at 18 h of age. Arch Dis Child Fetal Neonatal Ed 2014;99:F76–9.
62. Clark RH, Bloom BT, Spitzer AR, et al. Empiric use of ampicillin and cefotaxime, compared with ampicillin and gentamicin, for neonates at risk for sepsis is associated with an increased risk of neonatal death. Pediatrics 2006;117:67–74.

The Term Newborn
Congenital Infections

Amaran Moodley, MD[a], Kurlen S.E. Payton, MD[b,*]

KEYWORDS

• Term • Newborn • Congenital • Infection

KEY POINTS

- Congenital cytomegalovirus infection is the most common congenital infection worldwide; however, many infants remain undetected because of mild or asymptomatic infection.
- Perinatally acquired human immunodeficiency virus (HIV) infection can largely be prevented through early maternal HIV testing, initiation of effective maternal antiretroviral treatment, prompt initiation of neonatal antiretroviral prophylaxis, and avoidance of maternal breastmilk.
- Recognition, diagnosis, and management of infants with suspected congenital infection can be challenging for newborn care providers, especially when emerging pathogens that are not included in the TORCH pneumonic (toxoplasmosis, rubella, cytomegalovirus, and herpes simplex virus) are being considered.
- Recent advances in diagnostic testing, chemoprophylaxis, and treatment have led to improved outcomes in certain congenital infections.

INTRODUCTION

Maternal bacterial, viral, and parasitic pathogens can be transmitted across the placenta to the fetus, resulting in congenital infection with sequelae ranging from asymptomatic infection to severe debilitating disease and still birth.[1]

The TORCH pneumonic includes toxoplasmosis, rubella, cytomegalovirus (CMV), and herpes simplex virus; however, it provides a limited description of the expanding list of pathogens associated with congenital infection. Human immunodeficiency virus (HIV), syphilis, enterovirus, parvovirus, varicella virus, Chagas disease, and several emerging pathogens such as Zika virus and severe acute respiratory syndrome coronavirus 2 (SARS-CoV-2) have also been associated with intrauterine transmission and should be considered in infants with suspected congenital infection.[2] Newborn care

Disclosure: The authors have nothing to disclose.
[a] Department of Pediatrics, Rady Childrens Hospital & University of California San Diego, 3020 Children's Way, MC 5041, San Diego, CA 92123, USA; [b] David Geffen School of Medicine at University of California Los Angeles, Division of Neonatology, Cedars-Sinai Medical Center, 8700 Beverly Boulevard, NT Suite 4221, Los Angeles, CA 90048, USA
* Corresponding author.
E-mail address: kurlen.payton@cshs.org

Clin Perinatol 48 (2021) 485–511
https://doi.org/10.1016/j.clp.2021.05.004

providers frequently deviate from recommendations on the evaluation of infants with congenital infections.[3] Traditionally used tests such as TORCH titer screens and total immunoglobulin (Ig) M for infants with isolated growth restriction or who are small for gestational age have limited value based on current evidence.[4–6]

This article focuses on the evaluation and management of infants with common congenital infections such as CMV, and infections that warrant early diagnosis and treatment to prevent serious complications, such as toxoplasmosis, HIV, and syphilis. Zika virus and Chagas disease remain uncommon and are discussed briefly.

CONGENITAL CYTOMEGALOVIRUS INFECTION

Disease Overview

CMV is a ubiquitous double-stranded DNA virus that belongs to the herpesvirus family. Similar to varicella zoster virus and herpes simplex virus, CMV establishes latency after primary infection and can reactivate intermittently, including during pregnancy. In high-income countries, congenital CMV is a leading cause of sensorineural hearing loss (SNHL), and is the most common congenital infection, with an estimated incidence of 0.6% to 0.7% of all live births.[7,8] In the absence of universal newborn screening for CMV, most infants with congenital infection remain undetected because almost all remain asymptomatic at birth. Infants with symptomatic infection are important to recognize because recent clinical trials have shown that early antiviral treatment can decrease the risk of serious long-term sequelae such as hearing loss and neurodevelopmental delay.[9]

Transmission and Pathogenesis

CMV is transmitted by direct contact with infected body fluids, including saliva, urine, blood, breastmilk, semen, and genital tract secretions. Women with no prior history of CMV infection are susceptible to primary infection during pregnancy, which may occur after household or occupational exposure to young children or other symptomatic or asymptomatic individuals shedding CMV.[10] Intrauterine CMV transmission occurs when CMV crosses the placenta to infect the fetus during a primary or nonprimary maternal CMV infection.

The rate of CMV transmission to the fetus and the risk of symptomatic disease in infected infants is higher after primary maternal CMV infection compared with nonprimary infection.[7,11] Infants infected in the first trimester (<13 weeks) after primary maternal CMV infection have a much higher risk of SNHL (24%) and other long-term neurologic sequelae (32%) compared with infants infected later in pregnancy.[12] Because of the challenges in diagnosing nonprimary maternal CMV infection, it is unclear whether the timing of nonprimary infection during pregnancy is associated with risk of symptomatic disease or SNHL in infected infants.

Although the risk of vertical transmission following primary maternal CMV infection is high (30%–35%), the proportion of infants with congenital CMV infection attributable to primary maternal infection is low (22.6%). This difference occurs because only 1% to 4% of CMV seronegative women develop primary CMV infection during pregnancy. Furthermore, most women of reproductive age are CMV seropositive and therefore not susceptible to primary CMV infection.[13,14]

Epidemiology

CMV infection is common among women of reproductive age worldwide, with seroprevalence approaching 100% in some resource-limited countries.[15] Rates of infection vary widely by age, race, and socioeconomic factors.[16] In a large study of the

Table 1
Estimated burden of congenital infection attributable to type of maternal cytomegalovirus infection and rate of cytomegalovirus transmission

Type of Maternal CMV Infection	Description	Rate of Transmission to Fetus (%)	Proportion of All Congenital CMV Infections Attributable to Type of Maternal Infection in the United States (%)
Primary	CMV infection in women without prior CMV infection and with no preexisting immunity	30–35	22.6
Nonprimary	Reactivation of latent CMV infection or reinfection with a new strain of CMV in women with prior CMV infection and preexisting immunity	0.1–1.7	77.4

US population, the overall age-adjusted CMV seroprevalence for girls and women aged 6 to 49 years was estimated to be 55.5%. CMV seropositivity was associated with older age, non-Hispanic black race, Mexican American ethnicity, foreign place of birth, low household income and education level, and high crowding index. Although most non-Hispanic black women and Mexican American women develop primary CMV infection during the peak reproductive years between adolescence and their 30s, almost all infants with congenital CMV infection are born to CMV-seropositive women who develop nonprimary infections during pregnancy (**Table 1**).[16] As the mean age of primiparous mothers increases in the United States, a higher proportion will be CMV seropositive during pregnancy.[17] This point is important to consider because efforts to prevent primary maternal CMV infection through vaccines or behavioral measures may have a limited impact in older mothers who have already had CMV infection.

Clinical Presentation

Approximately 85 to 90% of infants with congenital CMV infection are asymptomatic at birth; however, approximately 13.5% of these infants may develop long-term complications. In symptomatic infants the risk is much higher with 40% to 58% developing permanent sequelae.[7,8] The clinical features and laboratory and imaging findings of infants with symptomatic infection are summarized in **Table 2**.[18] Infants with isolated hearing loss have been characterized as both symptomatic and asymptomatic subjects in clinical trials and are now considered a distinct cohort by many experts.

The overall mortality associated with congenital CMV infection is estimated to be 4%, with the highest mortality in infants who present with severe or fulminant disease at birth.[19]

Diagnosis

A significant challenge for health care providers is knowing which infants to test for evidence of congenital CMV infection. In infants with mild disease or nonspecific signs

Table 2
Clinical, laboratory, and imaging findings in symptomatic congenital cytomegalovirus infection

Clinical Features	Prematurity Small for gestational age (≤2 SD for gestational age) Microcephaly (≤2 SD for gestational age) Petechiae or purpura, blueberry muffin rash Jaundice Hepatosplenomegaly Lethargy, hypotonia, seizures, poor sucking reflex
Laboratory Abnormalities	Anemia Thrombocytopenia Leukopenia, isolated neutropenia Hepatitis (increased liver aminotransferase or bilirubin level) CSF abnormalities such as increased protein levels
Neuroimaging Abnormalities[a]	Intracranial calcifications, periventricular cysts, ventriculomegaly, white matter abnormalities, cortical atrophy, migration disorders, cerebellar hypoplasia, lenticulostriatal vasculopathy
Hearing Evaluation	SNHL affecting 1 or both ears
Ophthalmologic Examination	Chorioretinitis Retinal hemorrhage, optic atrophy, strabismus

Abbreviation: CSF, cerebrospinal fluid; SD, standard deviation.
[a] Head ultrasonography, magnetic resonance imaging or computed tomography.

and symptoms, a high index of suspicion is required. The following indications should prompt testing for CMV infection[18]:

- Infants born to women with a history of suspected or confirmed primary CMV infection during pregnancy
- Infants with signs and symptoms consistent with congenital CMV infection (**Table 2**)
- Infants with confirmed SNHL. Some experts recommend CMV testing in infants with suspected SNHL if a formal audiologic evaluation cannot be done before 3 weeks of life
- Infants with prenatal or postnatal neuroimaging findings consistent with congenital CMV infection

Infants with congenital CMV infection shed large amounts of virus in urine and saliva for prolonged periods. Historically, the gold-standard technique for establishing a diagnosis was standard or rapid (shell vial) viral culture of urine or saliva. However, recent clinical studies have shown that polymerase chain reaction (PCR) is more sensitive than viral culture and has lower costs and much shorter turnaround time.[20] In high-income countries, testing for congenital CMV by urine or saliva PCR is therefore preferred and should be done before the first 2 to 3 weeks of life, because detection of CMV beyond this period cannot reliably distinguish postnatal from congenital infection (**Table 3**). When congenital CMV infection is suspected in infants older than 3 weeks, a PCR assay can be performed on newborn dried blood samples (Guthrie cards) if available; however, a negative result does not rule out CMV infection because the sensitivity is much lower compared with PCR of urine or saliva.[21]

Although false-positive results are uncommon, all infants with a positive urine or saliva PCR or rapid viral culture result should have a confirmatory PCR test performed

Table 3
Diagnosis of congenital cytomegalovirus infection

Sample	Sample Method	Test Method	Sensitivity (%)	Specificity (%)	Advantages	Disadvantages
Saliva	Use a sterile swab to collect saliva from the inside of an infant's mouth between the cheek and lower gum before breastfeeding, or >1 h after breastfeeding. Place swab in a dry storage tube or transport medium	PCR	97.4–100	99.9	Sample collection is noninvasive, quick and can easily be performed at the bedside	False-positive results can occur when infant saliva is contaminated with maternal breast milk or maternal genital tract secretions during delivery
Urine	Use a sterile urine collection bag or place sterile cotton balls in the diaper[a]	PCR	93–100	99–100	—	Urine collection can be challenging, especially in preterm infants
Blood	CMV antigen CMV serology (IgG, IgM) Dried blood spot PCR Whole-blood or plasma quantitative CMV PCR[b]		Not routinely recommended for the diagnosis of congenital CMV			

[a] Urine obtained from sterile cotton balls placed in the diaper was reported to be less sensitive when rapid CMV culture was compared with PCR.
[b] Blood CMV PCR should not be used to rule out early CMV infection because not all infants with symptomatic disease have detectable viremia.

on either urine or saliva. A single negative urine CMV PCR result is sufficient to exclude congenital CMV infection.[18]

Management of Infants with Congenital Cytomegalovirus Infection

Asymptomatic infants with congenital CMV infection often do not require antiviral treatment or additional supportive care. A clinical trial is being conducted to determine whether antiviral treatment of asymptomatic neonates without hearing loss decreases the risk of delayed-onset hearing loss during the first 18 months of life (https://clinicaltrials.gov/ct2/show/NCT03301415).

The optimal management of asymptomatic infants with isolated hearing loss remains unclear; however, clinical trials are being conducted to evaluate the effectiveness of antiviral treatment on hearing and developmental outcomes (https://clinicaltrials.gov/ct2/show/NCT03107871). With little evidence to recommend routine antiviral treatment of asymptomatic infants, health care providers should discuss the risks and potential benefits of antiviral treatment with parents and caregivers.

Infants with symptomatic disease should have a comprehensive evaluation for associated complications, as summarized in **Table 4**.

Health care providers should observe universal or standard precautions when caring for infants with congenital CMV infection. Gloves should be worn with any potential exposure to blood, urine, saliva, or other body fluids. Although transmission of CMV from breast milk can lead to postnatal CMV infection in infants without congenital infection, maternal breastfeeding of infants with congenital CMV infection is not contraindicated. In infants who already have CMV infection, postnatal exposure to maternal CMV virus in breast milk is unlikely to lead to a new infection or worse outcome.

Table 4
Management of symptomatic infants with congenital cytomegalovirus infection

Physical Examination	Evaluate for clinical features of infection (**Table2**)
Laboratory Tests	CBCd LFTs Creatinine, BUN Blood CMV PCR viral load at baseline has been associated with adverse CNS Outcomes; however, routine monitoring is not recommended
Hearing Assessment	Evaluate with brain stem auditory evoked response to detect SNHL
Ophthalmologic Evaluation	Obtain ophthalmology eye examination to evaluate for chorioretinitis
Neuroimaging	Obtain head ultrasonography. MRI or computed tomography imaging is recommended when there are abnormalities on ultrasonography or when there are clinical features suggestive of CNS disease, such as microcephaly or seizures
Antiviral Treatment	Intravenous ganciclovir or oral valganciclovir
Supportive Care	Treatment of CNS complications such as seizures with antiepileptic drugs Management of hematologic abnormalities such as thrombocytopenia

Abbreviations: BUN, blood urea nitrogen; CBCd, complete blood count with differential; CNS, central nervous system; LFTs, liver function tests.

Antiviral treatment and monitoring

Infants with symptomatic congenital CMV should receive treatment with either intravenous ganciclovir or oral valganciclovir (**Table 5**) as soon as the diagnosis is confirmed and ideally before 30 days of life. Randomized controlled trials have shown that antiviral treatment improves hearing and neurodevelopmental outcomes up to 24 months of age, and that 6 months of treatment with oral valganciclovir is more effective than 6 weeks of the antiviral treatment.[9,22,23] Adverse effects associated with antiviral treatment are mostly hematologic and include neutropenia and thrombocytopenia. Increased levels of liver transaminases may also be observed.

Follow-up care of infants infected with cytomegalovirus

All symptomatic and asymptomatic infants with congenital CMV infection should have periodic hearing assessments performed because hearing loss can worsen or emerge during infancy and early childhood. Formal hearing assessments performed by an audiologist are recommended every 3 to 6 months in the first year, then every 6 months until 3 years of age, and then every 12 months until 6 years of age.[18] Follow-up with an ophthalmologist, an ear, nose, and throat specialist, and a developmental specialist may also be indicated based on disease severity.

Symptomatic infants who are discharged on oral valganciclovir treatment require follow-up with a pediatric infectious disease specialist for monitoring of physical growth and development and for management of valganciclovir dosing and treatment-related adverse effects.

PERINATAL HUMAN IMMUNODEFICIENCY VIRUS EXPOSURE AND INFECTION

Disease Overview

HIV-1 and HIV-2 are enveloped RNA retroviruses that are transmitted predominantly through contact with body fluids, such as blood, semen, vaginal secretions, and breast milk. In 2019, the World Health Organization (WHO) estimated that 38 million people worldwide were living with HIV infection, including approximately 1.8 million children less than 15 years of age.[24] High-income countries such as the United States have a much lower prevalence of HIV infection, with an estimated 1.2 million people living with HIV at the end of 2018,[25] including approximately 1918 children less than 13 years of age.[26]

The development of safe and effective antiretroviral (ARV) drugs for HIV treatment and prophylaxis, and improvements in access to HIV testing and treatment, have led to significant decreases in new HIV infections, HIV-related deaths, and in the rates of mother-to-child transmission (MTCT) worldwide.[24] HIV-2 infection is uncommon outside of western Africa and is not discussed further in this article.

Transmission and Pathogenesis

Infants can acquire HIV-1 infection from the mother during pregnancy (in utero), during labor and delivery, or postnatally through breastfeeding. Without interventions to prevent transmission, the risk of MTCT is approximately 25% to 30%, with higher rates up to 42% reported in resource-limited countries.[27] Most MTCT transmission occurred during pregnancy and labor (15%–30%), whereas 10% to 20% was attributed to breastfeeding.[27] In the United States and many high-income countries, the risk of MTCT has been reduced to approximately 1% to 2%.

Most Perinatal HIV transmission occurs during labor and delivery when infant mucosal surfaces are exposed to maternal blood and vaginal secretions containing HIV. In a large clinical trial conducted in resource-limited countries, the initiation of maternal ARV treatment during pregnancy reduced perinatal HIV transmission rates

Table 5
Antiviral treatment of symptomatic congenital cytomegalovirus infection

Antiviral Drug	Indication	Dose	Duration	Adverse Effects	Monitoring
Valganciclovir (oral suspension)	Mild disease	16 mg/kg/dose twice daily	6 mo	Neutropenia Thrombocytopenia Increased levels of transaminases	Obtain CBCd, LFTs, BUN, creatinine before treatment; then weekly for first 4 wk, then monthly until treatment completion
Ganciclovir (IV)[a]	Severe or life-threatening disease or when oral absorption is suboptimal	6 mg/kg/dose every 12 h	Up to 6 wk; may switch to oral valganciclovir once condition improves and oral feeds are tolerated	Neutropenia Thrombocytopenia Hepatotoxicity	

[a] Ganciclovir should be administered intravenously through a central venous catheter.

to less tthan 0.5% through the first week of life, underscoring the impact of early maternal HIV testing and effective ARV treatment on pregnancy outcomes.

The risk of HIV transmission through breastfeeding seems to be highest in the first few months of life and is associated with maternal viral load, degree of maternal immune suppression, presence of mastitis, and duration of breastfeeding. HIV-infected cells and cell-free virus can be detected in human breast milk. Although breastfeeding is discouraged in high-income countries, the risk of postnatal HIV transmission in breastfed infants in resource-limited countries can be reduced to less than 1% when effective antepartum ARV treatment is coupled with either prolonged infant ARV prophylaxis or extended maternal ARV treatment.

Epidemiology

The number of women living with HIV infection who give birth each year in the United States has gradually declined from approximately 8700 in 2006, to recent estimates of 5000 per year.[28] Although fewer women with HIV infection give birth each year, most of the reduction in MTCT has been attributed to several prenatal (universal HIV antibody testing of pregnant women, maternal antiretroviral treatment during pregnancy), intrapartum (antiretroviral treatment, elective cesarean section for women with high risk of HIV transmission), and postnatal (infant antiretroviral prophylaxis, avoidance of maternal breastfeeding) interventions.[29] It is estimated that the implementation of these measures resulted in 22,000 fewer cases of perinatal HIV transmission in the United States between the years 1994 and 2010.[30] Recent data indicate that, of the approximately 37,968 individuals newly diagnosed with HIV infection in the United States in 2018, only 65 (<1%) were attributed to infants with perinatally acquired HIV infection.[26] Although HIV infection occurs among all racial and ethnic groups, black/African American individuals are disproportionately affected in the United States, accounting for approximately 65% of perinatal HIV infections and 57% of new HIV infections in adults and adolescents in 2018.[26]

Clinical Presentation

Most infants with perinatal HIV exposure or infection remain asymptomatic at birth and have normal physical examinations during the neonatal period. Adverse pregnancy outcomes such as preterm birth and low birth weight have been associated with maternal HIV infection and use of combination ARVs during pregnancy.[31] Opportunistic infections such as disseminated candidiasis or *Pneumocystis jiroveci* pneumonia, and other clinical and laboratory abnormalities associated with HIV infection such as lymphadenopathy, hepatosplenomegaly, delayed developmental milestones, anemia, and leukopenia, tend to occur later in infancy.

Diagnosis

Newborn care providers have an important role in ensuring that every infant born to a mother with an unknown HIV status undergoes prompt maternal or infant testing with a US Food and Drug Administration (FDA)–approved rapid HIV antigen/antibody immunoassay that detects HIV-1 and HIV-2 antibodies, and HIV-1 p24 antigen. These tests are reported to have sensitivities and specificities that range from 99% to 100%.[32] In high-income countries, a positive rapid test result should lead to the initiation of infant antiretroviral prophylaxis as soon as possible, and to delayed maternal breastfeeding while confirmatory HIV testing is done.

All infants with known perinatal HIV exposure should have HIV RNA or HIV DNA nucleic acid tests (NATs) performed during the first few weeks of life (**Tables 6 and 7**).[33] Infants with higher risk of perinatal HIV transmission may require earlier and

Table 6
Perinatal human immunodeficiency virus transmission risk, timing of human immunodeficiency virus diagnostic testing, and selection of antiretroviral regimen

Risk Category	HIV Diagnostic Tests [a,b]	ARV Treatment Regimen	Duration of Treatment
Low risk of perinatal HIV transmission: • Infants born to mothers who received antiretroviral therapy during pregnancy and had sustained viral suppression at the time of delivery (HIV RNA level <50 copies/mL)	HIV RNA or DNA NATs should be obtained at the following ages: • 14–21 d • 1–2 mo • 4–6 mo	Single drug treatment with ZDV	4 wk
Higher risk of perinatal HIV transmission: • Mothers who received neither antepartum nor intrapartum ARV drugs • Mothers who received only intrapartum ARV drugs • Mothers who received antepartum and intrapartum ARV drugs but who have detectable viral loads near delivery, particularly when delivery was vaginal • Mothers with acute or primary HIV infection during pregnancy • Mothers with unconfirmed HIV status who have a positive HIV antibody test at delivery or postpartum	HIV RNA or HIV DNA NATs should be performed at the following ages: • Birth • 14–21 d • 1–2 mo • 2–6 wk after ARV prophylaxis is discontinued • 4–6 mo	Three-drug regimen: ZDV, lamivudine plus (nevirapine or raltegravir)	Consultation with a pediatric HIV expert is recommended

[a] Positive HIV NAT results should be confirmed with a repeat NAT as soon as possible.
[b] The exclusion of HIV infection in infants who are not breastfed requires 2 or more negative HIV NATs obtained at age greater than or equal to 1 month and age greater than or equal to 4 months respectively, or 2 negative HIV antibody tests obtained separately at age greater than or equal to 6 months.

Table 7
Antiretroviral drug dosages by gestational age at birth

Antiretroviral Drug (ARV)	Dosage
ZDV • Oral solution is available in 10 mg/mL	Oral: • GA ≥ 35 wk: 4 mg/kg/dose every 12 h • GA ≥ 30 to <35 wk: 2 mg/kg/dose every 12 h; increase to 3 mg/kg/dose every 12 h at PNA 15 d • GA<30 wk: 2 mg/kg/dose every 12 h Intravenous (75% of oral dose): • GA ≥ 35 wk: 3 mg/kg/dose every 12 h • GA ≥ 30 to <35 wk: 1.5 mg/kg/dose every 12 h; increase to 2.3 mg/kg/dose every 12 h at PNA 15 d • GA<30 wk: 1.5 mg/kg/dose every 12 h
Lamivudine (3TC) • Oral solution is available in 2 concentrations (10 mg/mL and 5 mg/mL)	Oral: • GA ≥ 32 wk: 2 mg/kg/dose twice daily; increase to 4 mg/kg/dose twice daily at 4 wk of age
Nevirapine • Oral solution available in 10 mg/mL	Oral: • GA ≥ 37 wk: 6 mg/kg/dose twice daily; increase to 200 mg/m^2 of BSA per dose twice daily at age >4 wk for infants with confirmed HIV infection • GA ≥ 34 to <37 wk: 4 mg/kg/dose twice daily during the first week of life; increase to 6 mg/kg/dose twice daily for age 1–4 wk; increase to 200 mg/m^2 of BSA per dose twice daily at age >4 wk for infants with confirmed HIV infection
Raltegravir • One packet can be used to prepare a suspension with a final concentration of 10 mg/mL	Oral: GA ≥ 37 wk and weight ≥2 kg: • Birth to 1 wk: 1.5 mg/kg/dose once daily Fixed dosing: 2 to <3 kg: 0.4 mL (4 mg) once daily 3to <4 kg: 0.5 mL (5 mg) once daily 4 to <5 kg: 0.7 mL (7 mg) once daily • 1–4 wk: 3 mg/kg/dose twice daily Fixed dosing: 2 to <3 kg: 0.8 mL (8 mg) twice daily 3 to <4 kg: 1 mL (10 mg) twice daily 4 to <5 kg: 1.5 mL (15 mg) twice daily • 4–6 wk: 6 mg/kg/dose twice daily Fixed dosing: 3 to <4 kg: 2.5 mL (25 mg) twice daily 4 to <6 kg: 3 mL (30 mg) twice daily 6 to <8 kg: 4 mL (40 mg) twice daily

Abbreviations: BSA, body surface area; GA, gestational age; PNA, postnatal age.

more frequent HIV testing.[33] The specificity of HIV RNA and DNA NATs approaches 100%, whereas the sensitivities range from 20% at birth to 100% by age 3 months.[34] A positive infant NAT result at or earlier than 48 hours of life suggests an intrauterine HIV infection, whereas infants with negative initial NATs who subsequently test positive likely developed an intrapartum HIV infection.

HIV antibody tests are not recommended for the diagnosis of HIV infection in infants less than 18 months of age because of transplacental transfer of maternal HIV antibodies. Umbilical cord blood should not be used for infant HIV testing because of the risk of contamination of the sample with maternal blood.

Management of Neonates with Perinatal Human Immunodeficiency Virus Exposure or Infection

All newborns with perinatal HIV exposure ideally should be treated with antiretroviral drugs within 6 to 12 hours of delivery.[33] The selection of a specific ARV regimen and dose should be determined by the gestational age of the infant and maternal and infant risk factors for HIV transmission (see **Table 6**). There is little evidence to guide changes in bathing practices or timing of circumcision for newborns with perinatal HIV exposure.[33]

Hepatitis B vaccine and all age-appropriate and weight-appropriate immunizations should be administered to infants with perinatal HIV exposure. Live, attenuated oral rotavirus vaccine can be safely administered to infants with HIV infection.

Women with HIV infection may be at increased risk of other sexually transmitted or opportunistic infections, such as hepatitis C, hepatitis B, syphilis, gonorrhea, chlamydia, toxoplasmosis, tuberculosis, or herpes simplex virus. A detailed maternal and obstetric history should be obtained and maternal test results for coinfections should be reviewed if available. Infants born to women with other infections should undergo appropriate diagnostic evaluations and may require additional treatment.

Universal or standard precautions should be observed when caring for infants with perinatal HIV exposure.[35] Gloves should be worn when handling newborns during and after birth and with any potential exposure to blood or body fluids.

Antiretroviral treatment and monitoring

Infants at low risk of MTCT should be treated with a 4-week course of oral or intravenous zidovudine (ZDV) prophylaxis (see **Table 6**). Infants with higher risk of MTCT or those with confirmed HIV infection may require treatment with a 3-drug ARV regimen recommended by a pediatric HIV expert.

A complete blood count with differential should be obtained before initiating antiretroviral drugs and after 4 weeks of treatment to evaluate for abnormalities such as anemia and neutropenia, which have been associated with ARV use in infants.

BREASTFEEDING AND FEEDING PRACTICES

In countries where safe water and affordable feeding alternatives such as infant formula are widely available, woman with HIV infection are strongly discouraged from breastfeeding their infants, regardless of maternal viral load. Although infant and maternal prophylaxis with antiretroviral drugs reduces the risk of postnatal HIV transmission, complete avoidance of maternal breast milk is the only effective way to prevent HIV transmission from breast milk to infants. Donor breast milk that has been pasteurized and adequately screened for infection may be a safe alternative for women who wish to feed their infants human breast milk. Occasionally, women with HIV infection on effective antiretroviral therapy and with undetectable viral loads may choose to breastfeed their infants, despite the risk of HIV transmission. In these circumstances, adult and pediatric HIV experts should be consulted to help minimize the risk of HIV transmission.[33]

Parents and caregivers with HIV infection should be advised to avoid feeding infants premasticated (prechewed or prewarmed) solid food, because this practice has been associated with HIV transmission.[36]

PROPHYLAXIS AGAINST *PNEUMOCYSTIS JIROVECI*

To prevent *P jiroveci* pneumonia, all infants with perinatal HIV exposure should begin trimethoprim-sulfamethoxazole prophylaxis at age 4 to 6 weeks, after completing infant ARV prophylaxis, unless HIV infection has been excluded presumptively with 2 or more negative NATs obtained at ages greater than or equal to 2 weeks and age greater than or equal to 4 weeks.

FOLLOW-UP OF INFANTS EXPOSED TO OR INFECTED WITH HUMAN IMMUNODEFICIENCY VIRUS

Infants with perinatal HIV exposure or infection may require additional HIV diagnostic testing and treatment and should follow up with a pediatric HIV expert after hospital discharge.

HELPFUL RESOURCES

In the United States, the http://nccc.ucsf.edu/clinician-consultation/perinatal-hiv-aids/ National Clinician Consultation Center provides consultations on the management of perinatal HIV infection (1-888-448-8765; 24 hours a day, 7 days a week).

SYPHILIS

Disease Overview

Congenital syphilis (CS) occurs when a mother with syphilis transmits the infection to the fetus. CS should always be considered in the evaluation of an infant with suspected congenital infection because the clinical presentation is highly variable, with significant overlap with other diseases.[2,37,38] CS is a preventable disease and is treatable if diagnosed early in the newborn period.

Epidemiology

CS incidence tends to follow trends of increasing primary and secondary syphilis cases in the adult population.[39] The United States and several other countries have reported marked increases in reported cases of CS in recent years. In the United States, the rate of reported CS cases was 33.1 cases per 100,000 live births in 2018 and this reflects a 185.3% increase compared with 2014 rates.[39] The increasing trend of adult syphilis cases is expected to continue, and reversing this increased incidence may not be possible without significant biomedical advancements or a vaccine.[40]

Transmission/Pathogenesis

CS occurs when the spirochete *Treponema pallidum* is transmitted from mother through the placenta to infect the fetus. Maternal primary and secondary syphilis infections are associated with higher rates of fetal and congenital infection than latent-stage syphilis.

Risk factors for transmission include:

- Limited prenatal care

- High treponemal titers
- Late or no maternal treatment

Clinical Presentation

CS presents with varying degrees of severity in fetuses and newborns, from asymptomatic infection to in utero demise, hydrops fetalis, and preterm birth (**Table 8**).[41,42,46] Undiagnosed and untreated infants with no apparent clinical signs at birth remain at risk for later sequelae and morbidity. Hepatomegaly is the most common fetal and postnatal clinical finding with CS.[38,43]

Diagnosis

The diagnosis of CS may be challenging in asymptomatic infants and is often first suspected after a detailed review of the maternal and prenatal history. Maternal treponemal and nontreponemal syphilis screening test results obtained during the pregnancy should be reviewed on all infants before discharge from the birth hospital.[44] Women who are at high risk for syphilis infection may benefit from repeat syphilis testing during the third trimester and at delivery because infections acquired later in pregnancy may be missed by first-trimester syphilis screening tests. A history of treated or untreated syphilis in the mother or a history of abnormal syphilis screening test results during pregnancy should prompt further evaluation in the infant. This

Table 8
Clinical, laboratory, and radiographic features of congenital syphilis

Clinical Pearls	1. Most infants with CS have no clinical signs at birth 2. Most common signs: hepatomegaly, syphilitic rhinitis (snuffles) jaundice, rash, lymphadenopathy, skeletal findings 3. Radiographic findings may be the only apparent feature, are commonly present at birth, and are usually bilateral and symmetric
Fetal[41–43]	In utero demise, IUGR, ascites, nonimmune hydrops fetalis, hepatomegaly, intrahepatic calcifications, increased middle cerebral artery dopplers, placentomegaly
Newborn Examination[37,38,44]	Fever, small for GA, rash, syphilitic rhinitis, cranial nerve palsies, seizure, hepatomegaly, splenomegaly, lymphadenopathy (may be generalized; palpable epitrochlear nodes) mucous patch, condylomata lata, pseudoparalysis of Parrot (presents as immobile extremity caused by pain), rectal bleeding
Ophthalmic[45]	Chorioretinitis, cataracts, glaucoma
Laboratory[38]	Hemolytic anemia, leukopenia, leukocytosis, thrombocytopenia, hypoglycemia, CSF pleocytosis, increased CSF protein level, increased liver transaminase levels, direct hyperbilirubinemia
Radiographic[44]	Periostitis, osteochondritis
Other	Pneumonia alba, nephrotic syndrome, pancreatitis, myocarditis, gastrointestinal malabsorption, hypopituitarism, diabetes insipidus

Abbreviation: IUGR, intrauterine growth restriction.

evaluation may include a detailed physical examination, nontreponemal blood tests such as reactive plasma regain (RPR) or venereal disease research laboratory (VDRL), and other laboratory and imaging studies based on risk of infection (**Table 9**).

Treatment

The evaluation, diagnosis, and treatment of CS is determined by the risk and severity of syphilis infection based on 4 categories of infection: proved or highly probable; possible; less likely; or unlikely[44] (see **Table 9**). Parenteral penicillin G is the only effective treatment of CS.[47,48]

Prevention

Preventing CS involves syphilis prevention for women and their partners as well as timely identification and treatment of pregnant women with syphilis. The WHO launched a global campaign for the elimination of CS in 2007, but several challenges have prevented significant reductions.[49,50]

Missed opportunities for prevention include limited prenatal care but also lack of adequate testing and inadequate or no treatment in some cases.[51] Repeat syphilis screening tests during the third trimester and at delivery can detect newly acquired infections in high-risk women.[39]

TOXOPLASMOSIS

Disease Overview

Congenital toxoplasmosis (CT) occurs when the obligate intracellular parasite, *Toxoplasma gondii*, is transmitted from mother to fetus. This infection is frequently asymptomatic in both mothers and newborns. Diagnosis may require testing at specialized laboratories, and treatment often includes agents unfamiliar to most newborn health care providers.[52]

Transmission and Pathogenesis

Cats are the definitive hosts, whereas humans and other animals serve as intermediate hosts. Humans become infected after ingestion of undercooked or raw meat, unpasteurized raw milk, and soil or water contaminated with oocytes from cat feces. Infection may also occur via blood transfusion and organ transplant.[52] The risk of maternal to fetal transmission varies greatly by region and country.[53]

Transmission of *T gondii* from mother to fetus may occur in 3 different scenarios of maternal infection:

1. Immunocompetent and seronegative mother who acquires acute primary infection 3 months before conception or during pregnancy
2. Pregnant mother who is immune to one strain and becomes infected with a new more virulent strain
3. Severely immunocompromised mother with reactivation of toxoplasmosis during pregnancy

Clinical Presentation

The presentation of congenital toxoplasmosis varies significantly, and different regions seem to have distinct clinical signs and severity that may reflect strain-related differences in phenotype. CT disease in the United States has been reported to be more severe than European disease.[54] Asymptomatic neonates are at risk of developing significant later sequelae.[55,56] **Table 10** describes the clinical features of CT.

Table 9
Evaluation and treatment of neonates born to women with reactive syphilis tests during pregnancy

Category	Clinical and Laboratory Findings	Evaluation	Treatment
Proven, highly probable CS	Abnormal physical examination Or Serum quantitative nontreponemal serologic titer, 4-fold higher than the mother's titer[a] Or A positive darkfield test or PCR assay of lesions or body fluids	CSF analysis (CSF VDRL, cell count, and protein) CBC with differential and platelet count Other tests (as clinically indicated): Long-bone radiographs, chest radiography, transaminases, neuroimaging, ophthalmologic examination, auditory brain stem response	Preferred treatment: Aqueous crystalline penicillin G, 50,000 U/kg, intravenously, every 12 h (during the first 7 d) then every 8 h (for infants older than 7 d) for a total of 10 d of therapy Or Alternative treatment: procaine penicillin G, 50,000 U/kg, IM in a single daily dose for 10 d
Possible CS	Normal examination And A serum quantitative nontreponemal serologic titer, ≤4-fold the maternal titer And one of the following: Mother was not treated, was inadequately treated, or had no documentation of receiving treatment Or Mother was treated with erythromycin or another nonrecommended regimen (ie a nonpenicillin regimen) Or Mother received recommended treatment <4 wk before delivery	CSF analysis (CSF VDRL, CBC count, and protein) CBC including differential and platelet count Long-bone radiography These evaluations may not be necessary if 10 d of parenteral therapy is administered	Preferred treatment: aqueous crystalline penicillin G, 50,000 U/kg, intravenously, every 12 h (1 wk or younger), then every 8 h for infants older than 1 wk, for a total of 10 d of therapy (preferred) Or Alternative treatment: Procaine penicillin G, 50,000 U/kg, IM (single daily dose for 10 d) Or Alternative treatment in select cases: benzathine penicillin G, 50,000 U/kg, IM, single dose (recommended by some experts, but only if all components of the evaluation are obtained and are normal, including normal CSF results and follow-up is certain)

CS less likely	Normal examination And A serum quantitative nontreponemal serologic titer equal to or less than 4-fold the maternal titer And Mother was treated during pregnancy (treatment was appropriate for stage of infection, and treatment was administered >4 wk before delivery) And Mother has no evidence of reinfection or relapse	No evaluation	Benzathine penicillin G, 50,000 U/kg, IM, single dose Alternative strategy[b]: Infants whose mother's nontreponemal titers decreased at least 4-fold after appropriate therapy for early syphilis or remained stable at low titer (eg, VDRL $\leq$ 1:2; RPR $\leq$ 1:4) may be followed every 2–3 mo without treatment until the nontreponemal test becomes nonreactive
CS is unlikely	Normal infant examination And A serum quantitative nontreponemal serologic titer equal to or less than 4-fold the maternal titer And Mother was treated adequately before pregnancy And Mother's nontreponemal serologic titer remained low and stable before and during pregnancy and at delivery (eg, VDRL $\leq$ 1:2; RPR $\leq$ 1:4)	—	No treatment required, but infants with reactive nontreponemal tests should be followed serologically to ensure test result returns to negative Recommended by some experts: benzathine penicillin G, 50,000 U/kg, IM, single dose can be considered if follow-up is uncertain and infant has a reactive test Neonates with a negative nontreponemal test result at birth and whose mothers were seroreactive at delivery should be retested at 3 months to rule out serologically negative incubating CS at the time of birth

Abbreviations: CBC, complete blood count; IM, intramuscularly.

[a] Absence of a 4-fold or greater title does not exclude CS.

[b] Nontreponemal antibody titers should decrease by 3 months of age and should be nonreactive by 6 mo of age whether the infant was infected and adequately treated or was not infected and initially seropositive because of transplacentally acquired maternal antibody. Patients with increasing titers or with persistent stable titers 6 to 12 months after initial treatment should be reevaluated. This evaluation should include a CSF examination. Treatment should include a 10-day course of parenteral penicillin G, even if they were treated previously.

Data from Centers for Disease Control and Prevention. Sexually Transmitted Diseases Treatment Guidelines. Congenital Syphilis. 2015; https://www.cdc.gov/std/tg2015/congenital.htm. and Kimberlin DW BM, Jackson MA, Long SS. *Red Book: 2018 Report of the Committee on Infectious Diseases*: American Academy of Pediatrics; 2018:773-788.

Table 10
Clinical features of congenital toxoplasmosis

Fetal	Fetal demise, hydrocephalus, intracranial calcifications/densities, intrahepatic calcifications, IUGR, ascites, pericardial effusions, increased placental thickness and placental densities, echogenic bowel
Neurologic	Hypotonia, macrocephaly or microcephaly, palsies, spasticity, seizures, CSF abnormalities, encephalopathy, intracranial calcifications, hydrocephalus, brain masses Nystagmus, cataracts, amblyopia, strabismus, optic nerve atrophy, amblyopia, chorioretinitis, microphthalmia, microcornea, pneumonitis
Ophthalmic	—
Other	Temperature instability, myocarditis, anemia, sepsislike syndrome, rash, hepatitis, jaundice, thrombocytopenia, hepatomegaly, splenomegaly, lymphadenopathy

Data from Maldonado YA, Read JS. Diagnosis, Treatment, and Prevention of Congenital Toxoplasmosis in the United States. *Pediatrics.* 2017;139(2):e20163860 and Feigin and Cherry's textbook of pediatric infectious diseases/[edited by] James D. Cherry, Gail J. Harrison, Sheldon L. Kaplan, William J. Steinbach, Peter J. Hotez. Eighth edition. ed. Philadelphia, PA: Elsevier; 2018.

DIAGNOSIS AND TREATMENT

Diagnosis of congenital toxoplasmosis is challenging because most women with toxoplasmosis remain asymptomatic. When maternal infection is suspected, early diagnosis, treatment, and evaluation of the fetus may help reduce the risks of infection and fetal complications. Evaluation of infants for CT should include multidisciplinary consultation with infectious disease specialists, retinal specialists, and neurologists. In 2017, Maldonado and colleagues[52] published a technical report with detailed recommendations on the evaluation, diagnosis, and treatment of CT. Clinicians

Table 11
Clinical and imaging findings associated with congenital Zika infection

Clinical Neurologic Signs	Severe microcephaly; hypertonia, dysphagia, hearing deficits
Neuroradiologic Signs	Lenticulostriate vasculopathy and germinolytic cysts; subcortical calcifications; ventriculomegaly, thin cortical mantle; fetal brain disruption sequence; brainstem hypoplasia
Eye	Microphthalmia; cataract; intraocular calcifications; coloboma, posterior ocular findings; focal macular pigment mottling, chorioretinal atrophy with a predilection for the macular area, congenital glaucoma and optical nerve hypoplasia, and optic disc abnormalities
Musculoskeletal	Arthrogryposis, clubfoot
Urologic	Cryptorchidism, hypospadias
Other	Craniofacial anomalies

Data from[45,66–68]

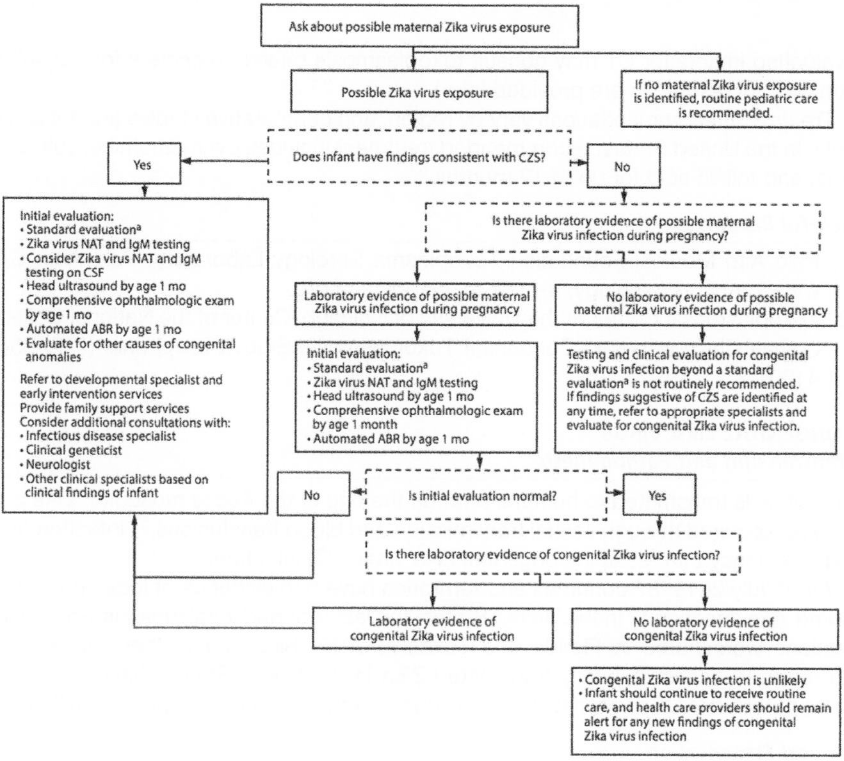

Ask about possible maternal Zika virus exposure
Possible Zika virus exposure
If no maternal Zika virus exposure is identified, routine pediatric care is recommended.
Does infant have findings consistent with CZS?
Yes
No
Initial evaluation:
• Standard evaluation[a]
• Zika virus NAT and IgM testing
• Consider Zika virus NAT and IgM testing on CSF
• Head ultrasound by age 1 mo
• Comprehensive ophthalmologic exam by age 1 mo
• Automated ABR by age 1 mo
• Evaluate for other causes of congenital anomalies
Refer to developmental specialist and early intervention services
Provide family support services
Consider additional consultations with:
• Infectious disease specialist
• Clinical geneticist
• Neurologist
• Other clinical specialists based on clinical findings of infant
Is there laboratory evidence of possible maternal Zika virus infection during pregnancy?
Laboratory evidence of possible maternal Zika virus infection during pregnancy
No laboratory evidence of possible maternal Zika virus infection during pregnancy
Initial evaluation:
• Standard evaluation[a]
• Zika virus NAT and IgM testing
• Head ultrasound by age 1 mo
• Comprehensive ophthalmologic exam by age 1 month
• Automated ABR by age 1 mo
Testing and clinical evaluation for congenital Zika virus infection beyond a standard evaluation[a] is not routinely recommended.
If findings suggestive of CZS are identified at any time, refer to appropriate specialists and evaluate for congenital Zika virus infection.
No
Is initial evaluation normal?
Yes
Is there laboratory evidence of congenital Zika virus infection?
Laboratory evidence of congenital Zika virus infection
No laboratory evidence of congenital Zika virus infection
• Congenital Zika virus infection is unlikely
• Infant should continue to receive routine care, and health care providers should remain alert for any new findings of congenital Zika virus infection

Fig. 1. Recommendations for the evaluation of infants with possible congenital Zika virus infection based on infant clinical findings,[a,b] maternal testing results,[c,d] and infant testing results[e,f] (United States, October 2017).[a] All infants should receive a standard evaluation at birth and at each subsequent well-child visit by their health care providers including (1) comprehensive physical examination, including growth parameters, and (2) age-appropriate vision screening and developmental monitoring and screening using validated tools. Infants should receive a standard newborn hearing screen at birth, preferably using auditory brainstem response. [b]Automated auditory brainstem response (ABR) by age 1 month if newborn hearing screen passed but performed with otoacoustic emission methodology. [c]Laboratory evidence of possible Zika virus infection during pregnancy is defined as (1) Zika virus infection detected by a Zika virus RNA NAT on any maternal, placental, or fetal specimen (referred to as NAT-confirmed); or (2) diagnosis of Zika virus infection, timing of infection cannot be determined or unspecified flavivirus infection, timing of infection cannot be determined by serologic tests on a maternal specimen (ie, positive/equivocal Zika virus IgM and Zika virus plaque reduction neutralization test [PRNT] titer $\geq$10, regardless of dengue virus PRNT value; or negative Zika virus IgM, and positive or equivocal dengue virus IgM, and Zika virus PRNT titer $\geq$10, regardless of dengue virus PRNT titer). The use of PRNT for confirmation of Zika virus infection, including in pregnant women, is not routinely recommended in Puerto Rico (https://www.cdc.gov/zika/laboratories/lab-guidance.html). [d]This group includes women who were never tested during pregnancy as well as those whose test results were negative because of issues related to timing or sensitivity and specificity of the test. Because the latter issues are not easily discerned, all mothers with possible exposure to Zika virus during pregnancy who do not have laboratory evidence of possible Zika virus infection, including those who tested negative with currently available technology, should be considered in this group. [e]Laboratory testing of infants for Zika virus should be performed as early as possible, preferably within the first few days after birth, and

evaluating infants for CT may consult toxoplasmosis reference centers for consultation (helpful resources are provided later).

Treatment recommendations vary by region, and comparative studies are not available. In the United States, recommended treatment includes pyrimethamine, sulfadiazine, and folinic acid for up to 12 months.[52]

Helpful Resources

(1) Palo Alto Medical Foundation Toxoplasma Serology Laboratory, Palo Alto, CA: www.pamf.org/serology; e-mail: toxolab@pamf.org.
(2) Toxoplasmosis Center at the University of Chicago (Center of the National Collaborative Chicago-based Congenital Toxoplasmosis Study): telephone, (773) 834-4130.

CONGENITAL ZIKA VIRUS

Transmission and Pathogenesis

Zika virus is transmitted to humans through the bite of the *Aedes* mosquito. Zika can also be acquired through sexual transmission and blood transfusions.[57] Infection during pregnancy can result in congenital Zika virus (CZ) infection.

As of July 2019, 87 countries and territories have had evidence of local mosquito-borne Zika infection.[58] In the United States, the last reported local mosquito-borne infections were noted in Florida and Texas in 2017. Since 2018, there have been no reported cases of locally transmitted Zika in the Unites States. Cases continue to be reported in US territories, but have significantly declined each year since 2017.[59]

Clinical Presentation

CZ can result in a range of clinical signs in the newborn.[60–64] Early reports describing CZ focused on microcephaly, but later studies revealed a wide range of associated anomalies in addition to microcephaly.[60] Clinicians should be aware that many newborns with CZ may have no clinical signs, including normal head circumference.[64] Exposed neonates without signs of CZ are still at risk for later neurodevelopmental delays and/or deficits despite normal clinical and imaging findings at birth.[65] Clinical and neuroimaging features of CZ are listed in **Table 11**.

Diagnosis and Treatment

The ideal strategy for laboratory evaluation and timing of diagnostic testing is unclear. Infants with signs of CZ have been noted to have negative laboratory evaluations.[60,67]

Fig. 1 provides guidance on evaluation of infants with possible CZ.[66]

No treatment is available for Zika virus and future epidemics are expected to expand into previously unaffected populations because of climate change, population growth, and population movement.[69,70]

includes concurrent Zika virus NAT in infant serum and urine, and Zika virus IgM testing in serum. If CSF is obtained for other purposes, Zika virus NAT and Zika virus IgM testing should be performed on CSF. [f]Laboratory evidence of congenital Zika virus infection includes a positive Zika virus NAT or a nonnegative Zika virus IgM with confirmatory neutralizing antibody testing, if PRNT confirmation is performed. CZS, congenital Zika syndrome. (From Adebanjo T, Godfred-Cato S, Viens L, et al. Update: Interim Guidance for the Diagnosis, Evaluation, and Management of Infants with Possible Congenital Zika Virus Infection - United States, October 2017. MMWR Morb Mortal Wkly Rep. 2017;66(41):1089-1099.)

Table 12
Clinical signs and features of congenital Chagas

More Common	Low birth weight Respiratory distress Hepatomegaly Splenomegaly
Less Common	Prematurity Cardiomyopathy/heart failure Sepsis Meningoencephalitis Petechiae Anemia

Data from[72–76]

Helpful Resources

1) Centers for Disease Control and Prevention (CDC) recommendations with detailed laboratory specimen guidance can be found at: https://www.cdc.gov/zika/hc-providers/test-specimens-at-time-of-birth.html

CHAGAS DISEASE

Transmission and Pathogenesis

Chagas disease, or American trypanosomiasis, is caused by infection with the protozoan parasite *Trypanosoma cruzi*. The parasite can be passed from mother to fetus, resulting in congenital infection. The prevalence of Chagas and congenital Chagas (CC) varies widely, and it is most prevalent in Mexico, Central America, and South America.[71]

Chagas is an underappreciated health concern in the United States, with 40,000 women of childbearing age estimated to have chronic Chagas disease. In the United States, it is estimated that up to 300 infants are born with CC each year.[71]

The CDC includes Chagas disease on its list of neglected parasitic infections, which includes parasitic disease based on numbers of infected individuals, disease severity, and ability to prevent and treat.[72]

Clinical Presentation, Diagnosis, Treatment, and Prevention

Women at risk for Chagas should be screened for infection before and during pregnancy.[71] Approximately half of infants with CC have no clinical signs. When clinical signs are present, they are similar to the nonspecific signs commonly associated with other congenital infections (**Table 12**). Both benznidazole and nifurtimox are used to treat infants with CC disease.[73,77] Early treatment of CC is well tolerated and is curative in 90% of cases.[77–79]

SUMMARY

Infants with congenital infections are often asymptomatic at birth or present with mild, nonspecific signs and symptoms, making diagnosis challenging. Newborn care providers should be aware of the wide range of traditional (TORCH) and emerging fetal and neonatal pathogens that can cause congenital infection. With the advancements in molecular and other diagnostic testing, a targeted, disease-specific evaluation for congenital infection is preferred rather than a broad search for infectious agents with comprehensive antibody panels. Although newborn care providers are critical in suspecting, diagnosing, and initiating early treatment, coordination among obstetric, perinatal, and pediatric infectious disease and other specialties is often required for the optimal diagnosis and management of infants with congenital infection.

CLINICS CARE POINTS

- Congenital HIV, CMV, syphilis, Zika, and Chagas all can be present in newborns with subtle or no apparent clinical signs.
- A single negative urine PCR is sufficient to exclude congenital CMV infection.
- Mother's can transmit HIV infection to an infant during pregnancy, during labor and delivery, or postnatally during breastfeeding.
- Hepatomegaly is the most common fetal and postnatal clinical finding with congenital syphilis
- Congenital syphilis is preventable and treatable if diagnosed early in the newborn period.
- Congenital toxoplasmosis is a challenging diagnosis because most women with toxoplasmosis are asymptomatic.
- Although congenital Zika is commonly associated with microcephaly, infected infants can have normal head circumference at birth and are still at risk for later neurologic sequalae.
- Early treatment of congenital Chagas is well tolerated and curative in 90% of cases.

BEST PRACTICES

What is the current practice?

- Newborn care providers frequently deviate from guidelines for evaluation of congenital infections
- Traditionally used tests such as TORCH titer screens and immunoglobulin M for infants who are small for gestational age have limited value based on current evidence.

What changes in current practice are likely to improved outcomes?

- Optimal collaboration among newborn, obstetric, perinatal, and pediatric infectious disease specialties.
- Awareness of subtle presentations of congenital infections
- Knowledge of advancements in diagnostic testing
- Disease specific evaluation

Major recommendations

- Targeted disease specific testing instead of "TORCH titer screens" and/or total IgM is the ideal approach to laboratory evaluation of congenital infections.(3,4)
- Urine or saliva PCR are the optimal tests for diagnosis of CMV because of superior sensitivity and rapid turn around time. The tests should be performed before 2-3 weeks of age to distinguish congenital from postnatal infection.
- Infants with symptomatic CMV infection should receive antiviral treatment as soon as the diagnosis is made and ideally before 30 days of life to decrease the risk of long term sequelae.(9,22,23)
- Mother's with unknown HIV status and their infants, should have prompt testing with a US Food and Drug Administration (FDA) approved rapid HIV antigen/antibody immunoassay that detects HIV-1 and HIV-2 antibodies, and HIV-1 p24 antigen.
- Mothers with high risk of syphilis should be screened during third trimester and at the time of delivery for to adequately rule out congenital infection.

- Consultation with toxoplasmosis reference centers and laboratories should be considered for optimal evaluation and management of congenital toxoplasmosis.(52)
- Women at risk for Chagas disease should be screened for infection before and during pregnancy.(71)

Summary Statement

- Newborn infants with congenital infections may not have apparent clinical signs at birth. Optimal collaboration and low index of suspicion among care providers with disease specific diagnostic evaluations may optimize outcomes.

WHAT ARE THE CURRENT BEST PRACTICES FOR CONGENITAL INFECTIONS RELATED TO HIV,CMV, TOXOPLASMOSIS, ZIKA, AND CHAGAS?

1. Optimal communication among obstetric and newborn care providers regarding maternal exposure, risk associated with congenital infections, and prenatal laboratory documentation.
2. Targeted disease-specific testing instead of TORCH titer screens and/or total IgM is the ideal approach to laboratory evaluation.
3. Urine or saliva PCR are the optimal tests for diagnosis of CMV because of superior sensitivity and rapid turnaround time. The tests should be performed before 2 to 3 weeks of age.
4. Infants with symptomatic CMV infection should be treated promptly with antiviral treatment to decrease the risk of long-term sequelae.
5. Mothers with unknown HIV status and their infants should have prompt testing with an FDA-approved rapid HIV antigen/antibody immunoassay that detects HIV-1 and HIV-2 antibodies, and HIV-1 p24 antigen.
6. Repeat syphilis screening should occur during the third trimester and at the time of delivery for high-risk mothers to adequately rule out congenital infection.
7. Consultation with toxoplasmosis reference centers and laboratories should be considered for optimal evaluation and management of congenital toxoplasmosis.
8. Newborn care providers should ask about the mother's potential Zika exposure for every newborn, because changes in interim guidance for maternal care may lead to lower numbers of mothers being tested.
9. Women at risk for Chagas disease should be screened for infection before and during pregnancy.

REFERENCES

1. Pereira L. Congenital viral infection: traversing the uterine-placental interface. Annu Rev Virol 2018;5(1):273–99.
2. Penner J, Hernstadt H, Burns JE, et al. Stop, think SCORTCH: rethinking the traditional 'TORCH' screen in an era of re-emerging syphilis. Arch Dis Child 2020; 106(2):117–24.
3. Hwang JS, Friedlander S, Rehan VK, et al. Diagnosis of congenital/perinatal infections by neonatologists: a national survey. J Perinatol 2019;39(5):690–6.
4. van der Weiden S, de Jong EP, te Pas AB, et al. Is routine TORCH screening and urine CMV culture warranted in small for gestational age neonates? Early Hum Dev 2011;87(2):103–7.
5. Khan NA. Screening small for gestational age babies for congenital infection. Am J Perinatol 2000;17(3):131–5.
6. Primhak RA. Screening small for gestational age babies for congenital infection. Clin Pediatr 1982;21(7):417–20.

7. Kenneson A, Cannon MJ. Review and meta-analysis of the epidemiology of congenital cytomegalovirus (CMV) infection. Rev Med Virol 2007;17(4):253–76.
8. Dollard SC, Grosse SD, Ross DS. New estimates of the prevalence of neurological and sensory sequelae and mortality associated with congenital cytomegalovirus infection. Rev Med Virol 2007;17(5):355–63.
9. Kimberlin DW, Jester PM, Sanchez PJ, et al. Valganciclovir for symptomatic congenital cytomegalovirus disease. N Engl J Med 2015;372(10):933–43.
10. Hyde TB, Schmid DS, Cannon MJ. Cytomegalovirus seroconversion rates and risk factors: implications for congenital CMV. Rev Med Virol 2010;20(5):311–26.
11. Demmler-Harrison GJ, Miller JA, Houston Congenital Cytomegalovirus Longitudinal Study G. Maternal cytomegalovirus immune status and hearing loss outcomes in congenital cytomegalovirus-infected offspring. PLoS One 2020; 15(10):e0240172.
12. Pass RF, Fowler KB, Boppana SB, et al. Congenital cytomegalovirus infection following first trimester maternal infection: symptoms at birth and outcome. J Clin Virol 2006;35(2):216–20.
13. Wang C, Zhang X, Bialek S, et al. Attribution of congenital cytomegalovirus infection to primary versus non-primary maternal infection. Clin Infect Dis 2011;52(2): e11–3.
14. Colugnati FA, Staras SA, Dollard SC, et al. Incidence of cytomegalovirus infection among the general population and pregnant women in the United States. BMC Infect Dis 2007;7:71.
15. Cannon MJ, Schmid DS, Hyde TB. Review of cytomegalovirus seroprevalence and demographic characteristics associated with infection. Rev Med Virol 2010;20(4):202–13.
16. Bate SL, Dollard SC, Cannon MJ. Cytomegalovirus seroprevalence in the United States: the national health and nutrition examination surveys, 1988-2004. Clin Infect Dis 2010;50(11):1439–47.
17. Mathews TJ, Hamilton BE. Mean age of mothers is on the rise: United States, 2000-2014. NCHS Data Brief 2016;(232):1–8.
18. Luck SE, Wieringa JW, Blazquez-Gamero D, et al. Congenital cytomegalovirus: a European expert consensus statement on diagnosis and management. Pediatr Infect Dis J 2017;36(12):1205–13.
19. Lopez AS, Ortega-Sanchez IR, Bialek SR. Congenital cytomegalovirus-related hospitalizations in infants <1 year of age, United States, 1997-2009. Pediatr Infect Dis J 2014;33(11):1119–23.
20. Boppana SB, Ross SA, Shimamura M, et al. Saliva polymerase-chain-reaction assay for cytomegalovirus screening in newborns. N Engl J Med 2011;364(22): 2111–8.
21. Boppana SB, Ross SA, Novak Z, et al. Dried blood spot real-time polymerase chain reaction assays to screen newborns for congenital cytomegalovirus infection. JAMA 2010;303(14):1375–82.
22. Oliver SE, Cloud GA, Sanchez PJ, et al. Neurodevelopmental outcomes following ganciclovir therapy in symptomatic congenital cytomegalovirus infections involving the central nervous system. J Clin Virol 2009;46(Suppl 4):S22–6.
23. Kimberlin DW, Lin CY, Sanchez PJ, et al. Effect of ganciclovir therapy on hearing in symptomatic congenital cytomegalovirus disease involving the central nervous system: a randomized, controlled trial. J Pediatr 2003;143(1):16–25.
24. UNAIDS. Global HIV &AIDS statistics - 2020 fact sheet 2020. Available at: https://www.unaids.org/en/resources/fact-sheet. Accessed 3 November 2020.

25. Centers for Disease Control and Prevention. Estimated HIV incidence and prevalence in the United States, 2014–2018. In: HIV surveillance supplemental report 202025. 2020. Available at: http://www.cdc.gov/hiv/library/reports/hiv-surveillance.html.
26. Centers for Disease Control and Prevention. HIV surveillance report, 2018 (Updated) 2020. Available at: http://www.cdc.gov/hiv/library/reports/hiv-surveillance.html. Accessed 15 October, 2020.
27. Rates of mother-to-child transmission of HIV-1 in Africa, America, and Europe: results from 13 perinatal studies. The working group on mother-to-child transmission of HIV. J Acquir Immune Defic Syndr Hum Retrovirol 1995;8(5):506–10.
28. Nesheim SR, FitzHarris LF, Lampe MA, et al. Reconsidering the number of women with HIV infection who give birth annually in the United States. Public Health Rep 2018;133(6):637–43.
29. Nesheim SR, FitzHarris LF, Mahle Gray K, et al. Epidemiology of perinatal HIV transmission in the United States in the era of its elimination. Pediatr Infect Dis J 2019;38(6):611–6.
30. Little KM, Taylor AW, Borkowf CB, et al. Perinatal antiretroviral exposure and prevented mother-to-child HIV infections in the era of antiretroviral prophylaxis in the United States, 1994–2010. Pediatr Infect Dis J 2017;36(1):66–71.
31. Fowler MG, Qin M, Fiscus SA, et al. Benefits and risks of antiretroviral therapy for perinatal HIV prevention. N Engl J Med 2016;375(18):1726–37.
32. Force USPST, Owens DK, Davidson KW, et al. Screening for HIV infection: US preventive services task force recommendation statement. JAMA 2019;321(23):2326–36.
33. Panel on treatment of pregnant women with HIV infection and prevention of perinatal transmission. In: Recommendations for the use of antiretroviral drugs in pregnant women with HIV infection and interventions to reduce perinatal HIV transmission in the United States. 2020. Available at: https://clinicalinfo.hiv.gov/sites/default/files/inline-files/pediatricguidelines.pdf. Accessed 15 October 2020.
34. Panel on antiretroviral therapy and medical management of children living with HIV. Guidelines for the use of antiretroviral agents in pediatric HIV infection. Available at: https://clinicalinfo.hiv.gov/sites/default/files/inline-files/pediatricguidelines.pdf. Accessed 26 October 2020.
35. Siegel JD, Rhinehart E, Jackson M, et al. Health care infection control practices advisory C. 2007 guideline for isolation precautions: preventing transmission of infectious agents in health care settings. Am J Infect Control 2007;35(10 Suppl 2):S65–164.
36. Gaur AH, Dominguez KL, Kalish ML, et al. Practice of feeding premasticated food to infants: a potential risk factor for HIV transmission. Pediatrics 2009;124(2):658–66.
37. Keuning MW, Kamp GA, Schonenberg-Meinema D, et al. Congenital syphilis, the great imitator—case report and review. Lancet Infect Dis 2020;20(7):e173–9.
38. Lago EG, Vaccari A, Fiori RM. Clinical features and follow-up of congenital syphilis. Sex Transm Dis 2013;40(2):85–94.
39. Centers for Disease Control and Prevention. Sexually Transmitted Disease Surveillance 2018. Atlanta: U.S. Department of Health and Human Services; 2019. https://doi.org/10.15620/cdc.79370.
40. Schmidt R, Carson PJ, Jansen RJ. Resurgence of syphilis in the United States: an assessment of contributing factors. Infect Dis 2019;12. 1178633719883282.
41. Hollier LM, Harstad TW, Sanchez PJ, et al. Fetal syphilis: clinical and laboratory characteristics. Obstet Gynecol 2001;97(6):947–53.

42. Nathan L, Twickler DM, Peters MT, et al. Fetal syphilis: correlation of sonographic findings and rabbit infectivity testing of amniotic fluid. J Ultrasound Med 1993; 12(2):97–101.
43. Rac MWF, Bryant SN, McIntire DD, et al. Progression of ultrasound findings of fetal syphilis after maternal treatment. Am J Obstet Gynecol 2014;211(4): 426.e421–6.
44. Kimberlin DW, Jackson MA, Long SS. Red Book: 2018 report of the committee on infectious diseases. Elk Grove (IL): American Academy of Pediatrics; 2018. p. 773–88.
45. Yepez JB, Murati FA, Pettito M, et al. Ophthalmic manifestations of congenital zika syndrome in Colombia and Venezuela. JAMA Ophthalmol 2017;135(5):440–5.
46. Rac MWF, Stafford IA, Eppes CS. Congenital syphilis: a contemporary update on an ancient disease. Prenatal Diagn 2020;40(13):1703–14.
47. Syphilis. Centers for Disease Control and Prevention (CDC). 2018. Available at: https://www.cdc.gov/std/stats18/syphilis.htm. Accessed November 25, 2020.
48. Centers for Disease Control and Prevention. Sexually transmitted diseases treatment guidelines. Congenital syphilis. 2015. Available at: https://www.cdc.gov/std/tg2015/congenital.htm. Accessed November 26, 2020.
49. The global elimination of congenital syphilis: rationale and strategy for action. Geneva: World Health Organization; 2007.
50. Taylor M, Gliddon H, Nurse-Findlay S, et al. Revisiting strategies to eliminate mother-to-child transmission of syphilis. Lancet Glob Health 2018;6(1):e26–8.
51. Kidd S, Bowen VB, Torrone EA, et al. Use of national syphilis surveillance data to develop a congenital syphilis prevention cascade and estimate the number of potential congenital syphilis cases averted. Sex Transm Dis 2018;45:S23–8.
52. Maldonado YA, Read JS. Diagnosis, treatment, and prevention of congenital toxoplasmosis in the United States. Pediatrics 2017;139(2):e20163860.
53. Bigna JJ, Tochie JN, Tounouga DN, et al. Global, regional, and country seroprevalence of Toxoplasma gondii in pregnant women: a systematic review, modelling and meta-analysis. Scientific Rep 2020;10(1):1–10.
54. Olariu TR, Remington JS, McLeod R, et al. Severe congenital toxoplasmosis in the United States: clinical and serologic findings in untreated infants. Pediatr Infect Dis J 2011;30(12):1056–61.
55. Peyron F, Wallon M, Liou C, et al. Treatments for toxoplasmosis in pregnancy. Cochrane Database Syst Rev 1999;(3):CD001684.
56. Cherry JD, Harrison GJ, Kaplan SL, et al, editors. Feigin and Cherry's textbook of pediatric infectious diseases. 8th edition. Philadelphia, PA: Elsevier; 2018.
57. Petersen LR, Baden LR, Jamieson DJ, et al. Zika Virus. N Engl J Med 2016; 374(16):1552–63.
58. Organization WH. Countries and territories with current or previous Zika virus transmission. 2019. Available at: https://www.who.int/emergencies/diseases/zika/countries-with-zika-and-vectors-table.pdf. Accessed November 20, 2020.
59. CDC) CfDCaP. Zika virus. Statistics and maps 2019. Available at: https://www.cdc.gov/zika/reporting/index.html. Accessed November 20, 2020.
60. Melo ASdO, Aguiar RS, Amorim MMR, et al. Congenital zika virus infection. JAMA Neurol 2016;73(12):1407.
61. Hoen B, Schaub B, Funk AL, et al. Pregnancy outcomes after ZIKV infection in French territories in the americas. N Engl J Med 2018;378(11):985–94.
62. Einspieler C, Utsch F, Brasil P, et al. Association of infants exposed to prenatal zika virus infection with their clinical, neurologic, and developmental status evaluated via the general movement assessment tool. JAMA Netw Open 2019;2(1): e187235.

63. Aragao MFVV, Holanda AC, Brainer-Lima AM, et al. Nonmicrocephalic infants with congenital zika syndrome suspected only after neuroimaging evaluation compared with those with microcephaly at birth and postnatally: How large is the zika virus "iceberg"? Am J Neuroradiol 2017;38(7):1427–34.
64. França GVA, Schuler-Faccini L, Oliveira WK, et al. Congenital Zika virus syndrome in Brazil: a case series of the first 1501 livebirths with complete investigation. Lancet 2016;388(10047):891–7.
65. Mulkey SB, Arroyave-Wessel M, Peyton C, et al. Neurodevelopmental abnormalities in children with in utero zika virus exposure without congenital zika syndrome. JAMA Pediatr 2020;174(3):269.
66. Adebanjo T, Godfred-Cato S, Viens L, et al. Update: interim guidance for the diagnosis, evaluation, and management of infants with possible congenital zika virus infection - United States, October 2017. MMWR Morb Mortal Wkly Rep 2017;66(41):1089–99.
67. de Araújo TVB, Rodrigues LC, de Alencar Ximenes RA, et al. Association between Zika virus infection and microcephaly in Brazil, January to May, 2016: preliminary report of a case-control study. Lancet Infect Dis 2016;16(12):1356–63.
68. Pool K-L, Adachi K, Karnezis S, et al. Association between neonatal neuroimaging and clinical outcomes in zika-exposed infants from rio de Janeiro, Brazil. JAMA Netw Open 2019;2(7):e198124.
69. Ryan SJ, Carlson CJ, Mordecai EA, et al. Global expansion and redistribution of Aedes-borne virus transmission risk with climate change. PLoS Negl Trop Dis 2019;13(3):e0007213.
70. Kraemer MUG, Reiner RC, Brady OJ, et al. Past and future spread of the arbovirus vectors Aedes aegypti and Aedes albopictus. Nat Microbiol 2019;4(5): 854–63.
71. Centers for Disease Control and Prevention. Congenital chagas disease 2019. Available at: https://www.cdc.gov/parasites/chagas/health_professionals/congenital_chagas.html%20. Accessed November 22, 2020.
72. Messenger LA, Gilman RH, Verastegui M, et al. Toward improving early diagnosis of congenital chagas disease in an Endemic setting. Clin Infect Dis 2017;65(2):268–75.
73. Edwards MS, Stimpert KK, Bialek SR, et al. Evaluation and management of congenital chagas disease in the United States. J Pediatr Infect Dis Soc 2019;8(5):461–9.
74. Freilij H, Altcheh J. Congenital chagas' disease: diagnostic and clinical aspects. Clin Infect Dis 1995;21(3):551–5.
75. Torrico F, Alonso-Vega C, Suarez E, et al. Maternal Trypanosoma cruzi infection, pregnancy outcome, morbidity, and mortality of congenitally infected and non-infected newborns in Bolivia. Am J Trop Med Hyg 2004;70(2):201–9.
76. Blanco SB, Segura EL, Cura EN, et al. Congenital transmission of Trypanosoma cruzi: an operational outline for detecting and treating infected infants in north-western Argentina. Trop Med Int Health 2000;5(4):293–301.
77. Carlier Y, Altcheh J, Angheben A, et al. Congenital chagas disease: updated recommendations for prevention, diagnosis, treatment, and follow-up of newborns and siblings, girls, women of childbearing age, and pregnant women. PLoS Negl Trop Dis 2019;13(10):e0007694.
78. Altcheh J, Moscatelli G, Moroni S, et al. Adverse events after the use of benznidazole in infants and children with chagas disease. Pediatrics 2010;127(1): e212–8.
79. Chippaux JP, Salas-Clavijo AN, Postigo JR, et al. Evaluation of compliance to congenital chagas disease treatment: results of a randomised trial in Bolivia. Trans R Soc Trop Med Hyg 2012;107(1):1–7.

Human Milk for the Term Newborn

Isabelle Von Kohorn, MD, PhD[a,b,*], Valerie Flaherman, MD, MPH[c,d]

KEYWORDS

• Human milk • Donor milk • Term newborn • Lactation • NICU • Mother's own milk

KEY POINTS

- Human milk is the gold standard for infant nutrition and should be actively supported and monitored, particularly in the first weeks after birth.
- Individual-level interventions effective at increasing lactation for term newborns have been identified.
- Some components of popular system-level interventions have been found ineffective or harmful.
- Term newborns admitted to the neonatal intensive care unit are at risk for not receiving human milk feedings, and little is known about how best to support lactation in this population.
- Public policies can help support lactation while promoting individual choice and equity.

INTRODUCTION

Human milk provides optimal nutrition for the term newborn. Breastfeeding is the ideal mode of feeding for most healthy mothers and term newborns and is promoted by all major organizations dedicated to the health and well-being of mothers and newborns in the United States and around the world.[1–3] That every term newborn is not breastfed is due to myriad reasons—medical, social, environmental, personal, and more. Nevertheless, breastfeeding is a public health priority and should be maximally promoted and facilitated.[1] Health care teams caring for mothers and newborns have an obligation to provide evidence-based, high-quality, effective support for breastfeeding; to eliminate barriers to breastfeeding; and to reduce disparities in breastfeeding.

This article reviews the benefits and risks of human milk for the term newborn and the unique factors associated with milk expression. Evidence regarding

[a] Department of Pediatrics, Holy Cross Health, 1500 Forest Glen Road, Silver Spring, MD 20910, USA; [b] Department of Pediatrics, The George Washington University School of Medicine & Health Sciences, Washington, DC, USA; [c] Department of Pediatrics, University of California, San Francisco, 3333 California Street, Box 0503, San Francisco, CA 94118, USA; [d] Department of Epidemiology and Biostatistics, University of California, San Francisco, San Francisco, CA, USA
* Corresponding author. 1500 Forest Glen Road, Silver Spring, MD 20910.
E-mail address: ivonkohorn@gmail.com

Clin Perinatol 48 (2021) 513–531
https://doi.org/10.1016/j.clp.2021.05.005 perinatology.theclinics.com

supplementation of breastfeeding with formula and donor breast milk (DBM) for the term newborn is discussed. Issues related to human milk for term newborns who require special or intensive care are considered and evidence outlined for interventions to reduce barriers and promote lactation, with a focus on purposeful reduction in disparities in breastfeeding.

EPIDEMIOLOGY OF HUMAN MILK FOR INFANTS

Human milk feeding rates have risen steadily in the United States during the twenty-first century. According to the Centers for Disease Control and Prevention (CDC), the proportion of infants in the United States who were ever breastfed rose from 76.7% in 2010 to 84.1% in 2017.[4] Over the same period, the percentage exclusively breastfed at 6 months of age rose from 17.2% to 25.6%.[4] Still, the United States falls short of international and national goals for breastfeeding initiation, exclusivity, and duration.[2,3,5] In reviewing the epidemiologic literature in this area, although the World Health Organization (WHO) defines "exclusive breastfeeding" as receiving only breast milk and no other food or fluid except vitamins, minerals, and medications, the term exclusive breastfeeding is not used consistently across studies.[6,7] In addition, epidemiologic studies of human milk consumption often do not distinguish between direct breastfeeding, feeding of mother's own milk (MOM) (either direct or expressed), and DBM feeding. This lack of consistent use of available definitions is a limitation of this, and any, review of the existing literature.

Mothers in the United States, as in other high-income countries, are less likely to breastfeed their infants than women in low-income and middle-income countries (LMICs).[8,9] In LMICs, breastfeeding may be inversely associated with wealth at the household level, with women from wealthier households breastfeeding less.[8] Conversely, in the United States and other high-income countries, women from higher-income households are more likely to breastfeed, and those from less wealthy households are less likely to breastfeed. For example, in the United States, women who receive or are eligible for the Special Supplemental Nutrition Program for Women, Infants, and Children (WIC) are less likely ever to breastfeed than those who are not eligible.[10] Researchers have postulated that lack of experience and training in breastfeeding techniques and lack of troubleshooting among health professionals and the lay public may contribute to lower breastfeeding rates in high-income countries.[11,12]

Other important disparities in breastfeeding rates exist in the United States. Across the country, breastfeeding rates vary by race and ethnicity with the lowest rates of breastfeeding experienced by women and infants who identify as non-Hispanic black/African American (**Fig. 1**). Because there are lifelong benefits to breastfeeding for both mothers and infants, different rates of breastfeeding may contribute to health disparities for generations. Reasons for lower breastfeeding rates among African American mothers include lower social support for breastfeeding,[13] higher acceptability of formula,[14,15] and racial disparities in maternity care.[16,17] Among Hispanic mothers, initiation of breastfeeding is high, but the prevalence of exclusive breastfeeding is much lower, with many mothers introducing formula in the first days of their infant's life.[18,19] To decrease US health disparities, interventions to address key racial and ethnic facilitators of and barriers to exclusive breastfeeding are needed.[13,20]

Extensive public health and health care efforts in the United States and worldwide seek to maximize breastfeeding for all mothers and infants. Goals well-aligned globally include exclusive breastfeeding through 6 months and continuation of breastfeeding through at least 1 year of life.[1,5,8] The WHO also recommends exclusive breastfeeding for 6 months and further defines optimal breastfeeding as "initiation within 1 hour of life

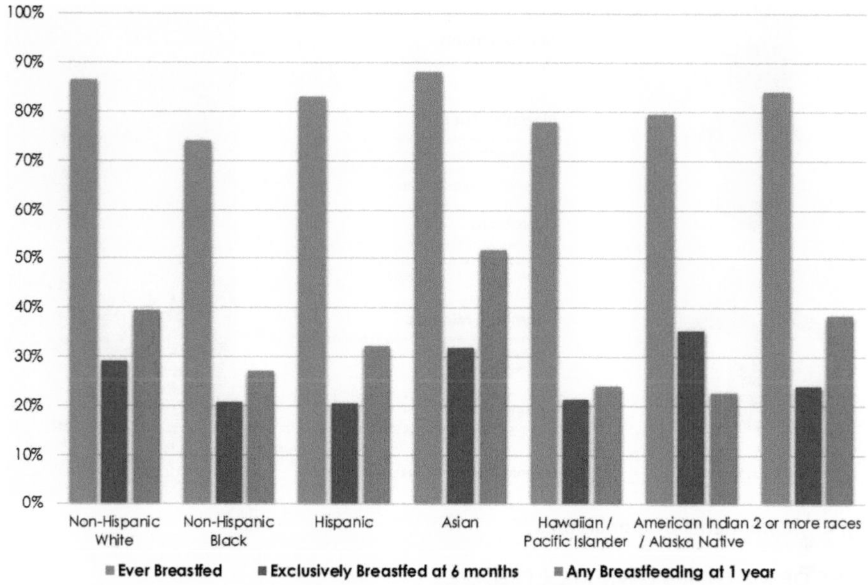
100%
90%
80%
70%
60%
50%
40%
30%
20%
10%
0%
Non-Hispanic White
Non-Hispanic Black
Hispanic
Asian
Hawaiian / Pacific Islander
American Indian / Alaska Native
2 or more races
Ever Breastfed
Exclusively Breastfed at 6 months
Any Breastfeeding at 1 year

Fig. 1. Breastfeeding in the United States by race, ethnicity; 2016 CDC data

and…for up to 2 years of age or beyond."[5] Healthy People 2030, the national US blueprint for improving health and well-being also has prioritized breastfeeding exclusivity and duration.[3]

Clinical Care Points

- Human milk feedings have increased in the United States during the twenty-first century.
- International and national goals for breastfeeding are aligned but often not met.
- There are important health disparities in breastfeeding rates.

BENEFITS OF MOTHER'S OWN MILK FEEDINGS

The benefits of MOM feedings are extensive for mothers and infants.[9,21–31] For infants, these benefits include decreased mortality,[21–23] improved cognitive function,[24,25] reduced rates of obesity,[26] acute otitis media,[27,28] and malocclusion of deciduous teeth.[29] For mothers, lactation is associated with a reduction in breast and ovarian cancer,[30] type 2 diabetes mellitus,[31] and mental health issues[32] and also is linked to increased birth spacing, mediated by lactational amenorrhea.[30] These benefits are proportional to the amount of MOM that makes up an infant's diet and the duration of MOM feedings, with improved outcomes associated with higher exclusivity and duration.[33,34]

The benefits of MOM feedings for the infant derive largely from the nutritional and bioactive components of human milk.[35–37] These include macronutrients and micronutrients specific to human milk, such as nutritional proteins, fats, and carbohydrates; bioactive components, such as immunoglobulins and maternal white blood cells; and prebiotics and probiotics, such as human milk oligosaccharides and milk microbiota. Although a detailed discussion of these is beyond the scope of this review, **Fig. 2** depicts the major known components of human milk.

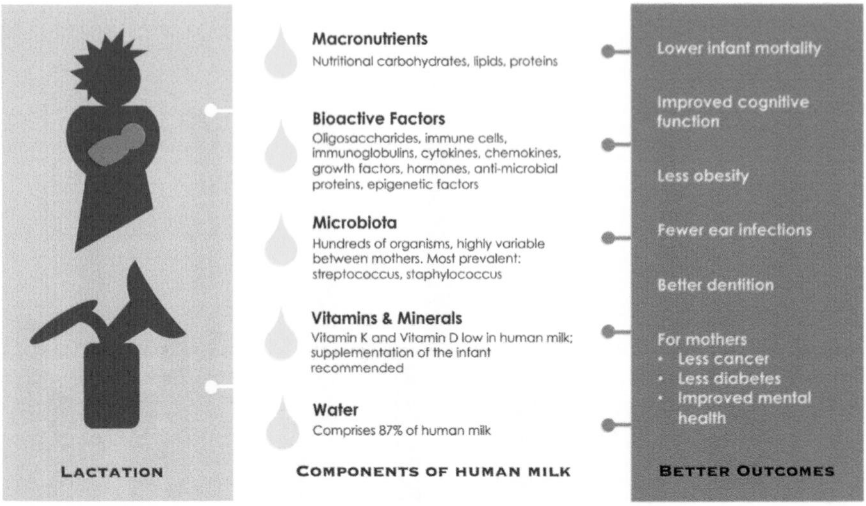
Macronutrients
Nutritional carbohydrates, lipids, proteins
Bioactive Factors
Oligosaccharides, immune cells, immunoglobulins, cytokines, chemokines, growth factors, hormones, anti-microbial proteins, epigenetic factors
Microbiota
Hundreds of organisms, highly variable between mothers. Most prevalent: streptococcus, staphylococcus
Vitamins & Minerals
Vitamin K and Vitamin D low in human milk; supplementation of the infant recommended
Water
Comprises 87% of human milk
Lower infant mortality
Improved cognitive function
Less obesity
Fewer ear infections
Better dentition
For mothers
Less cancer
Less diabetes
Improved mental health
LACTATION
COMPONENTS OF HUMAN MILK
BETTER OUTCOMES

Fig. 2. Components of human milk.

RISKS OF MOTHER'S OWN MILK FEEDINGS

Despite the many benefits of MOM feedings, there also are risks. For example, MOM is contraindicated for conditions, such as infant galactosemia or maternal treatment with chemotherapeutic agents. Other risks of MOM may derive from a disruption in lactogenesis, which is the 2-stage process of initiating and developing copious milk production. Maternal anatomic, physiologic, psychological, and emotional factors may inhibit lactogenesis, as may infant factors.[38,39] Any combination of problems may lead to inappropriate supply of milk to the infant with the consequence of inadequate nutrition and/or hydration for the infant, possibly resulting in

- Excessive weight loss and dehydration[40]
- Nutritional deficiency and growth failure[41]
- Severe hyperbilirubinemia[42]
- Hospital readmission[40]

The first 2 weeks after birth are a critical period for promoting exclusive MOM while limiting the risks of MOM feedings. Health care providers should screen for and address factors that may predispose to lactation failure, such as maternal or infant illness and anatomic problems (eg, infant with cleft lip/palate and maternal history of breast surgery). Health care providers then should actively monitor for problems with lactation and nursing. Providers should suspect insufficient lactogenesis if they observe signs indicating that there is too little transfer of milk from mother to newborn, including

- Hypoglycemia unresponsive to appropriate frequent breastfeeding[38]
- Clinical or laboratory evidence of significant dehydration[38]
- Weight loss
    - 8% to 10% by day 5 (120 hours) or later[38]
    - Greater than 75th percentile for age[43]
    - Failure to regain birth weight by 2 weeks of age[44]
- Delayed bowel movements, fewer than 4 stools on day 4 of life, or continued meconium stools on day 5 (120 hours)[38]

- Insufficient urination, possibly with urate crystals
- Excessive hyperbilirubinemia[38]
- Signs of medical illness
- Delayed secretory activation (lack of abundant milk production by days 4–7)[45,46]
- Hypoplastic breast shape or poor breast growth during pregnancy[38]
- Infrequent breastfeeding or milk expression
- Intolerable pain during feedings unrelieved by interventions[38]

Once suspected, insufficient lactogenesis should be evaluated and treated urgently with intensive, evidence-based interventions.[38,47–49]

Clinical Care Points

- The first 2 weeks after birth are a critical period for promoting MOM while limiting its risks.
- Health care providers should provide effective support for breastfeeding, screen for risk factors for insufficient lactation, observe closely for signs of milk transfer from mother to newborn, and treat lactation problems urgently.

CONSIDERATIONS FOR EXPRESSED BREAST MILK

When a newborn is not able to breastfeed effectively, mothers must express milk if they wish to provide it to their infants. Expression also may be used when mothers are separated from their infants or for maternal preference. The vast majority (85%) of breastfeeding mothers in the United States express milk to feed to their infants, and a quarter of breastfeeding mothers report routinely expressing milk.[50,51] Studies of outcomes associated with expressed milk feeding have been hampered by the fact that many data collection tools feature items that assess both direct breastfeeding and expressed milk feedings without distinguishing between them.[52–55] For this reason, it is difficult to assess the effects of expressed milk feeding compared with direct breastfeeding for term newborns. Some important differences between these 2 feeding approaches, however, have been identified. First, expressing, storing, and reheating milk may degrade its nutritional value, with documented decreases in antioxidant activity, immunologic factors and vitamin content from these processes.[35,56–58] Second, the process of expressing and storing human milk introduces the opportunity for contamination of milk,[51]given that mothers can and do express milk in many locations, including their cars, bathrooms, and office spaces; furthermore, mothers may store milk in myriad containers and unregulated cool storage devices.[51,59] Guidelines exist to help mothers make their milk expression as safe as possible and should be promoted by clinicians.[60] Third, separating milk expression from infant feeding introduces the potential for a mismatch between milk supply and demand. Some data indicate that mothers may overexpress milk to ensure their infants have sufficient milk in their absence.[61] To ensure adequate supply, mothers also may pump milk after they breastfeed, thereby feeding the infant a higher dose of foremilk during the breastfeeding session and storing the more fat-rich hindmilk for a subsequent feed.[51] The effects of this practice on infant macronutrient intake are unknown. Fourth, expressed milk may obviate some breastfeeding's benefits, including its reduction in risk of otitis media.[62] Finally, exclusive milk expression may be associated with shorter duration of MOM feedings.[63] This association may be mediated by a variety of factors; 1 study found that mothers who expressed their milk for voluntary reasons (eg, return to work) provided milk to their infants for longer than mothers who expressed their milk for involuntary reasons (eg, insufficient supply or infant unable to breastfeed due to illness).[64]

For the healthy term infant, the possible risks of expressed MOM feeding likely are small, particularly when infants receive a combination of direct breastfeeding and expressed milk feedings. The potential risks of expressed MOM feedings for sick term newborns are unknown but may be greater than for well term newborns.[65] For this reason, mothers expressing milk for sick term newborns must pay especially careful attention to hygiene and storage.

Clinical Care Points

- Expressed milk has risks compared with direct breastfeeding, including nutritional degradation, mismatch between supply and demand, and decreased breastfeeding duration.
- Clinicians caring for sick newborns should ensure that mothers expressing milk for such infants are knowledgeable about the importance of careful hygiene and storage.
- Understanding a mother's attitudes about and the circumstances related to milk expression may be key to prolonging MOM feedings.

SUPPLEMENTATION

Exclusive MOM not always is possible. Sometimes, MOM feedings are not a safe option; other times, MOM may not meet the nutritional or physiologic needs of the infant. Careful prevention of problems and evaluation of insufficient lactation are the first steps in supporting MOM feedings through early challenges.[38] Still, supplementation may be necessary for some infants.

Formula

Many studies about formula supplementation during the birth hospitalization indicate that availability and use of infant formula is associated with a reduction in MOM feedings.[66,67] In addition, there is some evidence that removing free samples and marketing of infant formula is associated with an increase in MOM feedings.[68] Organizations and nations committed to promoting breastfeeding actively discourage the marketing and use of breast milk substitutes.[69]

Although routine provision of infant formula may be problematic, there are medical indications for supplementation of MOM feedings. Recent studies indicate that treatment of potentially dangerous early breastfeeding problems with infant formula may help conserve lactation. A randomized controlled trial of early limited formula supplementation showed that among infants at risk for excessive weight loss, small volumes of formula to supplement breastfeeding until establishment of mature milk supply resulted in longer duration of breastfeeding.[47] A secondary analysis showed that the use of small volumes of infant formula ($\leq$4 oz daily) in the first month of life was not associated with earlier breastfeeding cessation, compared with larger volumes of supplementation.[70]

Donor Breast Milk

When supplementation of breastfeeding is needed, DBM is an alternative to infant formula. Although informal sharing of breast milk is unsafe and should be highly discouraged,[1] the use of DBM that has been pasteurized and distributed by a formal donor milk bank is believed to be safe and nutritious. Considerations related to DBM that has been pasteurized and provided by milk banks accredited by reliable regulatory institutions, such as the Human Milk Banking Association of North America, are discussed.

Although DBM has been demonstrated to be a safe source of nutrition and provides many components similar to MOM, DBM is not biologically equivalent to MOM. First, the composition of DBM is impacted by the process of pasteurization and storage, which may decrease the bioactivity of proteins and eliminate beneficial microbiota.[71–74] Second, the stage of lactation of DBM may not be an ideal match for the recipient infant and may be substantially different from MOM in its nutritional and bioactive composition.[75] Likely for these reasons, DBM has not been shown to provide the full range of beneficial effects conveyed by MOM.[75,76] Although it is not equivalent to MOM, DBM may be preferable to infant formula when MOM is not available.

The vast majority of research on the health benefits of DBM compared with formula has focused on very low birthweight (VLBW) infants born weighing less than 1500 g. There is moderately good evidence to support the use of DBM for VLBW infants when MOM is not available,[76–79] and its use appears to be cost-effective in that population.[80] The health and economic benefits of DBM in the VLBW population, however, are due largely to the beneficial association between exclusive human milk feedings and reduced incidence of necrotizing enterocolitis (NEC). Because NEC is infrequent for term newborns, the beneficial effects of DBM for term newborns cannot be entirely inferred from evidence available from the VLBW population. Some data suggest that DBM may be beneficial for sick term newborns, including those with congenital heart disease and gastroschisis,[81,82] but little to no evidence exists for healthy term infants, and the data are mixed about whether DBM supplementation supports lactation for mothers of term newborns.[83–85]

Nevertheless, DBM use for term newborns increasing, and institutions that provide DBM to term newborns report higher rates of exclusive breastfeeding than those who do not provide DBM.[53] These reported associations have the potential to be misleading, because metrics used by certifying organizations characterize any human milk (either MOM or DBM) delivered by breast, bottle, or other feeding method as "exclusive breastfeeding." For this reason, it is unclear to what extent an increase in "exclusive breastfeeding" resulting from DBM use is due to improved rates of lactogenesis.[53,54,86] The acceptability of DBM varies by maternal race and ethnicity, with nonwhite mothers and those with limited English proficiency less likely to agree to DBM for their infants.[87–89] Thus, the use of DBM may exacerbate rather than reduce existing disparities.

Clinical Care Points

1. If the supply of DBM is limited, its use should be targeted toward populations of mothers and infants for whom there is proven benefit.[77,90]
2. Interventions to prioritize DBM rather than formula for term infants should ensure that DBM does not displace MOM as the preferred feeding type for all infants.[91]
3. Research and interventions to increase the availability and acceptability of DBM should identify and address facilitators and barriers specific to different racial and ethnic groups.

HUMAN MILK FOR THE TERM NEWBORN IN THE NEONATAL INTENSIVE CARE UNIT

Although the vast majority (93%) of term infants receive routine care during the birth hospitalization, some require admission to a neonatal intensive care unit (NICU).[92] Term infants make up approximately 50% of NICU admissions in the United States, although their average length of stay (approximately 5 days) is dramatically shorter than for their preterm counterparts.[93] Term newborns admitted to the NICU are significantly less likely to breastfeed than their term counterparts who receive routine care.[92,94] A vast majority of term newborns admitted to the NICU have low to moderate acuity illness, indicating that they have an excellent prognosis.[95] Thus, for most term newborns admitted to the NICU, reduced lactation may be 1 of the most substantial lifetime risks associated with their NICU admission.

Hardly any data exist about the benefits of human milk specific to the sick term newborn or about how best to support lactation when a term infant is admitted to the NICU, although the benefits of human milk for preterm newborns have been described extensively.[96–102] Extensive, thoughtful research has identified facilitators of and barriers to providing MOM to premature infants, and quality improvement efforts targeting these factors have been quite successful in improving MOM feeds in the preterm population, as well as in reducing racial and ethnic disparities.[103–108] Similar research to understand facilitators and barriers related to provision of MOM for term infants in the NICU is needed.

Clinical Care Points

- Term newborns admitted to the NICU are substantially less likely to receive human milk than their healthy counterparts.
- Reduced lactation may be one of the most substantial lifetime risks associated with NICU admission for the term newborn.
- Evidence to inform the development of interventions to improve lactation for mothers of term newborns in the NICU is needed.

EVIDENCE-BASED SUPPORT FOR LACTATION FOR MOTHERS OF TERM NEWBORNS

Given the health benefits of breastfeeding and the substantial resources expended by the health care system to support it, woefully little evidence exists to evaluate the effectiveness of lactation support strategies for healthy mothers and their term newborns. The data that do exist indicate that the most effective interventions to promote lactation are individual-level interventions delivered directly to women, tailored to their individual needs, and informed by their culture, beliefs, and environment. System-level interventions (separate from routine provision of effective individual-level interventions) have not been shown to improve breastfeeding in high-income settings.

Individual-level Interventions

Primary care support and education provided to mothers

Recent reviews provide good evidence that a variety of individual-level interventions targeting lactation support and education during the pregnancy, peripartum, and postpartum periods can increase the initiation, duration, and exclusivity of MOM feedings.[11,109–111] Interventions implemented at multiple time points may be more effective than those at a single time point.[110–112] Interventions delivered only in the antepartum period may not be as effective as those delivered postpartum or with a postpartum component.[113] Interventions also may be more successful when implemented in settings with high rates of lactation initiation.[11] Features of successful lactation support include that it is

- A standard part of care
- Offered by personnel trained in lactation support
- Predictable in timing so women know when it will be available
- Tailored to the particular needs of a population
- Face-to-face[11]

Primary care practices associated with improved lactation
Some of the primary care interventions identified in the review underlying the US Preventive Services Task Force recommendations for lactation support[110] that contribute positively to improved lactation include

- Lactation consultation integrated into routine care[114]
- Electronically prompted guidance from health care providers[114]
- Peer counseling to support breastfeeding as a core service of the WIC program[115]
- Home-based prenatal and postnatal early intervention services that specifically promote breastfeeding[116]
- Daily feeding log[117]
- Antenatal breastfeeding education delivered by a health care professional[118,119]
- Postnatal lactation support[118]
- Motivational interviewing by nurses who have received formal training in breastfeeding management, counseling skills, motivational interviewing, and reflective practice and who use a standardized intervention tool[120]
- Professional breastfeeding telephone support provided early in the postnatal period, and continued for the first month postpartum[121]
- An individual, routine, preventive, outpatient visit within 2 weeks after the birth provided by a physician who received a 5-h training program on breastfeeding[122]

In-hospital practices associated with improved lactation but other potential risks
Skin-to-skin care in the early postnatal period has been shown to have multiple beneficial effects for mothers and newborns and to improve breastfeeding rates.[123] The practice has come under scrutiny, however, because it is associated with sudden unexpected postnatal collapse (SUPC) of the newborn—a life-threatening event occurring in the first few days of life.[124–126] Although rare (estimates range from 2.6 to 133/100,000 infants), more than one-third of SUPC events occur in the first 2 hours of life. Many risk factors for SUPC are associated with early skin-to-skin care, including prone position of the infant, first breastfeeding attempt, mother in episiotomy position, and parents being left alone with baby during first hours after birth.[125] Although rare, SUPC can be devastating; approximately 50% of SUPC events are fatal, with a majority of survivors suffering major neurologic consequences.[125] A focus on safety is critical for policies intended to support lactation.[126]

System-level Interventions

No recent review of well-controlled studies has found good evidence that system-level interventions are effective at increasing breastfeeding in a high-income country setting.[110,111] The most well-known system-level intervention is the Baby-Friendly Hospital Initiative (BFHI), best studied in a national trial in Belarus in the 1990s.[127] Other quasi-experimental and observational studies also have shown an association between implementation of the BFHI and an increase in breastfeeding.[128] More stringent analysis of the data from high-income countries indicate, however, that the BFHI may interfere with breastfeeding in some settings.[129] There is some indication that BFHI may have greater benefit for mothers who have lower education levels.[110–112,130]

The BFHI is composed of Ten Steps to Successful Breastfeeding.[131] These 10 steps were assembled in the twentieth century, and some now have been found to be either ineffective or potentially harmful. For example, a mother rooming in with her infant after delivery has not been shown to increase breastfeeding rates, although the practice has been adopted widely and may have other benefits for maternal-infant bonding.[132] Similarly, there are no studies regarding the benefit of infant-led, or on-demand, breastfeeding compared with scheduled feedings.[133] Avoidance of all supplemental nutrition actually may impede lactation.[43] Finally, avoidance of pacifier use has not been proved effective for increasing the initiation or duration of breastfeeding among mothers who are well-motivated to breastfeed.[134] Furthermore, pacifier use seems to be protective against sudden infant death syndrome, thereby making the avoidance of pacifier use a potentially dangerous practice.[112] Development of system-level interventions to support lactation that are evidence-based and subject to routine quality improvement are needed.[112,124,135]

A model for development of such system-level interventions accompanied by quality improvement can be found in the efforts to increase MOM for premature newborns.[104,106,107] An important common feature of these programs is that they are founded on qualitative research that sought to understand the perspectives of people who are experts in the issue being studied: in this case, mothers of preterm newborns. Future system-level interventions to increase breastfeeding among mothers and their term newborns may be most successful if they are underpinned by similar qualitative research that also identifies key racial and ethnic variation in perspectives.

Clinical Care Points

- Numerous individual-level interventions have been shown to improve lactation for mothers of term newborns.
- In contrast, no system-level interventions have yet been demonstrated to improve lactation for mothers of term newborns.
- Clinical guidance and quality measures should routinely incorporate new evidence regarding best practices and safety if "bundles" such as BFHI have not yet been updated.
- Future research urgently is needed to inform the development of system-level interventions effective for improving breastfeeding initiation and duration and should:
    - Be founded on qualitative research
    - Seek to decrease health disparities
    - Be modified routinely as new evidence becomes available

PUBLIC POLICIES TO IMPROVE HUMAN MILK FOR THE TERM NEWBORN

Public policies are an important driver of human milk for term newborns. In the United States, paid family leave policies are associated positively with lactation rates, although some policies may widen disparities by conferring greater benefit to already more advantaged mothers.[136] Internationally, longer paid family leave (up to 6–12 months) is associated with consistently improved infant health, including reduced infant mortality, with breastfeeding as a likely key factor.[137]

Women always will be disproportionately affected by attempts to increase lactation.[51,112,138] As the only person who can provide MOM to their infant, a woman must choose between or balance lactation and paid employment. Social policies are critical in helping to facilitate options regarding lactation and work.[139] More nuanced social policies are needed to make lactation and paid work possible at every stage of lactation, from prenatal preparation through at least 2 years after birth. Policymakers must pay special attention to the impact of policies on different groups of women, with the goal of implementing policies that reduce health disparities.

SUMMARY

Human milk is the gold standard for infant nutrition. The United States does not meet goals for provision of human milk to term newborns. Expressed milk, donor milk, or formula may be needed if early growth goals are not met. Expressed milk often is consumed by US infants and has its own specific benefits and risks compared with direct breastfeeding. Donor human milk as a supplement for term newborns is increasing in popularity but requires more study. Individual-level interventions, such as peer counseling and motivational interviewing, have been found to be effective at increasing human milk for term newborns, but no system-level interventions have yet been demonstrated effective in high-income settings, and some popular system-level interventions have not yet incorporated new evidence regarding safety. Term newborns admitted to the NICU are at special risk for not receiving human milk feedings, and little is known about how best to support lactation in this population. Nuanced public policies have the potential to address these deficits in evidence while helping increase lactation and promoting individual choice and equity.

Best Practices Box

Human milk for the term newborn

The benefits of human milk are extensive and are associated with higher exclusivity and duration.[33,34]

Best practices to increase human milk for term newborns

- Identification and prevention of barriers to breastfeeding[38]
- Individual-level interventions shown effective for the promotion of breastfeeding, both during pregnancy and after birth, such as peer counseling and electronic decision support[110,111]
- Rapid identification and treatment of insufficient lactation[38]
- Public policies to support lactation[112,138,139]

Practices that may be beneficial but require more study

- DBM as a supplement for term infants[53,82,84,85,91]
- Small-volume formula supplementation for term infants with pronounced weight loss[47,140,141]

Practice that should be implemented with safety precautions

- Skin-to-skin care after birth[135]

Practice that may need to be discontinued due to known side effects

- Avoidance of pacifiers[112]

Key areas for research

- Effective, modifiable system-level interventions to improve human milk for term newborns
- Interventions to improve lactation for term newborns admitted to the NICU
- Interventions and policies to decrease health disparities in lactation

DISCLOSURE

The authors have no conflicts of interest to disclose.

REFERENCES

1. American Academy of Pediatrics. Breastfeeding and the use of human milk. Pediatrics 2012;129(3):e827–41.
2. World Health Organization. Breastfeeding. Available at: https://www.who.int/health-topics/breastfeeding#tab=tab_1. Accessed: November 18, 2020.

3. Healthy People 2030. Improve the health and safety of infants. Available at: https://health.gov/healthypeople/objectives-and-data/browse-objectives/infants. Accessed November 18, 2020.
4. Centers for Disease Control and Prevention. National immunization survey, results: breastfeeding rates. Available at: https://www.cdc.gov/breastfeeding/data/nis_data/results.html. Accessed November 29, 2020.
5. World Health Organization. Global nutrition targets 2025: breastfeeding policy brief. Available at: https://apps.who.int/iris/bitstream/handle/10665/149022/WHO_NMH_NHD_14.7_eng.pdf. Accessed November 20, 2020.
6. Flaherman VJ, Chien AT, McCulloch CE, et al. Breastfeeding rates differ significantly by method used: a cause for concern for public health measurement. Breastfeed Med 2011;6(1):31–5.
7. McGrath JM, Brandon D. Why human milk and not breast milk among other changes: 2018 author guideline updates. Adv Neonatal Care 2017;17(5):325–6.
8. UNICEF. Breastfeeding: a mother's gift, for every child. https://www.unicef.org/publications/index_102824.html.
9. Victora CG, Bahl R, Barros AJ, et al. Breastfeeding in the 21st century: epidemiology, mechanisms, and lifelong effect. Lancet 2016;387(10017):475–90.
10. Centers for Disease Control and Prevention. National immunization survey, rates of any and exclusive breastfeeding by Sociodemographics among Children born in 2017. Available at: https://www.cdc.gov/breastfeeding/data/nis_data/rates-any-exclusive-bf-socio-dem-2017.html. Accessed November 29, 2020.
11. McFadden A, Gavine A, Renfrew MJ, et al. Support for healthy breastfeeding mothers with healthy term babies. Cochrane Database Syst Rev 2017. https://doi.org/10.1002/14651858.cd001141.pub5.
12. Renfrew MJ. Time to get serious about educating health professionals. Matern Child Nutr 2006;2(4):193–5.
13. Asiodu IV, Waters CM, Dailey DE, et al. Infant feeding decision-making and the Influences of social support persons among first-time African American mothers. Matern Child Health J 2017;21(4):863–72.
14. Nommsen-Rivers LA, Chantry CJ, Cohen RJ, et al. Comfort with the idea of formula feeding helps explain ethnic disparity in breastfeeding intentions among expectant first-time mothers. Breastfeed Med 2010;5(1):25–33.
15. McKinney CO, Hahn-Holbrook J, Chase-Lansdale PL, et al. Racial and ethnic differences in breastfeeding. Pediatrics 2016;138(2). https://doi.org/10.1542/peds.2015-2388.
16. Sipsma HL, Rabinowitz MR, Young D, et al. Exposure to hospital breastfeeding support by maternal race and ethnicity: a Pilot study. J Midwifery Womens Health 2019;64(6):743–8.
17. Lind JN, Perrine CG, Li R, et al. Racial disparities in access to maternity care practices that support breastfeeding - United States, 2011. MMWR Morb Mortal Wkly Rep 2014;63(33):725–8.
18. Centers for Disease Control and Prevention. Breastfeeding report card. Available at: https://www.cdc.gov/breastfeeding/data/reportcard.htm. Accessed November 18, 2020.
19. Linares AM, Rayens MK, Gomez ML, et al. Intention to breastfeed as a predictor of initiation of exclusive breastfeeding in Hispanic women. J Immigrant Minor Health 2015;17(4):1192–8.
20. Linares AM, Cartagena D, Rayens MK. Las dos Cosas versus exclusive breastfeeding: a Culturally and Linguistically Exploratory intervention study in Hispanic mothers Living in Kentucky. J Pediatr Health Care 2019;33(6):e46–56.

21. Ip S, Chung M, Raman G, et al. Breastfeeding and maternal and infant health outcomes in developed countries. Evid Rep Technol Assess (Full Rep 2007;(153):1–186.
22. WHO Collaborative Study Team on the Role of Breastfeeding on the Prevention of Infant Mortality. Effect of breastfeeding on infant and child mortality due to infectious diseases in less developed countries: a pooled analysis 2000;355(9202):451–5.
23. Sankar MJ, Sinha B, Chowdhury R, et al. Optimal breastfeeding practices and infant and child mortality: a systematic review and meta-analysis. Acta Paediatr 2015;104(467):3–13.
24. Horta BL, Loret de Mola C, Victora CG. Breastfeeding and intelligence: a systematic review and meta-analysis. Acta Paediatr 2015;104(467):14–9.
25. Heikkila K, Kelly Y, Renfrew MJ, et al. Breastfeeding and educational achievement at age 5. Matern Child Nutr 2014;10(1):92–101.
26. Horta BL, Loret de Mola C, Victora CG. Long-term consequences of breastfeeding on cholesterol, obesity, systolic blood pressure and type 2 diabetes: a systematic review and meta-analysis. Acta Paediatr 2015;104(467):30–7.
27. Bowatte G, Tham R, Allen KJ, et al. Breastfeeding and childhood acute otitis media: a systematic review and meta-analysis. Acta Paediatr 2015;104(467): 85–95.
28. Lodge CJ, Tan DJ, Lau MX, et al. Breastfeeding and asthma and allergies: a systematic review and meta-analysis. Acta Paediatr 2015;104(467):38–53.
29. Peres KG, Cascaes AM, Peres MA, et al. Exclusive breastfeeding and risk of Dental malocclusion. Pediatrics 2015;136(1):e60–7.
30. Chowdhury R, Sinha B, Sankar MJ, et al. Breastfeeding and maternal health outcomes: a systematic review and meta-analysis. Acta Paediatr 2015;104(467): 96–113.
31. Horta BL, de Lima NP. Breastfeeding and type 2 diabetes: systematic review and meta-analysis. Curr Diab Rep 2019;19(1):1.
32. Ritchie-Ewing G, Mitchell AM, Christian LM. Associations of maternal beliefs and distress in pregnancy and postpartum with breastfeeding initiation and early cessation. J Hum Lactation 2019;35(1):49–58.
33. Meier PP, Engstrom JL, Patel AL, et al. Improving the use of human milk during and after the NICU stay. Clin Perinatol 2010;37(1):217–45.
34. Kramer MS, Kakuma R. Optimal duration of exclusive breastfeeding. Cochrane Database Syst Rev 2012;(8):CD003517.
35. Ballard O, Morrow AL. Human milk composition: nutrients and bioactive factors. Pediatr Clin North Am 2013;60(1):49–74.
36. Lyons KE, Ryan CA, Dempsey EM, et al. Breast milk, a source of beneficial Microbes and associated benefits for infant health. Nutrients 2020;12(4):1039.
37. Fitzstevens JL, Smith KC, Hagadorn JI, et al. Systematic review of the human milk microbiota. Nutr Clin Pract 2017;32(3):354–64.
38. Kellams A, Harrel C, Omage S, et al. ABM clinical Protocol #3: supplementary feedings in the healthy term breastfed Neonate, Revised 2017. Breastfeed Med 2017;12(4):188–98.
39. Lee S, Kelleher SL. Biological underpinnings of breastfeeding challenges: the role of genetics, diet, and environment on lactation physiology. Am J Physiol Endocrinol Metab 2016;311(2):E405–22.
40. Escobar GJ, Gonzales VM, Armstrong MA, et al. Rehospitalization for neonatal dehydration. Arch Pediatr Adolesc Med 2002;156(2):155.

41. Rana R, McGrath M, Gupta P, et al. Feeding interventions for infants with growth failure in the first Six Months of life: a systematic review. Nutrients 2020;12(7): 2044.
42. Kuzniewicz MW, Escobar GJ, Wi S, et al. Risk factors for severe hyperbilirubinemia among infants with Borderline Bilirubin levels: a Nested case-Control study. The J Pediatr 2008;153(2):234–40.
43. Flaherman VJ, Schaefer EW, Kuzniewicz MW, et al. Early weight loss nomograms for exclusively breastfed newborns. Pediatrics 2015;135(1):e16–23.
44. Paul IM, Schaefer EW, Miller JR, et al. Weight Change nomograms for the first Month after birth. Pediatrics 2016;138(6). https://doi.org/10.1542/peds.2016-2625.
45. Hoban R, Bigger H, Schoeny M, et al. Milk volume at 2 Weeks Predicts mother's own milk feeding at neonatal intensive care Unit Discharge for very low birthweight infants. Breastfeed Med 2018;13(2):135–41.
46. Medina Poeliniz C, Engstrom JL, Hoban R, et al. Measures of secretory activation for research and practice: an integrative review. Breastfeed Med 2020; 15(4):191–212.
47. Flaherman VJ, Aby J, Burgos AE, et al. Effect of early limited formula on duration and exclusivity of breastfeeding in at-risk infants: an RCT. *Pediatr* Jun 2013; 131(6):1059–65.
48. Straňák Z, Feyereislova S, Černá M, et al. Limited amount of formula may facilitate breastfeeding: randomized, controlled trial to Compare standard clinical practice versus limited supplemental feeding. PLOS ONE 2016;11(2):e0150053.
49. Westerfield KL, Koenig K, Oh R. Breastfeeding: common Questions and Answers. Am Fam Physician 2018;98(6):368–73.
50. Labiner-Wolfe J, Fein SB, Shealy KR, et al. Prevalence of breast milk expression and associated factors. Pediatrics 2008;122(Suppl 2):S63–8.
51. Rasmussen KM, Geraghty SR. The quiet revolution: breastfeeding transformed with the use of breast pumps. Am J Public Health 2011;101(8):1356–9.
52. Wood NK, Woods NF. Outcome measures in interventions that Enhance breastfeeding initiation, duration, and exclusivity. MCN, The Am J Maternal/Child Nurs 2018;43(6):341–7.
53. Belfort MB, Drouin K, Riley JF, et al. Prevalence and Trends in donor milk Use in the well-baby nursery: a survey of Northeast United States birth hospitals. Breastfeed Med 2018;13(1):34–41.
54. The Joint Commission. Specifications Manual for Joint Commission national quality measures 2015. Available at: https://manual.jointcommission.org/releases/TJC2015B/DataElem0273.html. Accessed November 20, 2020.
55. O'Sullivan EJ, Geraghty SR, Cassano PA, et al. Comparing alternative breast milk feeding Questions to U.S. Breastfeeding Surveillance Questions. Breastfeed Med 2019;14(5):347–53.
56. Garza C, Johnson CA, Harrist R, et al. Effects of methods of collection and storage on nutrients in human milk. Early Hum Dev 1982;6(3):295–303.
57. Williamson MT, Murti PK. Effects of storage, time, temperature, and composition of containers on biologic components of human milk. J Hum Lact 1996; 12(1):31–5.
58. Hanna N. Effect of storage on breast milk antioxidant activity. Arch Dis Child - Fetal Neonatal Edition 2004;89(6):F518–20.
59. Geraghty SR, Rasmussen KM. Redefining "breastfeeding" initiation and duration in the age of breastmilk pumping. *Breastfeed Med* Jun 2010;5(3):135–7.

60. Centers for Disease Control and Prevention. Proper storage and preparation of breast milk. Available at: https://www.cdc.gov/breastfeeding/recommendations/handling_breastmilk.htm. Accessed November 29, 2020.
61. Geraghty SR, Sucharew H, Rasmussen KM. Trends in breastfeeding: it is not only at the breast anymore. Matern Child Nutr 2013;9(2):180–7.
62. Boone KM, Geraghty SR, Keim SA. Feeding at the breast and expressed milk feeding: associations with otitis media and Diarrhea in infants. J Pediatr 2016; 174:118–25.
63. Bai DL, Fong DY, Lok KY, et al. Practices, predictors and consequences of expressed breast-milk feeding in healthy full-term infants. Public Health Nutr 2017; 20(3):492–503.
64. Felice JP, Cassano PA, Rasmussen KM. Pumping human milk in the early postpartum period: its impact on long-term practices for feeding at the breast and exclusively feeding human milk in a longitudinal survey cohort. The Am J Clin Nutr 2016;103(5):1267–77.
65. Widger J, O'Connell NH, Stack T. Breast milk causing neonatal sepsis and death. Clin Microbiol Infect 2010;16(12):1796–8.
66. Chantry CJ, Dewey KG, Peerson JM, et al. In-hospital formula use increases early breastfeeding cessation among first-time mothers intending to exclusively breastfeed. J Pediatr 2014;164(6):1339–45.e5.
67. McCoy MB, Heggie P. In-hospital formula feeding and breastfeeding duration. Pediatrics 2020;146(1). https://doi.org/10.1542/peds.2019-2946.
68. Tarrant M, Lok KY, Fong DY, et al. Effect of a hospital policy of not accepting free infant formula on in-hospital formula supplementation rates and breast-feeding duration. Public Health Nutr 2015;18(14):2689–99.
69. World Health Organization. Marketing of breast milk substitutes: national implementation of the international code, status report 2020. Available at: https://www.who.int/publications/i/item/9789240006010. Accessed November 18, 2020.
70. Flaherman VJ, McKean M, Braunreuther E, et al. Minimizing the Relationship between early formula Use and breastfeeding cessation by limiting formula volume. Breastfeed Med 2019;14(8):533–7.
71. Demers-Mathieu V, Huston RK, Markell AM, et al. Differences in maternal immunoglobulins within mother's own breast milk and donor breast milk and across Digestion in preterm infants. Nutrients 2019;(4):11. https://doi.org/10.3390/nu11040920.
72. Paulaviciene IJ, Liubsys A, Eidukaite A, et al. The effect of prolonged Freezing and Holder pasteurization on the macronutrient and bioactive protein compositions of human milk. Breastfeed Med 2020;15(9):583–8.
73. Chang F-Y, Fang L-J, Chang C-S, et al. The effect of processing donor milk on its nutrient and Energy content. Breastfeed Med 2020;15(9):576–82.
74. Ford SL, Lohmann P, Preidis GA, et al. Improved feeding tolerance and growth are linked to increased gut microbial community diversity in very-low-birth-weight infants fed mother's own milk compared with donor breast milk. Am J Clin Nutr 2019;109(4):1088–97.
75. Meier P, Patel A, Esquerra-Zwiers A. Donor human milk update: evidence, mechanisms, and Priorities for research and practice. The J Pediatr 2017;180: 15–21.
76. Quigley M, Embleton ND, McGuire W. Formula versus donor breast milk for feeding preterm or low birth weight infants. Cochrane Database Syst Rev 2019;7:CD002971.

77. American Academy of Pediatrics. Donor human milk for the high-risk infant: preparation, safety, and usage options in the United States. Pediatrics 2017;139(1):e20163440.
78. Cristofalo EA, Schanler RJ, Blanco CL, et al. Randomized trial of exclusive human milk versus preterm formula diets in extremely premature infants. J Pediatr 2013;163(6):1592–5.e1.
79. Kantorowska A, Wei JC, Cohen RS, et al. Impact of donor milk availability on breast milk Use and necrotizing enterocolitis rates. Pediatrics 2016;137(3):e20153123.
80. Johnson TJ, Berenz A, Wicks J, et al. The economic impact of donor milk in the neonatal intensive care Unit. J Pediatr 2020;224:57–65.e4.
81. Hoban R, Khatri S, Patel A, et al. Supplementation of mother's own milk with donor milk in infants with gastroschisis or Intestinal Atresia: a Retrospective study. Nutrients 2020;24(2):12. https://doi.org/10.3390/nu12020589.
82. Bhatia A, Moellinger A, Abernathy S, et al. Donor breast milk improves feeding tolerance in infants with critical congenital heart disease. Pediatrics 2020;146(1 MeetingAbstract):125–6.
83. Parker MG, Burnham L, Mao W, et al. Implementation of a donor milk program is associated with greater consumption of mothers' own milk among VLBW infants in a US, level 3 NICU. J Hum Lact 2016;32(2):221–8.
84. Merjaneh N, Williams P, Inman S, et al. The impact on the exclusive breastfeeding rate at 6 months of life of introducing supplementary donor milk into the level 1 newborn nursery. J Perinatology 2020;40(7):1109–14.
85. Kair LR, Flaherman VJ, Colaizy TT. Effect of donor milk supplementation on breastfeeding outcomes in term newborns: a randomized controlled trial. Clin Pediatr (Phila) 2019;58(5):534–40.
86. Kair LR, Phillipi CA, Lloyd-McLennan AM, et al. Supplementation practices and donor milk Use in US well-newborn Nurseries. Hosp Pediatr 2020;10(9):767–73.
87. Kair LR, Nidey NL, Marks JE, et al. Disparities in donor human milk supplementation among well newborns. J Hum Lact 2020;36(1):74–80.
88. Brownell EA, Smith KC, Cornell EL, et al. Five-year Secular Trends and predictors of Nonconsent to receive donor milk in the neonatal intensive care Unit. Breastfeed Med 2016;11(6):281–5.
89. Pal A, Soontarapornchai K, Noble L, et al. Attitudes towards donor breast milk in an Inner city population. Int J Pediatr 2019;2019:3847283.
90. Taylor C, Joolay Y, Buckle A, et al. Prioritising allocation of donor human breast milk amongst very low birthweight infants in middle-income countries. Matern Child Nutr 2018;14(Suppl 6):e12595.
91. Brandstetter S, Mansen K, DeMarchis A, et al. A decision tree for donor human milk: an example tool to Protect, promote, and support breastfeeding. Front Pediatr 2018;6:324.
92. Colaizy TT, Morriss FH. Positive effect of NICU admission on breastfeeding of preterm US infants in 2000 to 2003. J Perinatology 2008;28(7):505–10.
93. March of Dimes Perinatal Data Center. Special care nursery admissions. Available at: https://www.marchofdimes.org/peristats/pdfdocs/nicu_summary_final.pdf. Accessed November 21, 2020.
94. Gertz B, Defranco E. Predictors of breastfeeding non-initiation in the NICU. Matern Child Nutr 2019;15(3):e12797.
95. Schulman J, Braun D, Lee HC, et al. Association between neonatal intensive care Unit admission rates and illness acuity. JAMA Pediatr 2018;172(1):17.

96. Boquien C-Y. Human milk: an ideal food for nutrition of preterm newborn. Front Pediatr 2018. https://doi.org/10.3389/fped.2018.00295.
97. Patel AL, Johnson TJ, Engstrom JL, et al. Impact of early human milk on sepsis and health-care costs in very low birth weight infants. J Perinatol 2013;33(7): 514–9.
98. Chen Y, Fantuzzi G, Schoeny M, et al. High-dose human milk feedings decrease Oxidative stress in premature infant. JPEN J Parenter Enteral Nutr 2019;43(1): 126–32.
99. Vohr BR, Poindexter BB, Dusick AM, et al. Persistent beneficial effects of breast milk ingested in the neonatal intensive care unit on outcomes of extremely low birth weight infants at 30 months of age. Pediatrics 2007;120(4):e953–9.
100. Meinzen-Derr J, Poindexter B, Wrage L, et al. Role of human milk in extremely low birth weight infants' risk of necrotizing enterocolitis or death. J Perinatol 2009;29(1):57–62.
101. Patel AL, Johnson TJ, Robin B, et al. Influence of own mother's milk on bronchopulmonary dysplasia and costs. Arch Dis Child Fetal Neonatal Ed 2017;102(3): F256–61.
102. Belfort MB, Anderson PJ, Nowak VA, et al. Breast milk feeding, Brain development, and Neurocognitive outcomes: a 7-year longitudinal study in infants born at less than 30 Weeks' Gestation. J Pediatr 2016;177:133–9.e1.
103. Patel AL, Meier PP, Canvasser J. Strategies to increase the use of mother's own milk for infants at risk of necrotizing enterocolitis. Pediatr Res 2020;88(Suppl 1):21–4.
104. Parker MG, Burnham LA, Melvin P, et al. Addressing disparities in mother's milk for VLBW infants through Statewide quality improvement. Pediatrics 2019; 144(1). https://doi.org/10.1542/peds.2018-3809.
105. Leeman KT, Barbas K, Strauss J, et al. Improving access to lactation consultation and early breast milk Use in an Outborn NICU. Pediatr Qual Saf 2019;4(1): e130.
106. Meier PP, Johnson TJ, Patel AL, et al. Evidence-based methods that promote human milk feeding of preterm infants: an expert review. Clin Perinatol 2017; 44(1):1–22.
107. Parker MG, Patel AL. Using quality improvement to increase human milk use for preterm infants. Semin Perinatol 2017;41(3):175–86.
108. Patel AL, Schoeny ME, Hoban R, et al. Mediators of racial and ethnic disparity in mother's own milk feeding in very low birth weight infants. Pediatr Res 2019; 85(5):662–70.
109. Balogun OO, O'Sullivan EJ, McFadden A, et al. Interventions for promoting the initiation of breastfeeding. Cochrane Database Syst Rev 2016. https://doi.org/10.1002/14651858.cd001688.pub3.
110. Patnode CD, Henninger ML, Senger CA, et al. Primary care interventions to support breastfeeding: updated evidence report and systematic review for the US preventive services Task Force. JAMA 2016;316(16):1694–705.
111. Bibbins-Domingo K, Grossman DC, Curry SJ, et al. Primary care interventions to support breastfeeding: US preventive services Task Force recommendation Statement. JAMA 2016;316(16):1688–93.
112. Flaherman V, Von Kohorn I. Interventions intended to support breastfeeding: updated Assessment of benefits and Harms. JAMA 2016;316(16):1685–7.
113. Lumbiganon P, Martis R, Laopaiboon M, et al. Antenatal breastfeeding education for increasing breastfeeding duration. Cochrane Database Syst Rev 2016. https://doi.org/10.1002/14651858.cd006425.pub4.

114. Bonuck K, Stuebe A, Barnett J, et al. Effect of primary care intervention on breastfeeding duration and intensity. Am J Public Health 2014;104(Suppl 1): S119–27.
115. Reeder JA, Joyce T, Sibley K, et al. Telephone peer counseling of breastfeeding among WIC participants: a randomized controlled trial. Pediatrics 2014;134(3): e700–9.
116. Wen LM, Baur LA, Simpson JM, et al. Effectiveness of an early intervention on infant feeding practices and "tummy time": a randomized controlled trial. Arch Pediatr Adolesc Med 2011;165(8):701–7.
117. Pollard DL. Impact of a feeding log on breastfeeding duration and exclusivity. Matern Child Health J 2011;15(3):395–400.
118. Su LL, Chong YS, Chan YH, et al. Antenatal education and postnatal support strategies for improving rates of exclusive breast feeding: randomised controlled trial. BMJ 2007;335(7620):596.
119. Mattar CN, Chong YS, Chan YS, et al. Simple antenatal preparation to improve breastfeeding practice: a randomized controlled trial. Obstet Gynecol 2007; 109(1):73–80.
120. Elliott-Rudder M, Pilotto L, McIntyre E, et al. Motivational interviewing improves exclusive breastfeeding in an Australian randomised controlled trial. Acta Paediatr 2014;103(1):e11–6.
121. Fu IC, Fong DY, Heys M, et al. Professional breastfeeding support for first-time mothers: a multicentre cluster randomised controlled trial. BJOG 2014;121(13): 1673–83.
122. Labarere J, Gelbert-Baudino N, Ayral AS, et al. Efficacy of breastfeeding support provided by trained clinicians during an early, routine, preventive visit: a prospective, randomized, open trial of 226 mother-infant pairs. Pediatrics 2005;115(2):e139–46.
123. Moore ER, Bergman N, Anderson GC, et al. Early skin-to-skin contact for mothers and their healthy newborn infants. Cochrane Database Syst Rev 2016. https://doi.org/10.1002/14651858.cd003519.pub4.
124. Gomez-Pomar E, Blubaugh R. The Baby Friendly Hospital Initiative and the ten steps for successful breastfeeding. a critical review of the literature. J Perinatol 2018;38(6):623–32.
125. Herlenius E, Kuhn P. Sudden unexpected postnatal collapse of newborn infants: a review of cases, definitions, risks, and preventive measures. Translational Stroke Res 2013;4(2):236–47.
126. Bass JL, Gartley T, Kleinman R. Unintended consequences of Current breastfeeding Initiatives. JAMA Pediatr 2016;170(10):923.
127. Kramer MS, Chalmers B, Hodnett ED, et al. Promotion of breastfeeding intervention trial (PROBIT). JAMA 2001;285(4):413.
128. Pérez-Escamilla R, Martinez JL, Segura-Pérez S. Impact of the Baby-friendly Hospital Initiative on breastfeeding and child health outcomes: a systematic review. Matern Child Nutr 2016;12(3):402–17.
129. Brodribb W, Kruske S, Miller YD. Baby-friendly hospital accreditation, in-hospital care practices, and breastfeeding. Pediatrics 2013;131(4):685–92.
130. Bass JL, Gartley T, Kleinman R. Outcomes from the Centers for disease Control and prevention 2018 breastfeeding report card: public policy Implications. J Pediatr 2020;218:16–21.e1.
131. World Health Organization. Ten steps to successful breastfeeding. Available at: https://www.who.int/activities/promoting-baby-friendly-hospitals/ten-steps-to-successful-breastfeeding. Accessed November 21, 2020.

132. Jaafar SH, Ho JJ, Lee KS. Rooming-in for new mother and infant versus separate care for increasing the duration of breastfeeding. Cochrane Database Syst Rev 2016;(8):CD006641.
133. Fallon A, Van Der Putten D, Dring C, et al. Baby-led compared with scheduled (or mixed) breastfeeding for successful breastfeeding. Cochrane Database Syst Rev 2016. https://doi.org/10.1002/14651858.cd009067.pub3.
134. Jaafar SH, Ho JJ, Jahanfar S, et al. Effect of restricted pacifier use in breastfeeding term infants for increasing duration of breastfeeding. Cochrane Database Syst Rev 2016;(8):CD007202.
135. Steinhorn RH. Breastfeeding, baby-friendly, and safety: Getting the balance Right. J Pediatr 2020;218:7–8.
136. Hamad R, Modrek S, White JS. Paid family leave effects on breastfeeding: a quasi-experimental study of US policies. Am J Public Health 2019;109(1):164–6.
137. Nandi A, Jahagirdar D, Dimitris MC, et al. The impact of parental and medical leave policies on Socioeconomic and health outcomes in OECD countries: a systematic review of the Empirical literature. Milbank Q 2018;96(3):434–71.
138. Flaherman VJ, Fuentes-Afflick E. Social and public health perspectives of promotion of breastfeeding. JAMA Pediatr 2014;168(10):877–8.
139. Rollins NC, Bhandari N, Hajeebhoy N, et al. Why invest, and what it will take to improve breastfeeding practices? Lancet 2016;387(10017):491–504.
140. Flaherman VJ, Cabana MD, McCulloch CE, et al. Effect of early limited formula on breastfeeding duration in the first year of life: a randomized clinical trial. JAMA Pediatr 2019;173(8):729–35.
141. Flaherman VJ, Narayan NR, Hartigan-O'Connor D, et al. The effect of early limited formula on breastfeeding, readmission, and intestinal microbiota: a randomized clinical trial. J Pediatr 2018;196:84–90.e1.

Hyperbilirubinemia in the Term Infant

Re-evaluating What We Think We Know

Cathy Hammerman, MD[a,b,*], Michael Kaplan, MBChB[b,c]

KEYWORDS

• Hyperbilirubinemia • Bilirubin • Term infant • Neurologic damage

KEY POINTS

- The clinical manifestations of bilirubin neurotoxicity, classically known as kernicterus, are now known to be many and varied, comprising what is newly defined as the kernicterus spectrum disorder.
- The kernicterus spectrum disorder continues to be rampant in developing countries with underdeveloped medical systems. Although rare, however, it also continues to be encountered in industrialized countries.
- Hemolytic conditions top the list of known etiologies of extreme hyperbilirubinemia and kernicterus, whereas genetic polymorphisms and mutations play a cardinal role in the conjugation and elimination of bilirubin.
- The absolute presumption of phototherapy safety may not be universally true, especially for the newer, high-intensity light-emitting diode units.
- In addition to its neurotoxic potential, bilirubin possesses antioxidant properties. Physiologic neonatal mild hyperbilirubinemia occurs precisely at a time in life when other physiologic antioxidant defenses are underdeveloped.

INTRODUCTION

In high concentrations, bilirubin is neurotoxic. If allowed to enter the brain, it binds avidly to cell membranes, especially to developing and myelinating membranes, rendering neurons in the newborn brain a prime target for irreversible bilirubin induced injury. It is the avoidance of this bilirubin-associated neurologic damage that is the motivating force behind the multifaceted efforts to understand, predict, prevent, diagnose, and treat hyperbilirubinemia. In this article, it is not the intention to

[a] Department of Neonatology, Shaare Zedek Medical Center; [b] The Faculty of Medicine of the Hebrew University, Jerusalem, Israel; [c] Department of Neonatology, Shaare Zedek Medical Center (Emeritus)

* Corresponding author. Department of Neonatology, Shaare Zedek Medical Center, POB 3235, Jerusalem 91031, Israel.

E-mail address: cathyh@ekmd.huji.ac.il

Clin Perinatol 48 (2021) 533–554
https://doi.org/10.1016/j.clp.2021.05.006 perinatology.theclinics.com

comprehensively review all aspects of neonatal hyperbilirubinemia in the term infant but, rather, to highlight contemporary issues and to focus attention on concepts with the potential for change in our approach to neonatal hyperbilirubinemia.

Some degree of neonatal jaundice, generally mild and transient,[1] affects up to 80% of otherwise healthy, term newborns.[2,3] It is a manifestation of immaturity of the bilirubin conjugating enzyme, Uridine 5'-diphospho-glucuronosyltransferase (UGT) (UGT) 1A1 coupled with increased red blood cell turnover. Rarely, the serum total bilirubin (STB) may progress to extreme levels, raising the potential danger of its deposition in vulnerable brain cells, resulting in severe and permanent sequelae.

THE WIDE CLINICAL SPECTRUM OF BILIRUBIN NEUROTOXICITY

Today it is recognized that there are many and varied aspects of the clinical manifestations of bilirubin neurotoxicity, classically known as kernicterus.[4] Although resulting from extreme neonatal hyperbilirubinemia, the most significant clinical neurologic features persist after resolution of the jaundice and may not be diagnosed until long after clinical jaundice has disappeared. Classic kernicterus, known as choreoathetotic cerebral palsy, relates to the persisting tetrad of (1) choreoathetosis, (2) auditory impairment, (3) paralysis of upward gaze, and (4) dental enamel dysplasia. The various components, however, also can exist independently, not as a tetrad, and still be attributable etiologically to prior hyperbilirubinemia. Thus, auditory manifestations of bilirubin neurotoxicity can manifest as varying degrees of hearing loss in combination with an auditory processing disturbance. The auditory nerve, and not the cochlear hair cells, is affected primarily by bilirubin neurotoxicity. Therefore, auditory neuropathy spectrum disorder (ANSD) includes absent or abnormal auditory brainstem response with intact otoacoustic emissions. The term, ANSD, is not synonymous with hearing loss but rather an abnormal processing of the auditory signal.

Another expression of bilirubin neurotoxicity has been described as subtle kernicterus. In this condition, neurodevelopmental disabilities similar to, but milder than, those seen in full-blown kernicterus exist in a previously severely hyperbilirubinemic newborn. Typical manifestations include isolated hearing loss not meeting the criteria of ANSD and/or mild motor involvement, including awkwardness or clumsiness. Once all other known etiologies have been excluded, they can be attributed to bilirubin neurotoxicity.

Kernicterus with additional neurologic dysfunctions not usually related to bilirubin neurotoxicity, for example, spasticity, epilepsy, microcephaly, or magnetic resonance imaging abnormalities not typically associated with kernicterus, is known as "kernicterus plus." Kernicteric children often also suffer from associated non-neurologic conditions, including gastroesophageal reflux, failure to thrive, sleep disorders, and neuro-orthopedic conditions.

Because of this wide spectrum of bilirubin neurotoxicity, Le Pichon and colleagues[4] have proposed using kernicterus spectrum disorder (KSD) as an all-encompassing term, including the many and varied clinical expressions of bilirubin neurotoxicity as well as their spectrum of severity.

IS KERNICTERUS SPECTRUM DISORDER STILL A PROBLEM?

Kernicterus in Developing Countries

KSD continues to be rampant in developing countries.[5,6] Data from the Global Burden of Disease Study demonstrate that neonatal hyperbilirubinemia accounted for 1309 deaths per 100,000 livebirths in 2016 and ranked seventh globally among all causes of neonatal deaths in the first week of life. The disease burden is greatest in South Asia and sub-Saharan Africa, where glucose-6-phosphate dehydrogenase (G6PD) deficiency may be a leading cause of extreme, unpredictable hyperbilirubinemia.[7] In a review of 134,000,000 late preterm and term neonates born in 2010,[8] 24,000,000 developed clinically significant jaundice; 481,000 extreme hyperbilirubinemia; 114,000 died, and greater than 63,000 survivors had significant long-term neurologic impairments. Zipursky and Paul[9] emphasize the lack of Rh disease preventive programs in the global burden of severe hyperbilirubinemia. **Box 1** presents potentially reversible factors contributing to the persistence of bilirubin neurotoxicity in developing countries.

Kernicterus in Industrialized Countries

That KSD continues to be widespread and uncontrolled in developing countries with underdeveloped medical systems and health organizations rendered ineffective by the ravages of war is not surprising. What is perhaps puzzling is its continued prevalence in industrialized countries.[10–21] Incidence of kernicterus reported in Western countries since 2000 ranges from 0.7/100,000 to 2.3/100,000 live births.[13,14,17,20,21] Readers should not be lulled into a state of complacency by the current low incidence of kernicterus in industrialized countries; rather, it must be remembered that many of these cases were preventable and that the neurologic consequences are irreversible leading to lifelong handicaps.[22]

Incidence of extreme hyperbilirubinemia in proxy of kernicterus

Because kernicterus is a rare condition, the incidence of extreme hyperbilirubinemia may be used as a proxy reflecting clinical challenge. A summary of the incidence of STB greater than or equal to 25 mg/dL and/or greater than or equal to 30 mg/dL (**Table 1**) demonstrates that extreme hyperbilirubinemia continues to occur in modern times in industrialized countries despite the availability of highly developed medical systems.

Etiology of Kernicterus

Table 1 presents the main etiologies for extreme hyperbilirubinemia when an etiology can be determined. In many reviews of kernicterus, an etiologic factor cannot be

Box 1
Some factors responsible for the persistence of kernicterus spectrum disorder in developing countries

- Home deliveries
- Long distances to be traveled to medical clinics
- Prolonged travel time to hospitals and poor transport facilities
- Lack of parental and medical caretaker education with regard to the dangers of severe neonatal hyperbilirubinemia
- Application of home remedies, some of which may have hemolytic properties (eg, menthol and henna)
- Absence of Rh isoimmunization prevention programs
- Inability to obtain serum or TcB testing
- Poor or erratic electricity supply
- Ineffective phototherapy equipment
- Inability to perform exchange transfusion

Table 1
Modern-day incidence of extreme hyperbilirubinemia per 100,000 deliveries in Western, industrialized countries/regions, demonstrating a wide range in incidence

Country/Region	Author/Year of Publication	Number of Newborns with Serum Total Bilirubin Greater than 25 mg/dL per 100,000 Deliveries	Number of Newborns with Serum Total Bilirubin Greater than 30 mg/dL per 100,000 Deliveries	Comment
Canada	Sgro et al,[13] 2006	40		STB ≥25 mg/dL or exchange transfusion
United Kingdom and Ireland	Manning et al,[14] 2007		7.1	
Denmark	Bjerre et al,[115] 2008	45		STB ≥26 mg/dL
Switzerland	Zoubir et al,[116] 2011	17		
Netherlands	Gotink et al,[117] 2013		10.4	STB ≥29 mg/dL or ≥20 + exchange transfusion
Utah, US	Christensen et al,[24] 2013	47.6	10.6	
California, US	Kuzniewicz et al,[118] 2014		8.6	
Australia	McGillivray et al,[119] 2015	9.4		STB ≥26 mg/dL
California	Bhutani et al,[23] 2016	21.3	4.2	
Canada	Sgro et al,[120] 2016	11.6		
Sweden	Alken et al,[121] 2019	50 (STB 25.0–29.9 mg/dL)	6.8	
Denmark	Donneborg et al,[21] 2020	42		

Note that all series included were published after the turn of the millennium (year 2000). Tabulation is in order of publication date.

determined. Recent reviews of extreme hyperbilirubinemia continue to report from 5% to 64% of cases have undetermined etiologies.[13,20,21]

Why Does Kernicterus Continue to Occur?

A systems failure was implicated in their assessment of what went wrong in the management of the newborns reported in the pilot USA Kernicterus Registry.[12] Despite publication of guidelines for the prevention and management of hyperbilirubinemia by authoritative institutions, such as the American Academy of Pediatrics (AAP),[25] Canadian Paediatric Society,[26] and others, published instructions not always are followed and parental concerns not always are taken seriously. Early discharge with inadequate postdischarge surveillance, poor breastfeeding, and incorrect information given to parents all may contribute. Delays in initiation of appropriate therapy, such as early phototherapy (during long transports) and appropriate transfers to centers able to perform exchange transfusions, may further exacerbate the damaging effects of severe hyperbilirubinemia.

What Can Be Done to Prevent Kernicterus Spectrum Disorder?

Bilirubin neurotoxicity can be prevented in term newborns by avoiding extreme hyperbilirubinemia. This objective is accomplished best through active surveillance of newborns for the development of jaundice, both during and after birth hospitalization. Hyperbilirubinemia is treated with phototherapy, and extreme hyperbilirubinemia, especially if accompanied by signs of acute bilirubin encephalopathy (ABE), by immediate performance of exchange transfusion.

Predischarge surveillance involves monitoring newborns for the development of jaundice throughout their birth hospitalization, noting especially those who become icteric during the first 24 hours after delivery, because this may be a sign of hemolysis. At least 1 predischarge bilirubin, either transcutaneous or via blood test, should be performed, and the result plotted on an hour specific bilirubin nomogram, such as that of Bhutani and colleagues.[3] The results should be evaluated in conjunction with risk factors for hyperbilirubinemia, notably gestational age.[27] Late preterm infants, and even early-term newborns (37–38 weeks gestation) are at higher risk for bilirubin neurotoxicity than full-term infants. Other risk factors include hemolytic diseases, G6PD deficiency, acidosis, and serum albumin less than 3.0 g/dL[28] (**Box 2**). Algorithms for the management of jaundice, dependent on the safety assessment of the bilirubin result should be consulted.[28] In the authors' practice, a transcutaneous bilirubin (TcB) is performed daily on all newborns during birth hospitalization. Plotting of the results on the nomogram allows for the bilirubin trajectory to be assessed and provides additional information beyond a single predischarge bilirubin result. Jumping tracks, or increasing at a rate higher than would be predicted by the nomogram, may suggest ongoing hemolysis. Adherence to this plan should facilitate detection of rapidly rising STB and prediction of postdischarge hyperbilirubinemia.

The efficacy of predischarge bilirubin screening in decreasing the incidence of extreme hyperbilirubinemia, and thereby the potential of bilirubin neurotoxicity, is well documented in general[29–31] as well as in ABO-incompatible newborns.[32] Nevertheless, despite successful in-hospital surveillance, extreme hyperbilirubinemia has not been eliminated.

Box 2
Major etiologic factors for extreme hyperbilirubinemia, extracted from recent series of extreme hyperbilirubinemia and kernicterus in Western countries, cited in Table 1

ABO blood group heterospecificity

G6PD deficiency

Isoimmunizations (other than Rh disease)

Late prematurity

Exclusive breastfeeding

Sepsis

Note: in developing countries, Rh disease is an additional important etiologic factor.

Postdischarge Surveillance: A Critical Timeframe

In many Western countries, the maternal/newborn dyad is discharged at approximately 48 hours. As is evident from perusal of the bilirubin nomogram, bilirubin continues rising at this age, peaking at approximately 4 days to 5 days. Concurrently, weight loss, itself associated with hyperbilirubinemia,[33] peaks at this time.[34] Recent studies have confirmed that shorter hospitalizations are associated with increased risk of readmission for neonatal hyperbilirubinemia.[35,36] Concomitantly, neonatal jaundice is the most frequent reason for readmission of a newborn infant.[37] Early follow-up is essential especially in populations with a high frequency of G6PD deficiency, which frequently results in unpredictable, sudden, and exponential increases in the STB to potentially neurotoxic levels.[38] Classically, these infants may have been discharged as nonjaundiced from their birth hospitalization and subsequently readmitted with extreme hyperbilirubinemia or bilirubin encephalopathy at or around postnatal day 5.[12–14,19,21] Clearly, a critical period ensues postdischarge at which time the baby already is at home and detached from ongoing in-hospital surveillance. It is essential, therefore, to develop methods of identifying neonates in whom jaundice may be developing or worsening postdischarge. The onus for identifying problems during this phase currently falls on the parents and community medical services.

Structuring Postdischarge Follow-up

In an attempt to minimize the development of severe hyperbilirubinemia, unrecognized by the parents at home, the Canadian Paediatric Society[39] and the AAP[25] have emphasized the need for newborn assessment by a qualified health care professional in the first few days after discharge "to assess infant well-being and the presence or absence of jaundice." The time frame generally coincides with the third to fifth postnatal day. The need for postdischarge follow-up was reemphasized by Maisels and colleagues,[28] who provide a schema as to what the physician should do at each follow-up visit regarding the evaluation of the infant and the need for repeat serum bilirubin or transcutaneous measurement.[40] Benitz and the Committee on Fetus and Newborn,[41] in an AAP Policy Statement, emphasized the need for an early postdischarge visit, including assessment of general health and the degree of jaundice.

Despite these recommendations, few studies have reported on the implementation of early postdischarge follow-up. Isolated reports from Houston, Texas; New York City; and Utah all found that a majority of newborns are not seen by a health care professional within a week of discharge.[42–44] The Israeli experience is interesting in this context. Although universal postdischarge community follow-up is recommended by the Israel Neonatal Society[45] and offered in local clinics in virtually every neighborhood, the attendance rate for early neonatal follow-up remains low (approximately 32%). Of those specifically instructed to return to hospital for a bilirubin blood test at a given time, however, the compliance rate was almost 100%.[46] These results suggest that it might be beneficial to provide parents with a specific date and venue for follow-up, rather than leaving it to the parents to initiate and organize contact with their local public health clinic.

CORONAVIRUS AND OTHER PANDEMICS

As this review is written, the world is suffering from a mass pandemic whose health, financial, and social ramifications have yet to be assessed. Although the authors are not aware of any direct effect of COVID-19 on neonatal jaundice, the combined drive toward even earlier hospital discharges together with the apprehension many mothers feel on entering any medical facility, aggravated by widespread quarantines restricting mobility, together impede access to even the best developed postdischarge follow-up care systems. Under such conditions, the risk of developing undiagnosed and, thereby, untreated extreme hyperbilirubinemia may be magnified. The medical community must develop creative solutions to prevent this with solutions aimed at increasing parental awareness. Home-based recognition of jaundice potentially can utilize smartphone applications.

HEREDITARY BACKGROUND TO NEONATAL HYPERBILIRUBINEMIA

In recent years, it has become increasingly clear that much of bilirubin metabolism is controlled genetically. A comprehensive review of the role of genes regulating the production and elimination of bilirubin is beyond the scope of this article. Some aspects of the UGT gene, however, are highlighted.

The *UGT1*A1 gene coding for the UGT1A1 enzyme plays a cardinal role in the conjugation and elimination of bilirubin. Polymorphisms and mutations of both coding (eg, *UGT1A1*6)* and noncoding areas (eg, *UGT1A1*28*) of the gene are associated with impaired enzyme function and, as a result, hyperbilirubinemia. Coexpression of *UGT1A1* abnormalities with additional hemolytic conditions, such as G6PD deficiency, may exacerbate hyperbilirubinemia.[47] UGT1A1 genetic aberrations also have been demonstrated to play a role in the pathophysiology of prolonged breast milk jaundice.[48,49]

EFFECT OF RACE, ETHNICITY, AND GEOGRAPHY ON NEONATAL HYPERBILIRUBINEMIA

The effect of heredity on the severity and/or incidence of jaundice is not limited to specific mutations or polymorphisms but varies among different ethnic groups. On the one hand, African American neonates have long been considered to be protected against hyperbilirubinemia.[50,51] For example, in a multinational, multiracial study involving 1370 newborns, 9% developed an STB greater than ninety-fifth percentile on the Bhutani nomogram.[3] When subdivided racially, 11% of white versus 5% of black neonates met jaundice criteria.[51] In the 2004 AAP hyperbilirubinemia guidelines, black race is listed as a factor decreasing the risk of significant jaundice.[25]

On the other hand, black neonates have a higher incidence of ABO incompatibility and of G6PD deficiency than whites.[52] African American G6PD-deficient newborns had a higher rate of hemolysis and of hyperbilirubinemia than G6PD-adequate controls (22% vs 7%, respectively; relative rate [RR] 3.27; 95% CI, 1.83–5.86).[53] Black infants also are at increased risk of kernicterus. Of 125 cases of kernicterus reported in the US-based Kernicterus Registry, 26% were black, overrepresented relative to the 12% overall black frequency in the US population.[12] Recently, in a Californian survey, Wickremasinghe and colleagues[54] confirmed that black infants were at greater risk than white infants of developing extreme hyperbilirubinemia levels greater than or equal to 30 mg/dL (RR 4.2; 95% CI, 1.33–13.2). Black newborns in the United Kingdom, Ireland,[14] and Central and West Africa also have been shown to have a high incidence of severe neonatal hyperbilirubinemia and kernicterus.[55,56]

The increased risk of extreme hyperbilirubinemia and kernicterus in black newborns may be explained in part by a higher incidence of G6PD deficiency[56] and a higher frequency of the *UGT1A1*28* promoter polymorphism in this population group.[57] Thus, there may be a subgroup(s) of neonates within the African or African American population at increased risk of developing kernicterus.

Asian newborns have higher mean maximal STB concentrations than do white and African American neonates. Autopsy-proved kernicterus is also higher in Asians than in the latter groups.[58,59] This may reflect the increased frequency of the Gly71Arg mutation of UGT1A1, associated with prolonged neonatal jaundice,[60] in Asian populations.

SHOULD BILIRUBIN NOMOGRAMS BE UNIVERSAL?

US-based guidelines recommend that bilirubin values, either serum or transcutaneous derived, be plotted on a nomogram[25,28] for interpretation and prediction of hyperbilirubinemia. The nomogram is an hour-specific plot of serum bilirubin values taken from term and late preterm newborns, greater than 35 weeks' gestational age, in Philadelphia (Bhutani and colleague.[3]). This nomogram, the only nomogram-based on serum bilirubin values, is used worldwide and TcB values frequently are plotted on the identical nomogram. This should be reliable for interpreting lower TcB values (<15 mg/dL), but, at higher bilirubin concentrations, it may be inaccurate. The ready availability of modern, painless, TcB devices has made construction of TcB nomograms feasible among differing population groups. TcB readings differ, however, between ethnic groups, as first demonstrated by De Luca and colleagues[61] and, more recently, by Kaplan and Bromiker.[62] The latter analyzed the ninety-fifth and seventy-fifth percentiles of 20 published TcB nomograms derived from 12 different countries. As seen in **Fig. 1**, a wide range of TcB readings was found through the first 5 postnatal days. The investigators speculated that the differences documented reflect dissimilarities in bilirubin metabolism, or differences in feeding practices and breastfeeding rates, between distinctive ethnic or racial groups. Interpretation of a TcB result, using either the serum-based nomogram or TcB nomograms constructed from a population group different from that of the specific newborn being tested, should be pursued with caution.

MODERN TECHNOLOGIES IN THE ASSESSMENT OF NEONATAL HYPERBILIRUBINEMIA

End-tidal Carbon Monoxide

Increased hemolysis is a risk factor for hyperbilirubinemia and thereby for bilirubin neurotoxicity.[63] Diverse laboratory measurements, including hemoglobin, hematocrit, reticulocyte count, lactic dehydrogenase, and haptoglobin, offer a reliable reflection of hemolysis in adults and older children. In newborns, however, there is greater overlap between hemolytic and nonhemolytic states, rendering these indices unreliable in neonatal hemolysis. Physiologically, heme degradation releases biliverdin, which subsequently is metabolized to bilirubin, carbon monoxide (CO), and iron. Accurate measurement of carboxyhemoglobin or end-tidal CO (ETCO), corrected for ambient CO, reflects endogenous CO production. Because most endogenous CO is derived from heme catabolism, endogenous CO accurately reflects heme catabolism and, by inference, bilirubin production secondary to hemolysis. ETCO measurement now is a clinically available, noninvasive, and painless point-of-care test. ETCO can be used to differentiate between hyperbilirubinemia resulting from increased hemolysis (increased ETCO) versus from diminished bilirubin conjugation (normal ETCO).[23]

Smartphone Apps for Bilirubin Estimation

Despite the availability of bilirubin measurement technologies in industrialized countries, geographic encumbrances, including very long distances to travel or severe weather conditions, may render availability unfeasible. In developing countries, geographic hinderances can be compounded by absent or inconsistent availability of bilirubin measurements. Visual estimation of the degree of jaundice is notoriously inaccurate.[64,65] In an attempt to overcome these obstacles, devices are being sought to enable parents

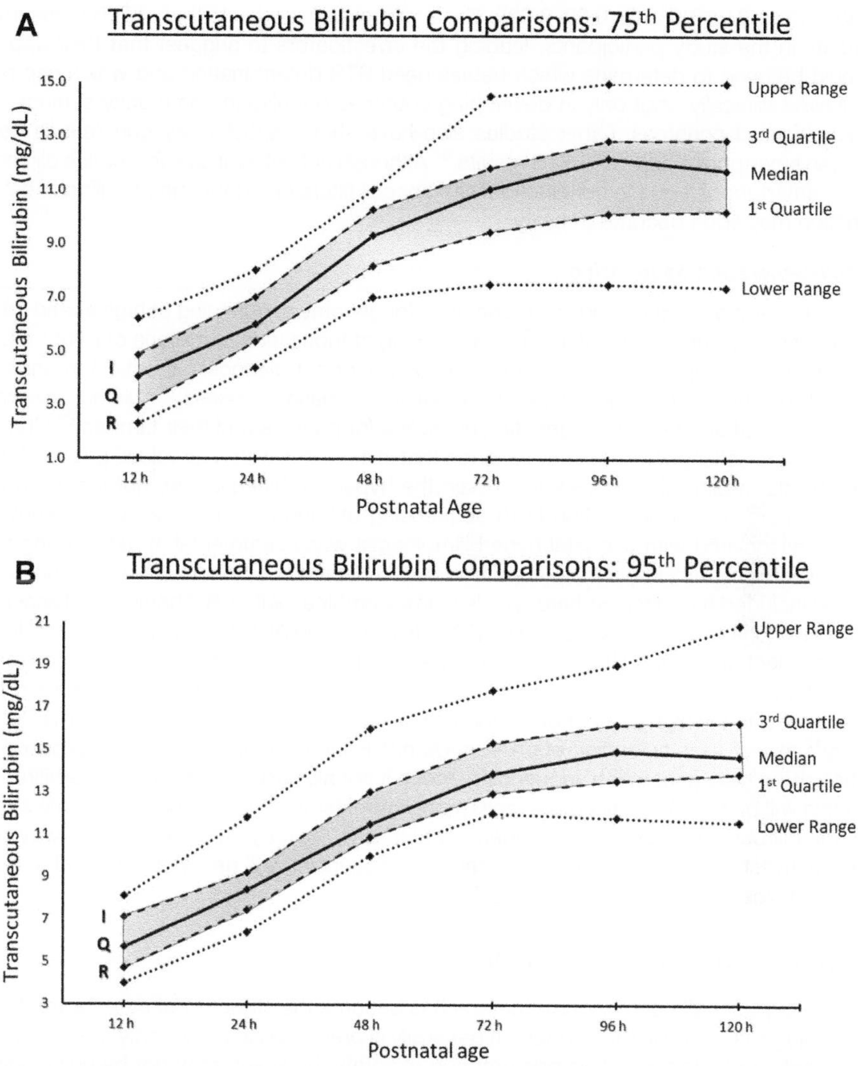
A
Transcutaneous Bilirubin Comparisons: 75th Percentile
Transcutaneous Bilirubin (mg/dL)
15.0
13.0
11.0
9.0
7.0
5.0
3.0
1.0
Upper Range
3rd Quartile
Median
1st Quartile
Lower Range
I
Q
R
12 h
24 h
48 h
72 h
96 h
120 h
Postnatal Age
B
Transcutaneous Bilirubin Comparisons: 95th Percentile
Transcutaneous Bilirubin (mg/dL)
21
19
17
15
13
11
9
7
5
3
Upper Range
3rd Quartile
Median
1st Quartile
Lower Range
I
Q
R
12 h
24 h
48 h
72 h
96 h
120 h
Postnatal age

Fig. 1. (*A, B*) Median TcB values, interquartile range, and upper and lower values for the range at each point studied, for the seventy-fifth (Panel A) and ninety-fifth (Panel B) percentiles, respectively, of the 20 nomogram studies analyzed. IQR, interquartile range. (*From* Kaplan M, Bromiker R. Variation in Transcutaneous Bilirubin Nomograms across Population Groups. J Pediatr 2019; 208:273-278.e1, with permission.)

or medical/nursing personnel to reliably estimate serum bilirubin measurements from home or distant community clinics. Although industrialized countries are at the forefront of smartphone-based medical technologies, acquisition of these devices is increasing rapidly among populations of low-income and middle-income countries as well.[65] In a recent study of greater than 500 newborns of diverse US ethnic subgroups, a technology based on the analysis of images obtained using an app on a commodity smartphone was successful in providing reasonably accurate estimates of STB values (correlation 0.91 [95% CI, 0.89–0.92)]. The accuracy was similar to that of TcB measurements in the study participants, leading the investigators to suggest that their app[66] could be used to determine which babies need STB determination and which can be followed clinically—not only in developing countries but also in community settings in industrialized countries. Other studies also have shown satisfactory correlations between smartphone apps and STB results.[67] Although not yet available for routine clinical use, smartphone apps in conjunction with special filters or algorithms for bilirubin estimation may soon become a reality.

Next-Generation Sequencing

Next-generation sequencing is a technology for genome sequencing at high speed and low cost, enabling the simultaneous sequencing of thousands to millions of DNA molecules, from multiple individuals simultaneously. Correct diagnosis is critical in understanding the pathologic hyperbilirubinemic disease process, guiding clinical management and facilitating genetic counseling for patients and their families.[68] Christensen and colleagues[69] recently reported that in neonates with STB values greater than 30 mg/dL, a clinical diagnosis to explain the hyperbilirubinemia was not identified in 66% whereas next-generation DNA sequencing utilizing a panel of 27 genes known to be associated with neonatal hyperbilirubinemia was instrumental in determining an etiology for hyperbilirubinemia in each of the 10 neonates studied. Etiologies encountered included hereditary spherocytosis (some combined with ABO hemolytic disease), pyruvate kinase deficiency, severe G6PD deficiency, and ABO hemolytic disease.[69] In a subsequent study of 7 Utah-based neonates with ABE, Christensen and colleagues[19] determined a diagnosis, based on this genetic technology, for all. These reports contrast with the high number of newborns labeled as idiopathic in the Kernicterus Registry[12] as well as in an earlier report from Utah.[70] Bahr and colleagues[71] have proposed that, using next-generation sequencing, most, if not all, cases of extreme hyperbilirubinemia will be found to have mutations or polymorphisms of genes encoding some step in the bilirubin production or conjugation processes. A study currently is under way by these investigators, in which next-generation sequencing will be used to study the genetic etiology of 100 US cases of ABE.

TREATMENT OF HYPERBILIRUBINEMIA

Over the past half century phototherapy has become the standard of care for treating pathologic jaundice in the neonate. It generally is presumed to be not only effective but also safe and harmless. This presumption of safety, however, may not be universally true, especially for the newer, high-intensity light-emitting diode (LED) units. The safety of phototherapy has not really been questioned or adequately tested when using these lights, and in recent years concerns have begun to emerge regarding potential damaging effects of phototherapy.[72]

In light of these concerns, the authors felt it important to review some of the basic underlying aspects of clinical phototherapy as well as their potential long-term risks. Although many of the side effects are both transient and controversial, awareness of the fact that phototherapy is not risk-free reinforces the need for a judicious clinical approach, aimed only at neonates who really need it, following recommended guidelines and always weighing risks versus benefits.

Phototherapy devices and intensity

Light intensity is defined by irradiance (number of photons delivered per square centimeter of exposed skin/nanometer [nm] of the wavelength). Phototherapy devices derive their efficacy from any of several different light sources, including fluorescent tubes, halogen spotlights, fiberoptic blankets/pads, and newer high-intensity blue LEDs. For decades, clinical phototherapy devices were limited to the first types, which provided irradiances of less than or equal to 20 $\mu W/cm^2/nm$. Conventional phototherapy reduces bilirubin by 6% to 20% within the first 24 hours. Recently, LEDs have transformed clinical phototherapy, offering irradiances of up to 50 $\mu W/cm^2/nm$ and reducing bilirubin levels by 30% to 40% within 24 hours.[73]

Early safety studies were done using the conventional devices. High-intensity LEDs have been assumed to be safe based on previous studies generally performed at irradiances below 30 $\mu W/cm^2/nm$. Safety studies have not been repeated at the higher intensities provided by LEDs.

Phototherapy dose response

Given that it now is possible to offer much higher doses of phototherapy than previously, it must be asked whether there is a concomitant increase in bilirubin degradation, that is, Is the dose-response curve linear? The existence of a dose-response relationship first was suggested by Tan,[74] who exposed term infants with nonhemolytic hyperbilirubinemia to 9 different irradiance levels using fluorescent lamps. He described a direct relationship between irradiance and the rate of in vivo total bilirubin decrease. Some have observed a plateau region, beginning at a spectral irradiance of approximately 30 $\mu W/cm^2/nm$, beyond which further increases in irradiance would not increase bilirubin degradation.[70] Using an LED light source, however, Vandborg and colleagues[75] observed a linear dose-response relationship between 20 $\mu W/cm^2/nm$ and 55 $\mu W/cm^2/nm$. They found no evidence of saturation up to 55 $\mu W/cm^2/nm$. Other investigators, however, have noted that the dose-response phototherapy curve does appear to plateau above 50 $\mu W/cm^2/nm$.[76]

Clinical implications of dose response

Although of intuitive importance, the intensity or quantity of phototherapy has not been included in most clinical recommendations. Although there are precise guidelines for the initiation and duration of phototherapy, as defined by a specific range of bilirubin values based on postnatal age and the potential risk for bilirubin neurotoxicity, recommendations regarding levels of irradiance are less precise. There is a general AAP recommendation of 30 $\mu W/cm^2/nm$ to 40 $\mu W/cm^2/nm$[25] as the target level for intensive phototherapy, with no details regarding etiology of jaundice, gestational age, or other risk factors. Given that the dose-response curve has been shown to be linear only up to 55 $\mu W/cm^2/nm$, it is possible—although not proved—that the dose-response curve plateaus above this level. The authors suggest, therefore, that there is little evidence of added clinical benefit to be derived from increasing spectral irradiance beyond this level. The authors propose, therefore, that this should be done only in specific high-risk cases and only after careful deliberation.

Subthreshold phototherapy

Despite the existence of precise therapeutic guidelines, a disturbing article[77] was published recently describing the benefits of administering subthreshold phototherapy to prevent readmission for jaundice. Phototherapy frequently was initiated in newborns with STB levels that were below the treatment threshold recommended by the AAP.[25] To obviate readmission for phototherapy, 14 newborns needed to remain hospitalized for an extra day receiving treatment of hyperbilirubinemia when their bilirubin levels were subthreshold, exposing them not only to unnecessary phototherapy but also to additional separation from their mothers.

Subclinical carcinogenicity

Big data analyses have enabled 2 extremely large epidemiologic surveys, which have raised the specter of a subclinical carcinogenic risk associated with neonatal phototherapy exposure.[78,79] They found a small but statistically significant increase in infantile cancers among those who were exposed to phototherapy. Infants who received phototherapy were 1.6-fold more likely to develop cancer, with 1 additional case per 10,638 infants treated. Cnattingius and colleagues[80] and Auger and colleagues[81] showed similar increases in infantile cancers in children who were exposed to neonatal phototherapy (2 times the risk of developing solid tumors compared with unexposed children). On the other hand, several studies seeking correlations between phototherapy and melanoma, basal cell carcinoma, and/or squamous cell carcinoma have not demonstrated evidence of any statistically significant risk.

The studies showing an increased cancer risk reviewed infants treated between 1995 and 2004—prior to the widespread introduction of the newer LED phototherapy units. The irradiance emitted by these earlier devices to which the infants in the study were exposed probably remained below 30 $\mu W/cm^2/nm$. Modern LED units can deliver levels of irradiance of up to 50 $\mu W/cm^2/nm$. Moreover, today's jaundiced neonates are often exposed to several such units concurrently. In such cases, irradiance levels can reach 100 $\mu W/cm^2/nm$.

Thus, although the increase in the absolute risk, if it even exists, is extremely small, it is sufficient to warrant caution in avoiding unnecessary and/or excessive use of phototherapy.

Genotoxicity

Exposure of cells to visible light can induce DNA strand breaks, sister chromatid exchanges, and mutations.[82–84] These DNA breaks cause DNA modifications that theoretically can contribute to oxidative stress-related diseases, such as necrotizing enterocolitis and retinopathy of prematurity and possibly increase the risk for future cancer development.[81,85]

Christensen and colleagues[84] demonstrated that phototherapy-induced single-strand DNA breaks were increased significantly when bilirubin solutions were added to cells in culture. Both Yahia and colleagues[87] and Mesbah-Namin and colleagues[88] studied hyperbilirubinemic infants with and without phototherapy, as well as nonjaundiced control infants, and both found increased genotoxic effects only in the phototherapy-treated infants.

Genotoxicity increases similarly with both conventional and intensive phototherapies.[86] Although few genotoxicity studies have been done with the newer LED light sources,[89] Kanmaz and colleagues[90] did study genotoxicity at different light intensities, including LED phototherapy, and found no intensity-related differences. A significant positive correlation has been demonstrated between the duration of phototherapy and increased genotoxicity.

Evidence indicates that the genotoxicity appears to be transient[91] and thus probably clinically irrelevant. Even the remote possibility of potential harm, however, supports the need for caution in adhering to therapeutic guidelines and avoiding excess phototherapeutic intensity and/or duration. In conclusion, the authors propose that phototherapy be considered a type of drug therapy and that irradiance levels be monitored clinically similarly to therapeutic drug levels monitoring. The goal should be to offer the lowest possible effective level of phototherapy—not the highest possible level.

Exchange transfusion: a lost art

Exchange transfusion was the first definitive treatment of extreme hyperbilirubinemia. Once the only treatment available, the technique was well known to earlier generations of pediatricians. With the advent of phototherapy, hyperbilirubinemia generally can be controlled essentially almost eliminating the need for exchange transfusions. Screening for Rh disease with antenatal and postnatal maternal Rho(D) immune globulin (RhoGAM) therapy as well as postnatal intravenous immune globulin therapy in immune-based hyperbilirubinemia has decreased the incidence of extreme hyperbilirubinemia further. As a result, exchange transfusion is becoming a lost art—rarely performed. A recent multicenter study found that among 1.25 million newborns born between 1997 and 2016, the rate of exchange transfusions decreased from a peak of 0.3% in 1997 to a nadir of 0.05% in 2016.[92]

Nevertheless, in cases in which the STB approaches AAP indications for exchange transfusion despite adequate phototherapy or in neonates who present with clinical features of ABE, it still should be performed, and it should be performed as quickly as possible. Unfortunately, newborns frequently need to be transferred to larger centers in order to have this procedure performed, often significantly postponing treatment. Organizing and performing the transfer may entail many hours' delay, prolonging exposure to potentially neurotoxic bilirubin concentrations with increased potential danger of developing KSD. In this respect, the Israeli model may be advantageous. In that country, there is a high level of awareness of neonatal jaundice among many sectors of the population, in part because of the need for an infant to be free of jaundice at the time of the eighth-day ritual circumcision.[93] Most hospitals with delivery services have neonatal intensive care services able to perform exchange transfusions, such that travel distances are short. In addition, the high frequency of G6PD deficiency in some ethnic subsets, may be responsible for heightened awareness of the potential problem, thereby shortening the time between recognition of the need for exchange transfusion and its actual performance.

Exchange transfusion is not a benign procedure and should be performed according to the indications of the AAP.[25] Reversible complications include thrombocytopenia and electrolyte disturbances, which frequently are asymptomatic and treatable.[92,94] More serious complications include seizures, necrotizing enterocolitis, and intraventricular hemorrhage, and even death.[92] In this multicenter study, 1% of term and near-term neonates died within 7 days of performance of exchange transfusion. Complications may be more frequent in preterm infants,[92,94] which is not surprising, considering that preterm infants often are hemodynamically unstable at the time of performing exchange transfusion.[95] Conversely, it may surprise readers to note that in the only published prospective, randomized controlled trial comparing phototherapy with exchange transfusion in premature neonates, there was a trend toward lower mortality in the exchange transfusion group. The lower mortality was noted entirely in the infants who were 501 g to 750 g.[96] At the very least, these findings imply that exchange transfusion did not increase the risk of mortality in the extremely low-birthweight subpopulation.

IS ACUTE BILIRUBIN ENCEPHALOPATHY INVARIABLY ASSOCIATED WITH SEVERE, CHRONIC NEUROLOGIC DYSFUNCTION?

ABE frequently is the forerunner of the kernicterus spectrum. Many of those affected progress to bilirubin neurotoxicity or even death despite having undergone exchange transfusion. However, There been reports of severely hyperbilirubinemic newborns with signs of ABE who were treated promptly and effectively with exchange transfusion and who subsequently had a good neurologic outcome.[14,21,97,98] It is a misconception that if an infant has signs of bilirubin encephalopathy, it is too late to justify treatment. All newborns with extreme hyperbilirubinemia, with or without signs of neurotoxicity, should be treated with a crash-cart approach.[12] Delays in transport to a center with the facilities for performing exchange transfusion should be avoided, whenever possible. Intense phototherapy must be provided while awaiting blood for exchange transfusion, even during transport! The need for urgent exchange transfusion in newborns presenting with ABE is emphasized by Donneborg and colleagues.[21] In their series of 12 infants with KSD, only 4 had undergone exchange transfusion. Citing a dramatic decrease in STB due to intense phototherapy, the remaining infants were not exchanged, a procedure that might have improved their outcome. These investigators cite, and support, Danish guidelines that infants with advanced ABE should receive an exchange transfusion, even if the STB is decreasing secondary to phototherapy.[99] The 2004 AAP guidelines also recommend immediate exchange transfusion in any infant showing signs of ABE.[25]

Bilirubin: a Double-Edged Sword

Although neonatal hyperbilirubinemia generally is a benign, transitory phenomena, bilirubin does have the ability to cross the blood-brain barrier and the potential to cause irreversible brain damage. As such, bilirubinemia in the neonate is known primarily for its neurotoxic potential. Bilirubin, however, also possesses antioxidant properties.[100] As such, it has been suggested that mild hyperbilirubinemia actually may offer the neonate some protective advantage.

The healthy human body maintains a physiologic equilibrium between the ongoing generation of pro-oxidants and the ability to neutralize them with antioxidants. Imbalance in this delicate equilibrium results in oxidative stress. At birth, the newborn is exposed to a relatively hyperoxic environment compared with the intrauterine environment and culminating in enhanced generation of reactive oxygen species. Furthermore, during early neonatal life many endogenous enzymatic antioxidant defense mechanisms are physiologically immature,[101,102] rendering neonates vulnerable to oxidative injury.

Unconjugated bilirubin can scavenge singlet oxygen molecules, quench free radical reactions, and serve as a reducing agent for certain peroxidases.[103,104] Serum bilirubin has been shown to be correlated significantly with in vivo total antioxidant status as measured by the peroxyl radical-trapping capability of human blood.[105]

Preliminary animal studies support a protective effect of hyperbilirubinemia. Dennery and colleagues[106] demonstrated that jaundiced Gunn rats exposed to hyperoxia developed less oxidative damage than did non-jaundiced rats. Hammerman and colleagues[107] showed that hyperbilirubinemia, acting as an antioxidant, ameliorated intestinal injury in a rat model of ischemia reperfusion injury.

Mildly elevated bilirubin levels have been shown to be protective against an array of human neonatal conditions associated with increased oxidative stress.[108] Benaron and colleagues[109] and Hegyi and colleagues[110] noted that infants suffering from conditions possibly associated with oxygen radical–mediated mechanisms had lower bilirubin levels than control, age-matched infants without proposed oxygen radical involvement. They, in turn, consider the possibility that bilirubin's antioxidant function in the face of greater antioxidant need could have led to increased bilirubin consumption.

Although many organ systems can be affected by oxidative injury, the neonatal brain is most vulnerable because of its rapid metabolic rate and increased oxygen consumption coupled with its high content of easily oxidized membrane lipids in the

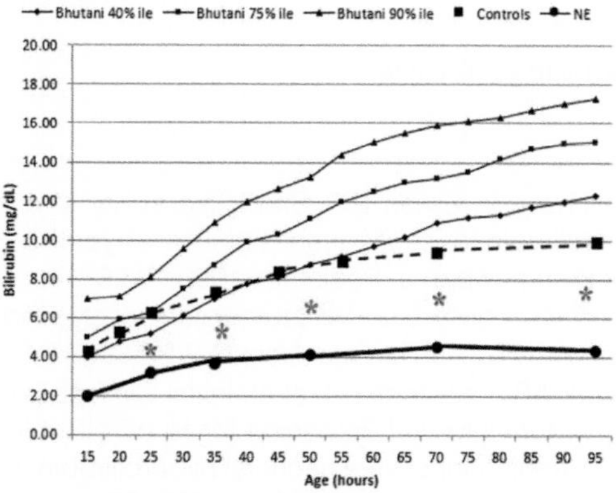
Bhutani 40% ile
Bhutani 75% ile
Bhutani 90% ile
Controls
NE
20.00
18.00
16.00
14.00
12.00
10.00
8.00
6.00
4.00
2.00
0.00
Bilirubin (mg/dL)
15 20 25 30 35 40 45 50 55 60 65 70 75 80 85 90 95
Age (hours)

Fig. 2. STB concentrations over time during the first 4 days of life in infants with and without neonatal encephalopathy. Mean serum bilirubin concentrations are plotted for neonatal encephalopathy (NE) babies, for local age matched controls, and for the fortieth, seventy-fifth, and ninety-fifth percentiles of the Bhutani nomogram over time. * indicates that The NE group is significantly lower than the controls at each time point measured. $p < 0.05$ for NE versus control bilirubin concentrations. None of the NE infants reached the fortieth percentile (%ile) of the Bhutani curve. (*From* Bin-Nun A, Mimouni FB, Kasirer Y, et al. Might bilirubin serve as a natural antioxidant in response to neonatal encephalopathy? Am J Perinatol 2018; 35:1107-12, with permission.)

face of limited antioxidant protective mechanisms.[111] In recent studies, both Hammerman and colleagues[112] (**Fig. 2**) and Dani and colleagues[113] observed that term neonates with neonatal encephalopathy also had lower serum bilirubin levels. The authors postulate that bilirubin is consumed for its antioxidant potential in the face of oxidative stress.

Further support for a protective effect of mild hyperbilirubinemia, albeit not in neonates, can be derived from the observation that in adult patients with Gilbert syndrome[114] with chronically mild hyperbilirubinemia have a substantially reduced risk of cardiovascular disease, cancer, and metabolic syndrome, again suggesting that bilirubin offers endogenous protection against oxidative stress related conditions.[1]

Serum bilirubin is naturally elevated during the first days of life in most neonates. The authors suggest that this mild neonatal bilirubinemia may offer a natural antioxidant protection precisely at a time in life when other physiologic antioxidant defenses are underdeveloped—while remaining cognizant of the delicate balance between the protective and potentially neurotoxic effects of bilirubin.

CLINICS CARE POINTS

- All neonates should be monitored vigilantly for the development of hyperbilirubinemia, both during birth hospitalization and during the first postdischarge days.
- There are emerging concerns regarding potentially damaging effects of phototherapy. Thus, phototherapy should be treated as a drug with clear guidelines regarding indications, durations, and dosages.
- Mild hyperbilirubinemia may offer the neonate some protective, antioxidant advantage. Clinicians always must remain cognizant of the delicate balance that exists between the protective and potentially neurotoxic effects of bilirubin.

DISCLOSURE

The authors have nothing to disclose.

REFERENCES

1. Bhutani VK, Johnson L, Sivieri EM. Predictive ability of a predischarge hour-specific serum bilirubin for subsequent significant hyperbilirubinemia in healthy term and near-term newborns. Pediatrics 1999;103:6–14.
2. Keren R, Tremont K, Luan X, et al. Visual assessment of jaundice in term and late preterm infants. Arch Dis Child Fetal Neonatal Ed 2009;94:F317–22.
3. Bhutani VK, Stark AR, Lazzeroni LC, et al, Initial Clinical Testing Evaluation and Risk Assessment for Universal Screening for Hyperbilirubinemia Study Group. Predischarge screening for severe neonatal hyperbilirubinemia identifies infants who need phototherapy. J Pediatr 2013;162:477–82.
4. Le Pichon JB, Riordan SM, Watchko J, et al. The neurological sequelae of neonatal hyperbilirubinemia: definitions, diagnosis and treatment of the kernicterus spectrum disorders. Curr Pediatr Rev 2017;13:199–209.
5. Olusanya BO, Kaplan M, Hansen TWR. Neonatal hyperbilirubinaemia: a global perspective. Lancet Child Adolesc Health 2018;2:610–20.
6. Hameed NN, Na' Ma AM, Vilms R, et al. Severe neonatal hyperbilirubinemia and adverse short-term consequences in Baghdad, Iraq. Neonatology 2011;100:57–63.
7. Olusanya BO, Teeple S, Kassebaum NJ. The contribution of neonatal jaundice to global child mortality: findings from the GBD 2016 study. Pediatrics 2018;141(2):e20171471.
8. Bhutani VK, Zipursky A, Blencowe H, et al. Neonatal hyperbilirubinemia and Rhesus disease of the newborn: incidence and impairment estimates for 2010 at regional and global levels. Pediatr Res 2013;74(Suppl 1):86–100.
9. Zipursky A, Paul VK. The global burden of Rh disease. Arch Dis Child Fetal Neonatal Ed 2011;96:F84–5.
10. Maisels MJ. Neonatal hyperbilirubinemia and kernicterus - not gone but sometimes forgotten. Early Hum Dev 2009;85:727–32.
11. Kaplan M, Bromiker R, Hammerman C. Severe neonatal hyperbilirubinemia and kernicterus: are these still problems in the third millennium? Neonatology 2011;100:354–62.
12. Johnson L, Bhutani VK, Karp K, et al. Clinical report from the pilot USA Kernicterus Registry1992 to 2004). J Perinatol 2009;29(Suppl 1):S25–45.
13. Sgro M, Campbell D, Shah V. Incidence and causes of severe neonatal hyperbilirubinemia in Canada. CMAJ 2006;175:587–90.
14. Manning D, Todd P, Maxwell M, et al. Prospective surveillance study of severe hyperbilirubinaemia in the newborn in the UK and Ireland. Arch Dis Child Fetal Neonatal Ed 2007;92:F342–6.
15. Dani C, Poggi C, Barp J, et al. Current Italian practices regarding the management of hyperbilirubinaemia in preterm infants. Acta Paediatr 2011;100:666–9.
16. Gotink MJ, Benders MJ, Lavrijsen SW, et al. Severe neonatal hyperbilirubinemia in The Netherlands. Neonatology 2013;104:137–42.
17. Sgro M, Campbell DM, Kandasamy S, et al. Incidence of chronic bilirubin encephalopathy in Canada, 2007-2008. Pediatrics 2012;130:e886–90.
18. McGillivray A, Polverino J, Badawi N, et al. Prospective surveillance of extreme neonatal hyperbilirubinemia in Australia. J Pediatr 2016;168:82–7.e3.

19. Christensen RD, Agarwal AM, George TI, et al. Acute neonatal bilirubin encephalopathy in the State of Utah 2009-2018. Blood Cells Mol Dis 2018;72:10–3.
20. Alkén J, Håkansson S, Ekéus C, et al. Rates of extreme neonatal hyperbilirubinemia and kernicterus in children and adherence to national guidelines for screening, diagnosis, and treatment in Sweden. JAMA Netw Open 2019;2: e190858.
21. Donneborg ML, Hansen BM, Vandborg PK, et al. Extreme neonatal hyperbilirubinemia and kernicterus spectrum disorder in Denmark during the years 2000-2015. J Perinatol 2020;40:194–202.
22. Brooks JC, Fisher-Owens SA, Wu YW, et al. Evidence suggests there was not a "resurgence" of kernicterus in the 1990s. Pediatrics 2011;127:672–9.
23. Bhutani VK, Srinivas S, Castillo Cuadrado ME, et al. Identification of neonatal haemolysis: an approach to predischarge management of neonatal hyperbilirubinemia. Acta Paediatr 2016;105:e189–94.
24. Christensen RD, Lambert DK, Henry E, et al. Unexplained extreme hyperbilirubinemia among neonates in a multihospital healthcare system. Blood Cells Mol Dis 2013;50:105–9.
25. American Academy of Pediatrics Subcommittee on Hyperbilirubinemia. Management of hyperbilirubinemia in the newborn infant 35 or more weeks of gestation. Pediatrics 2004;114:297–316.
26. Fetus and Newborn Committee, Canadian Paediatric Society. Guidelines for detection, management and prevention of hyperbilirubinemia in term and late preterm newborn infants (35 or more weeks' gestation). Paediatr Child Health 2007;12(Suppl B):1B–12B.
27. Keren R, Luan X, Friedman S, et al. A comparison of alternative risk-assessment strategies for predicting significant neonatal hyperbilirubinemia in term and near-term infants. Pediatrics 2008;121:e170–9.
28. Maisels MJ, Bhutani VK, Bogen D, et al. Hyperbilirubinemia in the newborn infant > or =35 weeks' gestation: an update with clarifications. Pediatrics 2009; 124:1193–8.
29. Eggert LD, Wiedmeier SE, Wilson J, et al. The effect of instituting a prehospital-discharge newborn bilirubin screening program in an 18-hospital health system. Pediatrics 2006;117:e855–62.
30. Kuzniewicz MW, Escobar GJ, Newman TB. Impact of universal bilirubin screening on severe hyperbilirubinemia and phototherapy use. Pediatrics 2009;124:1031–9.
31. Mah MP, Clark SL, Akhigbe E, et al. Reduction of severe hyperbilirubinemia after institution of predischarge bilirubin screening. Pediatrics 2010;125:e1143–8.
32. Christensen RD, Baer VL, MacQueen BC, et al. ABO hemolytic disease of the fetus and newborn: thirteen years of data after implementing a universal bilirubin screening and management program. J Perinatol 2018;38:517–25.
33. Miyoshi Y, Suenaga H, Aoki M, et al. Determinants of excessive weight loss in breastfed full-term newborns at a baby-friendly hospital: a retrospective cohort study. Int Breastfeed J 2020;15:191–8.
34. Flaherman VJ, Schaefer EW, Kuzniewicz MW, et al. Early weight loss nomograms for exclusively breastfed newborns. Pediatrics 2015;135:e16–23.
35. Lain SJ, Roberts CL, Bowen JR, et al. Early discharge of infants and risk of readmission for jaundice. Pediatrics 2015;135:314–21.
36. Jones E, Taylor B, Rudge G, et al. Hospitalisation after birth of infants: cross sectional analysis of potentially avoidable admissions across England using hospital episode statistics. BMC Pediatr 2018;18:390.

37. Battersby C, Michaelides S, Upton M, et al, Jaundice Working Group of the Atain Avoiding Term Admissions Into Neonatal unit programme, led by the Patient Safety team in NHS Improvement. Term admissions to neonatal units in England: a role for transitional care? A retrospective cohort study. BMJ Open 2017;7: e016050.
38. Kaplan M, Hammerman C, Bhutani VK. Parental education and the WHO neonatal G-6-PD screening program: a quarter century later. J Perinatol 2015; 35:779–84.
39. Lemyre B, Jefferies AL, O'Flaherty P. Facilitating discharge from hospital of the healthy term infant. Paediatr Child Health 2018;23:515–31.
40. Yonemoto N, Dowswell T, Nagai S, et al. Schedules for home visits in the early postpartum period. Cochrane Database Syst Rev 2017;(8):CD009326.
41. Benitz WE, Committee on Fetus and Newborn, American Academy of Pediatrics. Hospital stay for healthy term newborn infants. Pediatrics 2015;135: 948–53.
42. Profit J, Cambric-Hargrove AJ, Tittle KO, et al. Delayed pediatric office follow-up of newborns after birth hospitalization. Pediatrics 2009;124:548–54.
43. O'Donnell HC, Trachtman RA, Islam S, et al. Factors associated with timing of first outpatient visit after newborn hospital discharge. Acad Pediatr 2014;14: 77–83.
44. Shakib J, Buchi K, Smith E, et al. Timing of initial well-child visit and readmissions of newborns. Pediatrics 2015;13:469–74.
45. Kaplan M, Merlob P, Regev R. Israel guidelines for the management of neonatal hyperbilirubinemia and prevention of kernicterus. J Perinatol 2008;28:389–97.
46. Kaplan M, Zimmerman D, Shoob H, et al. Post-discharge neonatal hyperbilirubinemia surveillance. Acta Paediatr 2020;109:923–9.
47. Kaplan M, Renbaum P, Levy-Lahad E, et al. Gilbert syndrome and glucose-6-phosphate dehydrogenase deficiency: a dose-dependent genetic interaction crucial to neonatal hyperbilirubinemia. Proc Natl Acad Sci U S A 1997;94: 12128–32.
48. Monaghan G, McLellan A, McGeehan A, et al. Gilbert's syndrome is a contributory factor in prolonged unconjugated hyperbilirubinemia of the newborn. J Pediatr 1999;134:441–6.
49. Žaja O, Tiljak MK, Štefanović M, et al. Correlation of UGT1A1 TATA-box polymorphism and jaundice in breastfed newborns-early presentation of Gilbert's syndrome. J Matern Fetal Neonatal Med 2014;27:844–50.
50. Linn S, Schoenbaum SC, Monson RR, et al. Epidemiology of neonatal hyperbilirubinemia. Pediatrics 1985;75:770–4.
51. Stevenson DK, Fanaroff AA, Maisels MJ, et al. Prediction of hyperbilirubinemia in near-term and term infants. Pediatrics 2001;108:31–9.
52. Kirkman HN Jr. Further evidence for a racial difference in frequency of ABO hemolytic disease. J Pediatr 1977;90:717–21.
53. Kaplan M, Herschel M, Hammerman C, et al. Hyperbilirubinemia among African American, glucose-6-phosphate dehydrogenase-deficient neonates. Pediatrics 2004;114:e213–9.
54. Wickremasinghe AC, Kuzniewicz MW, Newman TB. Black race is not protective against hazardous bilirubin levels. J Pediatr 2013;162:1068–9.
55. Slusher TM, Vreman HJ, McLaren DW, et al. Glucose-6-phosphate dehydrogenase deficiency and carboxyhemoglobin concentrations associated with bilirubin-related morbidity and death in Nigerian infants. J Pediatr 1995;126: 102–8.

56. Olusanya B, Emokpae A, Zamora T, et al. Addressing the burden of neonatal hyperbilirubinaemia in countries with significant glucose-6-phosphate dehydrogenase deficiency. Acta Paediatr 2014;103:1102–9.
57. Kaplan M, Slusher T, Renbaum P, et al. (TA)n UDP-glucuronosyltransferase 1A1 promoter polymorphism in Nigerian neonates. Pediatr Res 2008;63(1):109–11.
58. Akaba K, Kimura T, Sasaki A, et al. Neonatal hyperbilirubinemia and mutation of the bilirubin uridine diphosphate-glucuronosyltransferase gene: a common missense mutation among Japanese, Koreans and Chinese. Biochem Mol Biol Int 1998;46:21–6.
59. Long J, Zhang S, Fang X, et al. Neonatal hyperbilirubinemia and Gly71Arg mutation of UGT1A1 gene: a Chinese case-control study followed by systematic review of existing evidence. Acta Paediatr 2011;100:966–71.
60. Weng YH, Cheng SW, Yang CY, et al. Risk assessment of prolonged jaundice in infants at one month of age: a prospective cohort study. Sci Rep 2018;8: 148241–6.
61. De Luca D, Jackson GL, Tridente A, et al. Transcutaneous bilirubin nomograms: a systematic review of population differences and analysis of bilirubin kinetics. Arch Pediatr Adolesc Med 2009;163:1054–9.
62. Kaplan M, Bromiker R. Variation in transcutaneous bilirubin nomograms across population groups. J Pediatr 2019;208:273–8.e1.
63. Kaplan M, Bromiker R, Hammerman C. Hyperbilirubinemia, hemolysis, and increased bilirubin neurotoxicity. Semin Perinatol 2014;38:429–37.
64. Riskin A, Kugelman A, Abend-Weinger M, et al. In the eye of the beholder: how accurate is clinical estimation of jaundice in newborns? Acta Paediatr 2003;92: 574–6.
65. Bastauerous A, Armstrong MJ. Mobile health use in low- and high-income countries: an overview of the peer-reviewed literature. J R Soc Med 2013;106: 130–42.
66. Taylor JA, Stout JW, de Greef L, et al. Use of a smartphone app to assess neonatal jaundice. Pediatrics 2017;140:e20170312.
67. Aune A, Vartdal G, Bergseng H, et al. Bilirubin estimates from smartphone images of newborn infants' skin correlated highly to serum bilirubin levels. Acta Paediatr 2020. https://doi.org/10.1111/apa.15287.
68. Rets A, Clayton AL, Christensen RD, et al. Molecular diagnostic update in hereditary hemolytic anemia and neonatal hyperbilirubinemia. Int J Lab Hematol 2019;41(Suppl 1):95–101.
69. Christensen RD, Nussenzveig RH, Yaish HM, et al. Causes of hemolysis in neonates with extreme hyperbilirubinemia. J Perinatol 2014;34:616–9.
70. Vreman H, Wong RJ, Stevenson DK. Phototherapy: current methods and future directions. Semin Perinatol 2004;28:326–33.
71. Bahr TM, Christensen RD, Agarwal AM, et al. The neonatal acute bilirubin encephalopathy registry: background, aims, and protocol. Neonatology 2019; 115:242–6.
72. Faulhaber FRS, Procianoy RS, Silveira RC. Side effects of phototherapy on neonates. Am J Perinatol 2019;36:252–7.
73. Bhutani VK, Committee on Fetus and Newborn, American Academy of Pediatrics. Phototherapy to prevent severe neonatal hyperbilirubinemia in the newborn infant 35 or more weeks of gestation. Pediatrics 2011 Oct;128(4):e1046–52.
74. Tan KL. The pattern of bilirubin response to phototherapy for neonatal hyperbilirubinaemia. Pediatr Res 1982;16:670–4.

75. Vandborg PK, Hansen BM, Greisen G, et al. Dose response relationship of phototherapy for hyperbilirubinemia. Pediatrics 2012;130:e352–7.
76. Maisels MJ, Stevenson DK, Watchko JF, et al. Phototherapy and other treatments. In: Stevenson DK, Maisels MJ, Watchko JF, editors. Care of the jaundiced neonate. McGraw Hill; 2012. p. 199.
77. Wickremasinghe AC, Kuzniewicz MW, McCulloch CE, et al. Efficacy of subthreshold newborn phototherapy during the birth hospitalization in preventing readmission for phototherapy. JAMA Pediatr 2018;172:378–85.
78. Wickremasinghe AC, Kuzniewicz MW, Grimes BA, et al. Neonatal phototherapy and infantile cancer. Pediatrics 2016;137 [pii:e20151354].
79. Newman TB, Wickremasinghe AC, Walsh EM, et al. Retrospective cohort study of phototherapy and childhood cancer in northern California. Pediatrics 2016; 137 [pii:e201513541-8].
80. Cnattingius S, Zack M, EkbomA, et al. Prenatal and neonatal risk factors for childhood myeloid leukemia. Cancer Epidemiol Biomarkers Prev 1995;4:441–5.
81. Auger N, Laverdière C, Ayoub A, et al. Neonatal phototherapy and future risk of childhood cancer. Int J Cancer 2019;145:2061–9.
82. Tatli MM, Minnet C, Kocyigit A, et al. Phototherapy increases DNA damage in lymphocytes of hyperbilirubinemic neonates. Mutat Res 2008;654:93–5.
83. Rosenstein BS, Ducore JM. Enhancement by bilirubin of DNA damage induced in human cells exposed to phototherapy light. Pediatr Res 1984;18:3–6.
84. Christensen T, Reitan JB, Kinn G. Single-strand breaks in the DNA of human cells exposed to visible light from phototherapy lamps in the presence and absence of bilirubin. J Photochem Photobiol B 1990;7:337–46.
85. Gathwala G, Sharma S. Oxidative stress, phototherapy and the neonate. Indian J Pediatr 2000;67:805–8.
86. Aycicek A, Kocyigit A, Erel O, et al. Phototherapy causes DNA damage in peripheral mononuclear leukocytes in term infants. J Pediatr (Rio J) 2008;84(2): 141–6.
87. Yahia S, Shabaan AE, Gouida M, et al. Influence of hyperbilirubinemia and phototherapy on markers of genotoxicity and apoptosis in full-term infants. Eur J Pediatr 2015;174:459–64.
88. Mesbah-Namin SA, Shahidi M, Nakhshab M. An increased genotoxic risk in lymphocytes from phototherapy-treated hyperbilirubinemic neonates. Iran Biomed J 2017;21:182–9.
89. Ramy N, Ghany EA, Alsharany W, et al. Jaundice, phototherapy and DNA damage in full-term neonates. J Perinatol 2016;36:132–6.
90. Kanmaz HG, Okur N, Dilli D, et al. The effect of phototherapy on sister chromatid exchange with different light density in newborn hyperbilirubinemia. Turk Pediatri Ars 2017;52:202–7.
91. Kahveci H, Dogan H, Karaman A, et al. Phototherapy causes a transient DNA damage in jaundiced newborns. Drug Chem Toxicol 2013;36(1):88–92.
92. Wolf MF, Childers J, Gray KD, et al. Exchange transfusion safety and outcomes in neonatal hyperbilirubinemia. J Perinatol 2020. https://doi.org/10.1038/s41372-020-0642-0.
93. Kaplan M, Bromiker R, Schimmel MS, et al. Evaluation of discharge management in the prediction of hyperbilirubinemia: the Jerusalem experience. J Pediatr 2007;150:412–7.
94. Patra K, Storfer-Isser A, Siner B, et al. Adverse events associated with neonatal exchange transfusion in the 1990s. J Pediatr 2004;144:626–31.

95. Kaplan M, Eidelman AI. Post factum imposition of exchange transfusion criteria: in defense of neonatologists. Acta Paediatr 2011;100:479–81.
96. Arnold C, Pedroza C, Tyson JE. Phototherapy in ELBW newborns: does it work? Is it safe? The evidence from randomized clinical trials. Semin Perinatol 2014;38: 452–64.
97. Harris MC, Bernbaum JC, Polin JR, et al. Developmental follow-up of breastfed term and near-term infants with marked hyperbilirubinemia. Pediatrics 2001; 107:1075–80.
98. Hansen TW, Nietsch L, Norman E, et al. Reversibility of acute intermediate phase bilirubin encephalopathy. Acta Paediatr 2009;98:1689–94.
99. Danish Paediatric Society. Guideline for treatment of neonatal hyperbilirubinemia. 2012. Available at: http://www.paediatri.dk/images/pdf_filer/dps_vejl/neo/008neo.pdf.
100. Perrone S, Negro S, Tataranno ML, et al. Oxidative stress and antioxidant strategies in newborns. J Matern Fetal Neonatal Med 2010;23(Suppl 3):63–5.
101. Friel JK, Friesen RW, Harding SV, et al. Evidence of oxidative stress in full-term healthy infants. Pediatr Res 2004;56:878–82.
102. Wilinska M, Borszewska-Kornacka MK, Niemiec T, et al. Oxidative stress and total antioxidant status in term newborns and their mothers. Ann Agric Environ Med 2015;22:736–40.
103. Stevens B, Small RD Jr. The photoperoxidation of unsaturated organic molecules—XV. O2 1Δg quenching by bilirubin and biliverdin. Photochem Photobiol 1976;23:33–6.
104. Stocker R, Yamamoto Y, McDonagh A, et al. Bilirubin is an antioxidant of possible physiological importance. Science 1987;235:1043–6.
105. Hammerman C, Goldstein R, Kaplan M, et al. Bilirubin in the premature: toxic waste or natural defense? Clin Chem 1998;44:2551–3.
106. Dennery PA, McDonagh AF, Spitz DR, et al. Hyperbilirubinemia results in reduced oxidative injury in neonatal Gunn rats exposed to hyperoxia. Free Radic Biol Med 1995;19:395–404.
107. Hammerman C, Goldschmidt D, Caplan MS, et al. Protective effect of bilirubin in ischemia-reperfusion injury in the rat intestine. J Pediatr Gastroenterol Nutr 2002;35:344–9.
108. Gazzin S, Vitek L, Watchko J, et al. A novel perspective of the biology of bilirubin in health and disease. Trends Mol Med 2016;22:758–68.
109. Benaron DA, Bowen FW. Variation of initial serum bilirubin rise in newborn infants with type of illness. Lancet 1991;338:78–81.
110. Hegyi T, Goldie E, Hiatt M. The protective role of bilirubin in oxygen radical diseases of the preterm infant. J Perinatol 1994;14:296–300.
111. Dohi K, Satoh K, Ohtaki H, et al. Elevated plasma levels of bilirubin in patients with neurotrauma reflect its pathophysiological role in free radical scavenging. In Vivo 2005;19:855–60.
112. Bin-Nun A, Mimouni FB, Kasirer Y, et al. Might bilirubin serve as a natural antioxidant in response to neonatal encephalopathy? Am J Perinatol 2018;35: 1107–12.
113. Dani C, Poggi C, Fancelli C, et al. Changes in bilirubin in infants with hypoxic-ischemic encephalopathy. Eur J Pediatr 2018. https://doi.org/10.1007/s00431-018-3245.
114. Vitek L, Bellarosa C, Tiribelli C. Induction of mild hyperbilirubinemia: hype or real therapeutic opportunity? Clin Pharmacol Ther 2019;106:568–75.

115. Bjerre JV, Petersen JR, Ebbesen F. Surveillance of extreme hyperbilirubinaemia in Denmark. A method to identify the newborn infants. Acta Paediatr 2008;97: 1030–4.
116. Zoubir S, Mieth RA, Berrut S, et al. Swiss Paediatric Surveillance Unit. Incidence of severe hyperbilirubinaemia in Switzerland: a nationwide population-based prospective study. Arch Dis Child Fetal Neonatal Ed 2011;96:F310–1.
117. Gotink MJ, Benders MJ, Lavrijsen SW, et al. Severe neonatal hyperbilirubinemia in the Netherlands. Neonatology 2013;104:137–42.
118. Kuzniewicz MW, Wickremasinghe AC, Wu YW, et al. Incidence, etiology, and outcomes of hazardous hyperbilirubinemia in newborns. Pediatrics 2014;134: 504–9.
119. McGillivray A, Polverino J, Badawi N, et al. Prospective Surveillance of Extreme Neonatal Hyperbilirubinemia in Australia. J Pediatr 2016;168:82–7.e3.
120. Sgro M, Kandasamy S, Shah V, et al. Severe Neonatal Hyperbilirubinemia Decreased after the 2007 Canadian Guidelines. J Pediatr 2016;171:43–7.
121. Alkén J, Håkansson S, Ekéus C, et al. Rates of Extreme Neonatal Hyperbilirubinemia and Kernicterus in Children and Adherence to National Guidelines for Screening, Diagnosis, and Treatment in Sweden. JAMA Netw Open 2019;2: e190858.

The Term Newborn

Postnatal Screening and Testing

Kathryn A. Johnson, MD, MS[a,*], Valerian Catanzarite, MD, PhD[b]

KEYWORDS

- Newborn screening • Newborn hearing screening • Newborn physical examination
- Critical congenital heart disease screening • Genetic screening in pregnancy
- Prenatal ultrasonography • Prenatal diagnosis

KEY POINTS

- Prenatal genetic screening has 3 components: evaluation for inherited genetic disorders, risk assessment for common aneuploidies, and sonographic assessment for structural anomalies and variants.
- Abnormal prenatal screening prompts additional evaluation, either prenatal or postnatal.
- The prenatal record should be reviewed by the newborn provider after delivery for abnormalities on prenatal screening, ultrasonography, or family history that require postnatal follow-up.
- A complete newborn examination, including growth parameters, can identify indications for additional evaluation.
- Recommended standard newborn screening includes blood, hearing, and critical congenital heart disease screening.

INTRODUCTION

Major birth defects occur in 1% of newborns, and minor ones occur in 3%. Fortunately, with advances in prenatal diagnosis, most major anomalies are detected before birth. One goal of prenatal care is to minimize undetected anomalies, so that the surprises after delivery will be pleasant ones! However, prenatal assessment leaves unresolved screening issues in 5% to 10% of pregnancies, to be addressed postnatally.

Prenatal genetic screening and testing are quite complex, and follow-up of prenatal findings is an integral part of newborn evaluation. The prenatal record should communicate the results of prenatal screening requiring postnatal follow-up. After delivery, a thorough newborn examination, combined with standard newborn screening, including blood, hearing, and congenital heart disease screening, can reveal

[a] University of California, San Diego, 9300 Campus Point Drive, La Jolla, CA 92037-7774, USA; [b] San Diego Perinatal Center, Rady Children's Specialists of San Diego, 7910 Frost Street Suite 130, San Diego, CA 92131, USA
* Corresponding author.
E-mail address: kajohnson@health.ucsd.edu

Clin Perinatol 48 (2021) 555–572
https://doi.org/10.1016/j.clp.2021.05.007

additional conditions requiring further evaluation. Coordination of care between obstetric and pediatric care providers is essential to ensure optimal neonatal outcomes.

PRENATAL GENETIC SCREENING

Prenatal genetic screening has 3 components—evaluation for inherited genetic disorders, aneuploidy risk assessment, and sonographic assessment. Diagnostic tests include karyotyping, microarray DNA testing, and specialized studies of amniocentesis and chorionic villus sampling (CVS) specimens, and imaging includes targeted sonography, fetal echocardiography, and MRI.

Screening for Inherited Genetic Disorders

Maternal screening for cystic fibrosis and spinal muscular atrophy are universally recommended. Additional screening may be indicated based on ancestry or family history, for example, hemoglobinopathy or Tay-Sachs screening.[1] Expanded carrier screening—inexpensive, simultaneous screening for hundreds of genetic disorders—is increasingly popular.[2] Screening of both parents would be optimal, but usually only the mother is screened, with contingent paternal screening. Diagnostic testing (CVS or amniocentesis), if indicated, permits prenatal diagnosis; some parents defer diagnostic testing until after delivery. Standard newborn screening may not include all conditions included in expanded carrier panels. The prenatal record should include positive screening results, and recommended newborn testing should be arranged before hospital discharge.

Screening for Aneuploidy

Prenatal aneuploidy screening is routine but not standardized. Screens in common use include maternal biochemical analyses (65%–80% trisomy 21 [T21] detection, 5% false-positives); combined nuchal translucency and biochemical screening, improving detection to greater than 85% and reducing false-positives; and NIPT based on assay of fetal cell-free DNA in maternal blood, sensitivity greater than 99% and false-positives less than 1%.[3–5]

Standard Noninvasive prenatal testing (NIPT) screens for T21, trisomy 18 (T18), and trisomy 13 (T13): Many laboratories include sex chromosome aneuploidies and microarray conditions such as DiGeorge syndrome (22q11.2 deletion).[6] Women with positive screens are offered CVS or amniocentesis. If parents decline, appropriate postnatal evaluation should be performed. CVS or amniocentesis may show microarray "variants of uncertain significance," potentially an indication for a dysmorphology evaluation.

Sonographic Screening

The first prenatal diagnosis of a birth defect, anencephaly, was reported nearly 50 years ago. Today prenatal ultrasonography is routine and conditions including central nervous system (CNS) and spinal defects, cardiac anomalies, diaphragmatic hernia, abdominal wall defects, renal anomalies, skeletal dysplasias, and movement disorders can be detected.[7] A national quality assurance program is administered by the American Institute for Ultrasound in Medicine (AIUM); sonography should be performed in accordance with AIUM guidelines and preferably in AIUM-certified centers.

Sonography, unlike laboratory assessment, is operator dependent. Experienced centers report detection rates greater than 30% for major birth defects at 11 to 14 weeks and greater than 60% at 18 to 22 weeks. For example, at 11 to 14 weeks, anencephaly, abdominal wall defects, and limb reduction defects are readily diagnosed. At 18 to 22 weeks, a more detailed examination of the fetus can be carried out. Expectations for experienced centers include greater than 98% detection of open spina bifida, greater than 70% for major congenital heart defects, and greater than 80% for major renal anomalies.

The sonographic diagnosis of a fetal anomaly typically prompts genetic counseling, consideration of CVS or amniocentesis if warranted, and arrangements for subspecialty evaluation and care after delivery. Sonography is also used for antenatal screening for aneuploidy risk, and to assess for anatomic variants that may be associated with anomalies.

Increased nuchal translucency. There is visible fluid within the skin of back of the fetal neck at 11 to 14 weeks, the nuchal translucency (NT). NT measurement, in an exact imaging plane and with strict quality control, is used in T13, T18, and T21 risk assessment. Measurements greater than 3.5 mm are associated with cardiac and other fetal malformations, genetic syndromes, and microarray DNA abnormalities.[8,9] Measurement greater than 3.5 mm should prompt a detailed newborn examination for anomalies. If not performed in utero, microarray DNA testing and echocardiography for the newborn should be considered.

Soft markers for aneuploidy are findings at 16 to 22 weeks that show increased risk for chromosomal abnormalities. Thickened nuchal skinfold, nonossified nasal bone, left ventricular echogenic focus, pyelectasis, and relatively short femur or humerus increase T21 risk.[10,11] Choroid plexus cysts flag increased T18 risk.[12] These findings may steer a family toward NIPT or amniocentesis. If the newborn does not have aneuploidy, these are considered to be normal anatomic variants, but parents may have persistent concerns after delivery. Soft markers and their implications are summarized in **Table 1**.

Table 1
Soft markers for aneuploidy and recommended postnatal follow-up

Soft Marker	Frequency at 16–22 wk	Risk Adjustment	Postnatal Follow-up
Choroid cyst[12]	0.5%–2%	T18: 9× increase	Detailed PE and reassurance. Choroid cysts resolve by 30 wk and do not affect neurodevelopment
Increased nuchal skinfold >5 mm[10,11]	0.5%–1%	T21: 11–21× increase	Consider echocardiography if nuchal skinfold >6 and detailed heart screening not done prenatally
Nonossified nasal bone[13]	Varies with ethnicity; <1%–9%	T21: 40–60× increase	Detailed PE
Echogenic focus[10,11]	5%–10%	T21: 2× increase	For multiple echogenic foci, consider echocardiography if not done prenatally
Pyelectasis[10,11]	1.5%–3%	T21: 1.5–2× increase	Renal ultrasonography if pyelectasis does not resolve prenatally
Humerus <90% of expected[10,11]	1.5%	T21: 5× increase	Detailed PE
Femur <90% of expected[10,11]	5%	T21: 2x increase	Detailed PE

Abbreviation: PE, physical examination.

Anatomic variants are sonographic findings not diagnostic of an abnormality, but can be associated with anomalies or congenital infections.

Brain

- *Mild and moderate ventriculomegaly.* The brain ventricles are routinely assessed by sonography. After 16 weeks the lateral ventricles should measure less than 10 mm. Measurements of 10 to 12 mm and 13 to 15 mm occur in 0.5% of sonograms and are classified as mild and moderate ventriculomegaly, respectively. When ventriculomegaly is present, even when no other abnormalities are seen, targeted sonography and consideration of amniocentesis are warranted, because 5% have aneuploidy, an additional 10% to 15% have an abnormal microarray, and 5% have cytomegalovirus (CMV) or toxoplasmosis. Structural CNS abnormalities not suspected by ultrasonography are diagnosed in 5% to 15% either by prenatal MRI or postnatal images. Among otherwise normal newborns with isolated mild ventriculomegaly, neurologic outcomes are similar to the general population, but with isolated moderate ventriculomegaly up to 25% of newborns have significant neurodevelopmental issues.[14–16]

  Postnatal evaluation: Careful physical examination, assessment for CMV and toxoplasomosis, and head ultrasonography; if amniocentesis was not performed prenatally, consider microarray DNA testing.
- *Prominent cisterna magna.* The cerebellum and posterior fossa are routinely imaged prenatally. The posterior fossa anteroposterior (AP) measurement should be less than 10 mm. A larger measurement may be associated with intracranial abnormalities or aneuploidy. However, measurements in the 10 to 12 mm range in the third trimester, if not associated with visible intracranial abnormalities, are likely physiologic.[17]

  Postnatal evaluation: Careful physical examination; head ultrasonography and MRI if other intracranial abnormalities present.

Heart

- *Linear valve insertions.* There is normally an offset between the mitral and tricuspid valves. Linear arrangement of the valves indicates increased risk for trisomy 21 and fetal inlet ventricular septal defects (VSDs).[18]

  Postnatal evaluation: Assessment for T21; fetal echocardiography if not completed prenatally.
- *Fetal VSDs* are the most common form of congenital heart disease, but VSDs, particularly muscular VSDs, are common in utero and occur in 1% of scans. Isolated muscular VSDs are not associated with aneuploidy and commonly close in utero or during the first year of life. Inlet and membranous VSDs may also close, but are associated with aneuploidy and microarray abnormalities (eg, DiGeorge 22q11.2 deletion in membranous VSDs).

  Postnatal evaluation: Echocardiography to confirm closure; consider microarray DNA analysis in cases of membranous or inlet VSDs.

Abdomen

- *Echogenic bowel* occurs in 0.4% of pregnancies. In about 90% of babies, it is not associated with pathologic condition. Echogenic bowel is a marker for Down syndrome (3% risk), cystic fibrosis (CF) (2% risk), CMV, and parvovirus B19 infections (2% risk) and is associated with increased rates of fetal growth impairment and bowel issues for the newborn.

  Postnatal evaluation: Verify normal CF, CMV, and parvovirus maternal screening and careful assessment for these conditions.[19]

- *Intra-abdominal echogenicities* are seen in about 1% of ultrasonographies; they commonly resolve during pregnancy. If multiple, they may indicate congenital viral infection such as CMV and warrant prenatal or postnatal evaluation. If isolated, they are not of pathologic significance; no specific postnatal evaluations are recommended.[20,21]
  Postnatal evaluation: Assess for CMV if multiple echogenicities.
- *Fetal gallbladder sludge and/or gallstones* are identified in 0.1% to 1% of pregnancies and typically resolve after birth; they are a variant of normal anatomy.
  Postnatal evaluation: Careful clinical evaluation.[21]
- *Fetal pyelectasis and hydronephrosis.* Pyelectasis, fetal renal collecting systems measuring ≥4 mm in the anteroposterior view, are seen in 1.5% to 3% of pregnancies at 16 to 22 weeks and are a low-level T21 soft marker (see **Table 1**). If pyelectasis is present, follow-up sonography in the third trimester is recommended. The upper range of normal increases later in pregnancy. The Society of Fetal Urology recommends a 10-mm cutoff after 28 weeks for diagnosis of fetal hydronephrosis. This cutoff represents a balance between sensitivity and specificity[22,23]; some centers recommend thresholds as low as 7 mm to increase sensitivity. If hydronephrosis is unresolved by the last prenatal sonography, further evaluation after birth is indicated.
  Postnatal evaluation: Renal ultrasonography, within 48 hours of delivery for severe or bilateral hydronephrosis, or hydronephrosis with associated ultrasonographic findings, such as contralateral renal agenesis, hydroureter, or bladder thickening; otherwise within 3 to 14 days of birth.
- *Ovarian cysts* occur in about 1:1300 female fetuses. Most are functional and more than half—particularly unilocular cysts less than 4 cm in diameter—resolve either during pregnancy or after delivery. In utero and postnatal torsion and hemorrhage into cysts are relatively common.[24]
  Postnatal evaluation: Abdominal ultrasonography and pediatric surgical consultation unless resolved in utero.
- *Hydroceles* occur in 15% or more of males. The majority resolve before birth or during the first year of life.[25]
  Postnatal evaluation: Careful physical examination, including transillumination of the scrotal sac; ultrasonography if indicated.

Umbilical cord

- *Variants of umbilical circulatory anatomy* including single umbilical artery, persistent right umbilical vein, and umbilical vein varix are readily detected by ultrasonography[26–28]; these are variants of normal circulatory anatomy, but have high rates of association with anomalies (**Table 2**) and carry increased risks for obstetric complications.
  Postnatal evaluation: Careful physical examination; consider an echocardiography if a complete set of screening heart views (4 chambers, great vessels, aortic and pulmonic outflows, and aortic and pulmonic outflows) or a fetal echocardiography was not done before birth.

Incomplete Sonographic Screening for Anomalies

A common question encountered by pediatric care providers is follow-up when detailed fetal anatomic evaluation was not possible by prenatal ultrasonography. Ascertainment of congenital anomalies is operator dependent and may be limited by maternal body habitus, abdominal wall scarring, or fetal position. The 3 organs that most commonly show abnormalities not apparent on newborn examination are the brain, heart, and kidneys.

Table 2
Variants of umbilical circulatory anatomy

Variant	Frequency at 16–22 wk	Associated Anomalies	Postnatal Follow-up
Single umbilical artery[24]	0.5%–1%	11% have at least 1 major or minor anomaly, including cardiac, GI, and renal defects, and trisomies 13 and 18	Careful PE. Consider echocardiography if a full set of cardiac screening views (or fetal echocardiography) was not done prenatally
Persistent right umbilical vein[25]	0.1%–0.3%	24%, including CNS, cardiac, and genitourinary as well as aneuploidy. Midline gallbladder is common	As for single umbilical artery. No adverse developmental effects
Intra-abdominal umbilical vein varix[26]	0.1%–0.2%	15% have major anomalies, including cardiac	As for single umbilical artery. Varices involute after delivery. No adverse developmental effects

Abbreviation: GI, gastrointestinal.

CNS examination by ultrasonography includes demonstration of the intracranial midline, cavum septum pellucidum, lateral ventricles, cerebellum, and posterior fossa. If views of intracranial anatomy were limited, a head ultrasonography of the newborn may be considered. Cardiac screening is the most technically demanding part of prenatal sonography. Population studies show rates of prenatal diagnosis ranging from 13% to 87%.[29] Even in an institution with excellent (74%) ascertainment of cardiac anomalies by ultrasonography, the addition of protocol-based postnatal evaluation adds another 20% ascertainment by hospital discharge.[30] The kidneys are readily demonstrated on ultrasonography. If both were not documented, then the fetus may have unilateral renal agenesis or an ectopic kidney. Neonatal renal sonography, preferably before hospital discharge, is indicated.

NEWBORN ASSESSMENT

The first newborn examination should occur within 24 hours of birth, and include a thorough head-to-toe assessment and attention to growth parameters.[31] The presence of any minor malformation on physical examination should prompt a careful examination for additional anomalies. Some benign physical examination findings, when detected in isolation, require no additional evaluation, whereas other findings require testing or referral to a pediatric specialist. A careful review of family history including the presence of congenital heart disease, hip dysplasia, childhood hearing loss, infant deaths, or other childhood conditions may prompt additional newborn screening and evaluation. A summary of common newborn examination findings, incidence, associations or risk factors, recommended evaluation, and follow-up appears in **Table 4**. Most newborn skin findings are benign and can be monitored by the pediatric care provider. Some newborn skin findings, however, warrant additional evaluation and referral to a pediatric dermatologist (**Table 5**).

Ear Pits and Tags

Ear pits and tags, found in 5 to 10 per 1000 newborns, are classically associated with an increased risk for hearing loss. When present, the newborn should undergo a routine hearing screening. A renal ultrasonography should be performed if other malformations are found and considered if there is a family history of hearing loss, maternal gestational diabetes, or teratogen exposure.[32]

Congenital Muscular Torticollis

Congenital muscular torticollis (CMT) affects 3.9% to 16%[33,34] of infants and is characterized by unilateral shortening of the sternocleidomastoid muscle resulting in cervical flexion and rotation. Careful examination, including visual inspection for ear cupping or jaw tilt, passive cervical rotation, and lateral flexion, can detect cervical range asymmetries that should prompt referral to physical therapy. CMT can be associated with other disorders of in utero crowding, such as developmental dysplasia of the hip (DDH) and metatarsus adductus. Outcomes are best when infants are diagnosed early and start physical therapy by 3 months of age, and duration of physical therapy can be reduced if initiated before 1 month of age.[35]

Cardiac Murmurs

The evaluation of cardiac murmurs varies greatly with the skill level of the examiner. In general, infants with asymptomatic murmurs in an unusual location or louder than 2/6 should be evaluated with an echocardiography before discharge. Electrocardiography, chest radiograph, and 4-limb blood pressures have low diagnostic potential and are not recommended for the evaluation of an asymptomatic murmur.[36] A postnatal echocardiography should also be considered for poorly controlled maternal diabetes mellitus (particularly first-trimester hemoglobin A_{1C} value >8%), family history of congenital heart disease requiring surgery in a first-degree relative, or an abnormal nuchal translucency measurement, especially if a fetal echocardiography was not completed.[37]

Developmental Dysplasia of the Hip

DDH encompasses hip joint abnormalities, including dysplasia, subluxation, and dislocation. The incidence is approximately 1 in 1000 live births. DDH risk factors include breech presentation, family history, female sex, and first-born infants. The left hip is more commonly affected than the right. Other associations include postmaturity, higher birth weight, and oligohydramnios.[38] When DDH is detected in the first months of life, treatment is unlikely to involve surgery and is more successful. Current guidelines support serial hip examinations to detect DDH, beginning with the initial newborn examination.[39] A careful hip examination, including visual inspection for leg length discrepancy (Galeazzi sign), symmetry of gluteal folds, and Barlow (adduction of hip with gentle posterior force) and Ortolani (abduction of hip with gentle anterior force) maneuvers can identify subluxation, dislocation, or a dislocated hip that may or may not be reducible.[40]

Infants with risk factors for DDH including breech positioning in utero beyond the 34 weeks, a family history of DDH, or a history of clinical hip instability warrant both periodic surveillance examinations and postnatal hip imaging. Hip clicks without instability detected on the newborn examination do not require follow-up.[41] Ultrasonography is the preferred imaging modality in infants younger than 4 months and should occur around 6 weeks of life.[40] Pediatric orthopedic follow-up should be arranged for infants with a dislocated or unstable hip (positive Ortolani), but initial observation may be appropriate for milder instability (positive Barlow or subluxation only).[39] There is currently not strong evidence to support the practice of double diapering to support an unstable hip. Parents should be counseled to avoid tight swaddling with the hips in an adducted position and should swaddle to allow for flexion and abduction of the hips.[39]

Polydactyly

Polydactyly ranges from a fully formed digit containing bone and a nail to a partially formed remnant of skin. Postaxial polydactyly (ulnar) is rarely associated with other anomalies, can be inherited in an autosomal dominant pattern, and is more common in African Americans (1 in 143 newborns).[42] Preaxial (radial) polydactyly is less common (1 in 3000 newborns) and is associated with anomalies such as Fanconi anemia, chromosomal abnormalities, and VACTERL association.[32] The presence of other minor anomalies should prompt consultation with a dysmorphologist and evaluation with chromosomal breakage studies and a chromosomal microarray.

Sacral Dimples

Sacral dimples are common (2%–4% of newborns)[43] and are only rarely associated with an underlying occult spinal dysraphism (OSD) such as tethered cord, spinal cord lipoma, or dermal sinus tract. Most OSDs are associated with skin findings such as a patch or tuft of hair, skin tag, hemangioma, lipoma, or large or atypical sacral dimple. A simple sacral dimple (single dimple less than 5 mm in diameter and <25 mm from the anal verge without cutaneous markers) warrants no further evaluation or imaging.[44] An atypical dimple (large, multiple, or associated with overlying skin findings) should prompt further evaluation and imaging and potential consultation with a pediatric neurosurgeon.[43]

Delaying spinal ultrasonography for an atypical dimple until 1 month of life, when both nerve root motion and philum thickness ultrasonographies are better visualized, can yield more accurate results.[45] Spinal ultrasonographies are generally the preferred study until after 3 to 6 months of age. MRI is preferred thereafter, or if neurologic symptoms are present.

STANDARD NEWBORN SCREENING

Standardized newborn screening in the United States originated in 1963 with testing for phenylketonuria. In 1968, Wilson and Jungner described standard criteria for the development of screening tests, which have served as a guide for expansion of newborn screening—the condition should be an important health problem, have a readily available test and treatment, and have a latent stage during which treatment prevents worsening of the disease.[46] Newborn screening was largely organized and regulated at the state level until the Newborn Screening Saves Lives Act of 2007 established a national collaborative overseeing newborn screening, created Web-accessible resources for patients and health care providers, and established quality oversight through the Department of Health and Human Services. The Act also established the Recommended Uniform Screening Panel (RUSP) and the process by which conditions are nominated and approved for addition to the panel.

Technologic advances in tandem mass spectrometry have allowed for screening for an increasing number of conditions with a small sample of blood. Advances in treatment modalities have made it possible to offer screening for previously untreatable conditions such as spinal muscular atrophy, the most recent addition to the RUSP in 2018. The RUSP presently includes 35 core and 26 secondary conditions, including pulse oximetry screening for critical congenital heart disease (CCHD) and newborn hearing screening. Of the 4 million newborns screened annually, approximately

12,500 are diagnosed with one of the core conditions on the RUSP, most commonly hearing loss, congenital hypothyroidism, cystic fibrosis, sickle cell disease, and medium-chain acyl-coenzyme A dehydrogenase deficiency.[47]

Newborn Screening

Newborn screening is performed by collecting multiple blood spots on a sample card and assessing for core and secondary conditions using tandem mass spectrometry, hemoglobin electrophoresis, or other individual tests. Most states screen for most disorders in the RUSP, and some states screen for additional disorders. Variation also exists between states in the timing of screening and the need for a second screening. Most newborn screening protocols recommend sample collection at 24 to 48 hours of life, after the initiation of feeding and before any blood transfusions (which can affect the results of hemoglobin electrophoresis, galactosemia, and biotinidase deficiency).[48] State-specific information about conditions screened for, details about screening programs, and parent education materials are all accessible via the Web site *Baby's First Test*.[49]

Out-of-hospital deliveries, transitions of care during the first 48 hours of life, or use of total parental nutrition can affect the collection and interpretation of newborn screening results.[48] Care should be taken that all newborns have an appropriately collected newborn screen and the results of the screening, whether positive or negative, are reviewed in a timely manner. State newborn screening programs are responsible for coordinating the careful follow-up required for an abnormal testing result, including any diagnostic testing required. The American College of Medical Genetics has developed action (ACTion) sheets to guide pediatricians in responding to abnormal newborn screening results.[50] Diagnostic testing and evaluation should be performed with the assistance of metabolic, endocrinologic, neurologic or immunologic specialists. In addition, infants born to parents with abnormal prenatal expanded carrier screening increasing the risk for certain conditions should have expedited newborn screening and follow-up with pediatric specialists as indicated.[51] Careful communication between obstetricians and newborn care providers ensures timely screening is completed.

Newborn Hearing Screening

Universal newborn hearing screening (UNHS) has led to the timely diagnosis of hearing impairment, earlier speech and language intervention, and prompt hearing aid fitting or cochlear implantation when indicated.[52] Current goals of the Early Hearing Detection and Intervention program include newborn hearing screening by 1 month of age, diagnostic hearing testing by 3 months of age for any newborn failing the UNHS, and hearing intervention by 6 months of age.[53] Unfortunately, the loss to follow-up rate after failed screening remains high, making patient education surrounding a failed screen and database management systems priorities to ensure program goals are met.

Hearing screening can be performed with either transient evoked otoacoustic emissions (OAEs) or automated auditory brainstem response (AABR). The OAE evaluates the function of the cochlea by measuring low-intensity sounds produced by hair cells in response to an acoustic stimulus. OAEs have a higher false-positive rate, especially when performed in the first 48 hours of life.[54] OAEs do not evaluate the entire auditory pathway and thus do not diagnose auditory neuropathies. The AABR evaluates the entire auditory pathway through the detection of response to transient acoustic stimuli using surface electrodes placed on the forehead and near the ears. AABRs can take longer to complete and are costlier, but are capable of detecting sensorineural hearing loss, and are therefore the recommended screening modality for the neonatal intensive care unit population and the preferred follow-up test for an abnormal OAE.[53]

A pass result on the newborn hearing screening does not exclude the possibility of future hearing loss.[55] All newborns should be evaluated for the presence of risk factors for hearing loss and referred for diagnostic follow-up at the recommended interval (**Table 3**). Infants who fail the newborn hearing screening should be referred for

Table 3
Risk factors for early childhood hearing loss

	Risk Factor	Recommended Diagnostic Follow-up
1	Family history of early, progressive, or delayed onset permanent childhood hearing loss	By 9 mo
2	Neonatal intensive care of more than 5 d	By 9 mo
3	Hyperbilirubinemia with exchange transfusion regardless of length of stay	By 9 mo
4	Aminoglycoside administration for more than 5 d	By 9 mo
5	Asphyxia or hypoxic-ischemic encephalopathy	By 9 mo
6	Extracorporeal membrane oxygenation	No later than 3 mo after occurrence
7	In utero infections, such as herpes, rubella, syphilis, and toxoplasmosis	By 9 mo
	In utero infection with CMV	No later than 3 mo after occurrence
	Mother positive for Zika and infant with no laboratory evidence & no clinical findings	Standard
	Mother positive for Zika and infant with laboratory evidence of Zika with or without clinical findings	AABR by 1 mo
8	Certain birth conditions or findings: • Craniofacial malformations including microtia/atresia, ear dysplasia, oral facial clefting, white forelock, or microphthalmia • Congenital microcephaly, congenital or acquired hydrocephalus • Temporal bone abnormalities	By 9 mo
9	Syndrome associated with hearing loss	By 9 mo
10	Culture-positive infections associated with sensorineural hearing loss, including confirmed bacterial and viral (especially herpes viruses and varicella) meningitis or encephalitis	No later than 3 mo after occurrence
11	Events associated with hearing loss: • Significant head trauma especially basal skull/temporal bone fractures • Chemotherapy	No later than 3 mo after occurrence
12	Caregiver concern regarding hearing, speech, language, developmental delay, and/or developmental regression	Immediate referral

Abbreviation: AABR, automated auditory brainstem response.

Table 4
Summary of newborn examination findings

Finding	Incidence	Associations/Risk Factors	Additional Evaluation	Outpatient Follow-up
Microcephaly (<third percentile)	8.7/10,000	Aneuploidy; growth restriction; CMV; Zika	CMV testing, head US, consider Zika testing	As needed
Ear pit or tag	5–10/1000	Hearing loss	Newborn hearing screening; consider renal US if other minor anomalies on PE, maternal DM or teratogen exposure	None required
CMT	40–160/1000	In utero crowding; DDH, metatarsus adductus	Examination for DDH or metatarsus adductus	PT f/u by 1 mo of age
Cardiac murmur	6–770/1000	Congenital heart disease	Echocardiography for louder than 2/6 or unusual location; consider maternal DM with elevated HbA_{1C}, abnormal NT, or FH of CHD requiring surgery (especially if no fetal echocardiography done)	As needed based on echocardiographic findings
DDH	1/1000	Breech presentation beyond 34 wk, family history of DDH, female; CMTs, metatarsus adductus	Careful hip examination including inspection for leg length discrepancy (Galeazzi sign), gluteal fold symmetry, Barlow and Ortolani maneuvers; check for CMT or metatarsus adductus	Close pediatric orthopedic f/u for unstable or dislocated hip; hip US at 6 wk of age for FH of DDH, breech presentation beyond 34 wk, or instability on later examination
Polydactyly	0.6–2.3/1000	Postaxial: none Preaxial: VACTERL, Fanconi anemia	Postaxial: none required Preaxial: careful PE for other minor anomalies; consider chromosomal microarray and breakage studies	Postaxial: none required Preaxial: consider genetics f/u
Sacral dimple	20–40/1000	Simple: none Atypical: OSD	Simple dimples (<5 mm diameter, <25 mm from anal verge, no skin findings): none required Atypical dimple: careful neurologic examination; spinal US or MRI (if neurologic examination abnormalities)	Simple dimple: none required Atypical dimple: neurosurgery f/u for MRI (if neurologic examination abnormalities) or spinal US
Hernia	Inguinal: 10–50/1000	Male; Right side more common		Inguinal: pediatric surgery f/u Umbilical: observation only

(*continued on next page*)

Table 4
(continued)

Finding	Incidence	Associations/Risk Factors	Additional Evaluation	Outpatient Follow-up
Undescended testis	20–50/1000	Preterm or early term	Unilateral: none Bilateral: consider evaluation for congenital adrenal hyperplasia, abdominal US	Pediatric urology f/u by 6 mo if still undescended
Metatarsus adductus	30/1000	In utero crowding; DDH, CMT	Examination for CMT or DDH	PT f/u by 1 mo of age if not resolving

Abbreviations: CHD, congenital heart disease; CMT, congenital muscular torticollis; DDH, developmental hip dysplasia; DM, diabetes mellitus; FH, family history; f/u, follow-up; HbA1c, hemoglobin A_{1C}; OSD, occult spinal dysraphism; US, ultrasonography; VACTERL, Vertebral anomalies, anorectal malformations, cardiovascular anomalies, tracheoesophageal fistula, esophageal atresia, renal and/or radial anomalies, and limb defects.

Table 5
Newborn skin findings

Skin Finding	Evaluation
• Slate gray patches (congenital dermal melanocytosis) • Salmon patches (nevus simplex) • Erythema toxicum • Transient neonatal pustular melanosis • Congenital melanocytic nevus	No evaluation needed
Port-wine stain	Evaluate for Sturge-Weber syndrome (face), Klippel-Trénaunay-Weber syndrome (extremity), or occult spinal dysraphism (back)
Subcutaneous fat necrosis (extensive)	Measure serum calcium level
Petechiae (widespread) or purpura	Check platelet count
IH	Referral to pediatric dermatology for: • Facial, frontal neck (beard distribution), breast, fingers/toes, or area of chronic irritation (diaper area) • >5 IHs in at least 2 different locations (need abdominal US to rule out hepatic involvement) • Segmental IH of face or scalp (PHACES syndrome) or lumbosacral area (LUMBAR syndrome)
Sebaceous nevus of Jadassohn	Observation, referral to pediatric dermatology in childhood
Café au Lait spot	No evaluation needed if <0.5 cm and fewer than 6; otherwise evaluate for neurofibromatosis

*Abbreviation:*IH, infantile hemangioma; PHACES, Posterior fossa brain malformations, Hemangioma, Arterial lesions, Cardiac abnormalities, and Eye abnormalities; LUMBAR, Lower body hemangioma and other cutaneous defects, Urogenital anomalies, Myelopathy, Bone deformities, Anorectal malformations and Arterial anomalies, and Renal anomalies.

outpatient retesting and diagnostic audiology evaluation in a timely manner. The family should be educated on the importance of repeat testing, and discharge communication to the outpatient pediatric care provider should include the results of the failed screen.

Targeted Congenital Cytomegalovirus Screening

Congenital CMV is one of the leading causes of sensorineural hearing loss in infants.[56] Targeted CMV screening for infants with a failed UNHS, performed either with salivary or urine viral DNA detection via polymerase chain reaction (PCR) or culture before 3 weeks of age, facilitates early diagnosis of congenital CMV and allows for more frequent hearing assessments, improved interventions, and better outcomes for these infants.[57] For this reason, many hearing screening programs perform targeted CMV screening using salivary PCR swabbing, completed at least 90 minutes after breastfeeding to avoid false-positive results. Positive salivary testing is usually confirmed with urine PCR or culture to further reduce false-positives. Other indications for targeted CMV screening include microcephaly, growth restriction, hepatosplenomegaly, elevated transaminases, petechiae, thrombocytopenia, or intracranial abnormalities.[52]

Critical Congenital Heart Disease Screening

CCHD screening was added to the US RUSP in 2011, and by July 2018 all states were screening for CCHD.[58] Legislation mandating screening has reduced the rates of cardiac death from CCHD by 33%.[59] The current model for screening, endorsed by the American Academy of Pediatrics, American Heart Association, and the American College of Cardiology recommends measurement of oxygen saturation in the right hand (preductal) and either foot (postductal).[60] Oxygen saturations should be 95% or greater in the hand and the foot, and there should not be more than a 3% difference between the two.[58] Typically, screening is performed after 24 hours of life. Earlier screening can be done but results in an increased false-positive rate.[58]

If the first CCHD screen is abnormal the screen should be repeated within a short time frame and the infant should be assessed carefully for other symptoms of cyanotic heart disease. Other potential causes of hypoxemia include pneumonia, persistent pulmonary hypertension of the newborn, or sepsis, so evaluation should include noncardiac causes. Updated strategies for screening recommend that failure of a second CCHD screening should immediately prompt further evaluation with an echocardiography and close monitoring.[58]

CCHD screening is not definitive. A negative result of CCHD screen does not exclude congenital heart disease. Coarctation of the aorta is the most commonly missed abnormality, and other forms of congenital heart disease that may require surgery such as atrial septal defect or VSD are not detected with CCHD screening. Therefore, close follow-up with an outpatient pediatric provider after discharge is essential during the first few weeks of life. Symptoms such as poor feeding, shortness of breath, cyanosis, loud or harsh murmur, or poor perfusion should warrant immediate referral to a pediatric cardiologist.

SUMMARY

Results of newborn screening should be communicated to the primary care provider and the parents, and abnormalities should prompt referral for additional diagnostic testing and pediatric specialist consultation. Anomalies or genetic disorders not suspected prenatally and the results of prenatally recommended postnatal imaging should be relayed to the prenatal care team. Metabolic or genetic conditions or the diagnosis of CCHD may require additional parental screening for carrier status or specialized imaging in future pregnancies. Closed-loop communication leads to a better understanding of the detection and management of newborn conditions and ultimately results in better quality care.

Best practices

What is the current practice?

- Prenatal ultrasonography
- Maternal serum aneuploidy screening and screening for inherited genetic disorders
- Diagnostic imaging or testing as indicated by maternal history or results of screening tests
- Detailed newborn physical examination and assessment of family and pregnancy history
- Newborn screening (including blood, hearing, and congenital heart disease) and, when indicated, diagnostic imaging and testing

- Follow-up of concerns raised by prenatal screening or testing and communication with pediatric and obstetric providers

What changes in current practice are likely to improve outcomes?

- As technology advances and costs decline, routine use of expanded carrier screening and NIPT.
- Require universal accreditation and quality assurance for prenatal anatomic screening sonography.
- Mechanisms to ensure communication of prenatal flags to pediatric care provider and closed-loop feedback from pediatric to obstetric care providers.
- Ensure abnormal newborn screening results receive appropriate follow-up and communication with family and pediatric care provider.

Major recommendations

- Abnormal prenatal or newborn screening results should prompt additional diagnostic testing guided by maternal fetal medicine, perinatal genetics, or pediatric specialists

Bibliographic sources:

- Benitz WE; Committee on Fetus and Newborn, American Academy of Pediatrics. Hospital stay for healthy term newborn infants. *Pediatrics.* 2015;135(5):948-953.
- Carrier screening for genetic conditions. Committee Opinion No. 691.American College of Obstetricians and Gynecologists. Obstet Gynecol 2017;129:e41–55.
- Carrier screening in the age of genomic medicine. Committee Opinion No. 690. American College of Obstetricians and Gynecologists. Obstet Gynecol 2017;129:e35–40.
- Committee on Practice Bulletins—Obstetrics and the American Institute of Ultrasound in Medicine. Practice Bulletin No. 175: Ultrasound in Pregnancy. Obstet Gynecol. 2016 Dec;128(6):e241-e256.
- Warren JB, Phillipi CA. Care of the well newborn. Pediatr Rev. 2012;33(1):4-18.

DISCLOSURE

The authors have nothing to disclose.

REFERENCES

1. Carrier screening for genetic conditions. Committee Opinion No. 691. American College of obstetricians and Gynecologists. Obstet Gynecol 2017;129:e41–55.
2. Carrier screening in the age of genomic medicine. Committee Opinion No. 690. American College of obstetricians and Gynecologists. Obstet Gynecol 2017; 129:e35–40.
3. Nicolaides KH. Screening for fetal aneuploidies at 11 to 13 weeks. Prenat Diagn 2011;31:7–15.
4. Alldred SK, Takwoingi Y, Guo B, et al. First and second trimester serum tests with and without first trimester ultrasound tests for Down's syndrome screening. Cochrane Database Syst Rev 2017;3(3):CD012599.
5. Norton ME, Jacobsson B, Swamy GK, et al. Cell-free DNA analysis for noninvasive examination of trisomy. N Engl J Med 2015;372(17):1589–97.
6. Di Renzo GC, Bartha JL, Bilardo CM. Expanding the indications for cell-free DNA in the maternal circulation: clinical considerations and implications. Am J Obstet Gynecol 2019;220(6):537–42.

7. Committee on practice Bulletins—Obstetrics and the American Institute of ultrasound in medicine. Practice Bulletin No. 175: ultrasound in pregnancy. Obstet Gynecol 2016;128(6):e241–56.
8. Souka AP, Krampl E, Bakalis S, et al. Outcome of pregnancy in chromosomally normal fetuses with increased nuchal translucency in the first trimester. Ultrasound Obstet Gynecol 2001;18(1):9–17.
9. Grande M, Jansen FA, Blumenfeld YJ, et al. Genomic microarray in fetuses with increased nuchal translucency and normal karyotype: a systematic review and meta-analysis. Ultrasound Obstet Gynecol 2015;46(6):650–8.
10. Nyberg DA, Souter VL, El-Bastawissi A, et al. Isolated sonographic markers for detection of fetal Down syndrome in the second trimester of pregnancy. J Ultrasound Med 2001;20(10):1053–63.
11. Smith-Bindman R, Hosmer W, Feldstein VA, et al. Second-trimester ultrasound to detect fetuses with Down syndrome: a meta-analysis. JAMA 2001;285:1044–55.
12. DiPietro JA, Cristofalo EA, Voegtline KM, et al. Isolated prenatal choroid plexus cysts do not affect child development. Prenat Diagn 2011;31(8):745–9.
13. Cicero S, Sonek JD, McKenna DS, et al. Nasal bone hypoplasia in trisomy 21 at 15-22 weeks' gestation. Ultrasound Obstet Gynecol 2003;21(1):15–8.
14. Fox NS, Monteagudo A, Kuller JA, et al. Mild fetal ventriculomegaly: diagnosis, evaluation, and management. Am J Obstet Gynecol 2018;219(1):B2–9.
15. Pagani G, Thilaganathan B, Prefumo F. Neurodevelopmental outcome in isolated mild fetal ventriculomegaly: systematic review and meta-analysis. Ultrasound Obstet Gynecol 2014;44(3):254–60.
16. Thorup E, Jensen LN, Bak GS, et al. Neurodevelopmental disorder in children believed to have isolated mild ventriculomegaly prenatally. Ultrasound Obstet Gynecol 2019;54(2):182–9.
17. Heard AJ, Urato AC. The isolated mildly enlarged cisterna magna in the third trimester: much ado about nothing? J Ultrasound Med 2011;30(5):591–3.
18. Grace D, Eggers P, Glantz JC, et al. Mitral valve-tricuspid valve distance as a sonographic marker of trisomy 21. Ultrasound Obstet Gynecol 2010;35(2):172–7.
19. D'Amico A, Buca D, Rizzo G, et al. Outcome of fetal echogenic bowel: a systematic review and meta-analysis. Prenat Diagn 2020. https://doi.org/10.1002/pd.5638.
20. Ji EK, Lee EK, Kwon TH. Isolated echogenic foci in the left upper quadrant of the fetal abdomen: are they significant? J Ultrasound Med 2004;23(4):483–8.
21. McNamara A, Levine D. Intraabdominal fetal echogenic masses: a practical guide to diagnosis and management. Radiographics 2005;25(3):633–45.
22. Cohen-Overbeek TE, Wijngaard-Boom P, Ursem NT, et al. Mild renal pyelectasis in the second trimester: determination of cut-off levels for postnatal referral. Ultrasound Obstet Gynecol 2005;25(4):378–83.
23. Arora M, Prasad A, Kulshreshtha R, et al. Significance of third trimester ultrasound in detecting congenital abnormalities of kidney and urinary tract-a prospective study. J Pediatr Urol 2019;15(4):334–40.
24. Bascietto F, Liberati M, Marrone L, et al. Outcome of fetal ovarian cysts diagnosed on prenatal ultrasound examination: systematic review and meta-analysis. Ultrasound Obstet Gynecol 2017;50(1):20–31.
25. Pretorius DH, Halsted MJ, Abels W, et al. Hydroceles identified prenatally: common physiologic phenomenon? J Ultrasound Med 1998;17(1):49–52.
26. Ebbing C, Kessler J, Moster D, et al. Single umbilical artery and risk of congenital malformation: population-based study in Norway. Ultrasound Obstet Gynecol 2020;55(4):510–5.

27. Lide B, Lindsley W, Foster MJ, et al. Intrahepatic persistent right umbilical vein and associated outcomes: a systematic review of the literature. J Ultrasound Med 2016;35:1–5.
28. di Pasquo E, Kuleva M, O'Gorman N, et al. Fetal intra-abdominal umbilical vein varix: retrospective cohort study and systematic review and meta-analysis. Ultrasound Obstet Gynecol 2018;51(5):580–5.
29. Bakker MK, Bergman JEH, Krikov S, et al. Prenatal diagnosis and prevalence of critical congenital heart defects: an international retrospective cohort study. BMJ Open 2019;9(7):e028139.
30. Levy DJ, Pretorius DH, Rothman A, et al. Improved prenatal detection of congenital heart disease in an integrated health care system. Pediatr Cardiol 2013;34(3):670–9.
31. Warren JB, Phillipi CA. Care of the well newborn. Pediatr Rev 2012;33(1):4–18.
32. Jones KL, Adam MP. Evaluation and diagnosis of the dysmorphic infant. Clin Perinatol 2015;42(2):243–viii.
33. Chen MM, Chang HC, Hsieh CF, et al. Predictive model for congenital muscular torticollis: analysis of 1021 infants with sonography. Arch Phys Med Rehabil 2005;86(11):2199–203.
34. Stellwagen L, Hubbard E, Chambers C, et al. Torticollis, facial asymmetry and plagiocephaly in normal newborns. Arch Dis Child 2008;93(10):827–31.
35. Petronic I, Brdar R, Cirovic D, et al. Congenital muscular torticollis in children: distribution, treatment duration and outcome. Eur J Phys Rehabil Med 2010;46(2):153–7.
36. Shenvi A, Kapur J, Rasiah SV. Management of asymptomatic cardiac murmurs in term neonates. Pediatr Cardiol 2013;34(6):1438–46.
37. Clur SA, Ottenkamp J, Bilardo CM. The nuchal translucency and the fetal heart: a literature review. Prenat Diagn 2009;29(8):739–48.
38. Chan A, McCaul KA, Cundy PJ, et al. Perinatal risk factors for developmental dysplasia of the hip. Arch Dis Child Fetal Neonatal Ed 1997;76(2):F94–100.
39. Shaw BA, Segal LS, SECTION ON ORTHOPAEDICS. Evaluation and referral for developmental dysplasia of the hip in infants. Pediatrics 2016;138(6):e20163107.
40. Clinical practice guideline: early detection of developmental dysplasia of the hip. Committee on quality Improvement, Subcommittee on developmental dysplasia of the hip. American Academy of pediatrics. Pediatrics 2000;105(4 Pt 1):896–905.
41. Bond CD, Hennrikus WL, DellaMaggiore ED. Prospective evaluation of newborn soft-tissue hip "clicks" with ultrasound. J Pediatr Orthop 1997;17(2):199–201.
42. Guo B, Lee SK, Paksima N. Polydactyly: a review. Bull Hosp Jt Dis 2013;71(1):17–23.
43. Zywicke HA, Rozzelle CJ. Sacral dimples. Pediatr Rev 2011;32(3):109–51.
44. Kucera JN, Coley I, O'Hara S, et al. The simple sacral dimple: diagnostic yield of ultrasound in neonates. Pediatr Radiol 2015;45(2):211–6.
45. Cho HH, Lee SM, You SK. Optimal timing of spinal ultrasound evaluations for sacral dimples in neonates: earlier may not Be better. J Ultrasound Med 2019;38(5):1241–7.
46. Wilson JM, Jungner JF. Principles and practice of screening for disease. Geneva (Switzerland): World Health Organization; 1968. Public Health Papers, no 34.
47. Centers for Disease Control and Prevention (CDC). CDC Grand Rounds: newborn screening and improved outcomes. MMWR Morb Mortal Wkly Rep 2012;61(21):390–3.
48. Berry SA. Newborn screening. Clin Perinatol 2015;42(2):441–x.

49. Genetic Alliance. Baby's first test. 2020. Available at: http://www.babysfirsttest.org. Accessed November 30, 2020.
50. American College of Medical Genetics and Genomics. ACT sheets and Algorithms. Available at: https://www.acmg.net/ACMG/Medical-Genetics-Practice-Resources/ACT_Sheets_and_Algorithms.aspx. Accessed November 30, 2020.
51. American Academy of Pediatrics Newborn Screening Authoring Committee. Newborn screening expands: recommendations for pediatricians and medical homes–implications for the system. Pediatrics 2008;121(1):192–217.
52. Dedhia K, Graham E, Park A. Hearing loss and failed newborn hearing screen. Clin Perinatol 2018;45(4):629–43.
53. The Joint Committee on Infant Hearing, The Journal of Early Hearing Detection and Intervention, 2019; 4(2):1–44.
54. van Dyk M, Swanepoel de W, Hall JW 3rd. Outcomes with OAE and AABR screening in the first 48 h--Implications for newborn hearing screening in developing countries. Int J Pediatr Otorhinolaryngol 2015;79(7):1034–40.
55. Weichbold V, Nekahm-Heis D, Welzl-Mueller K. Universal newborn hearing screening and postnatal hearing loss. Pediatrics 2006;117(4):e631–6.
56. Fowler KB. Congenital cytomegalovirus infection: audiologic outcome. Clin Infect Dis 2013;57(Suppl 4):S182–4.
57. Diener ML, Zick CD, McVicar SB, et al. Outcomes from a hearing-targeted cytomegalovirus screening program. Pediatrics 2017;139(2):e20160789.
58. Martin GR, Ewer AK, Gaviglio A, et al. Updated strategies for pulse oximetry screening for critical congenital heart disease. Pediatrics 2020;146(1):e20191650.
59. Abouk R, Grosse SD, Ailes EC, et al. Association of US state implementation of newborn screening policies for critical congenital heart disease with early infant cardiac deaths. JAMA 2017;318(21):2111–8 [published correction appears in JAMA. 2018;320(12):1288].
60. Kemper AR, Mahle WT, Martin GR, et al. Strategies for implementing screening for critical congenital heart disease. Pediatrics 2011;128(5):e1259–67.

Perinatal Cardiovascular Physiology and Recognition of Critical Congenital Heart Defects

Yogen Singh, MD, MA (Cantab)[a,*], Satyan Lakshminrusimha, MD[b]

KEYWORDS

• Perinatal cardiovascular physiology • Critical • Congenital heart defect (CHD)
• Neonate • Infant • Transitional circulation

KEY POINTS

- Understanding perinatal cardiovascular physiology is essential for timely diagnosis and management of congenital heart defects (CHDs).
- The signs and symptoms of critical congenital heart defects are often nonspecific soon after birth.
- A high degree of suspicion is warranted in critical CHDs in infants presenting with shock or hypoxia.
- Timely recognition and therapy with prostaglandin E1 infusion can be lifesaving in neonatal cardiac emergencies.

INTRODUCTION

The incidence of congenital heart defects (CHDs) is reported in 7 to 9 out of 1000 live births, of which 25% are critical congenital heart conditions.[1] Critical CHD is defined as a congenital heart condition needing surgery/intervention or leading to death within 1 month after birth.[1,2] Around 50% to 60% of the critical CHDs are detected on fetal anomaly screening.[1,2] The routine newborn physical examination often fails to detect many of these critical CHDs during the transitional circulation because of lack of signs soon after birth. Routine pulse oximetry screening at 24 to 48 hours after birth may help in detecting cyanotic heart conditions; however, noncyanotic CHDs such as

Funding: None.
Disclosure: None.
Authors' contribution: Y. Singh and S. Lakshminrusimha contributed equally to the article.
[a] Department of Pediatrics - Division of Neonatology, Loma Linda University Children's Hospital and Loma Linda University School of Medicine, 11175 Coleman Pavillion, Loma Linda, CA 92374, USA; [b] Department of Pediatrics, UC Davis Children's Hospital, UC Davis Health, Sacramento, CA 95817, USA
* Corresponding author.
E-mail address: Yogen.Singh@nhs.net

Clin Perinatol 48 (2021) 573–594
https://doi.org/10.1016/j.clp.2021.05.008

coarctation of aorta may go undetected on pulse oximetry screening in asymptomatic infants.[2] Some infants may deteriorate while waiting for pulse oximetry screening if it is not performed early to detect critical congenital heart conditions. Delay in diagnosis of CHDs has been reported to be associated with poor outcomes, and hence, it is extremely important to detect them in asymptomatic well-infants.[3–7]

The clinical presentation of CHDs depends on their underlying pathology and perinatal cardiovascular physiology, which is complex and involves rapid changes soon after birth. Therefore, a comprehensive understanding of cardiovascular physiology and hemodynamics is essential to understand the presentation of infants with critical CHDs, to initiate early specific management and optimize the cardiorespiratory management in the neonatal intensive care unit, and to plan the timing for cardiac intervention or surgery.[8] The neonatologists and pediatricians are at the forefront to review these infants in the delivery room, postnatal ward, and emergency room, who may not possess echocardiography skills. Hence, it is crucial for them to have a good understanding of perinatal cardiovascular physiology, changes that take place during fetal to neonatal circulation, and how to recognize critical CHDs.[8,9]

This article is focused on understanding perinatal cardiovascular physiology and transition of fetal to neonatal circulation with particular emphasis on recognition and initial management of critical CHDs in term infants by neonatal and pediatric providers.

FETAL CARDIOVASCULAR SYSTEM

As compared to the adult cardiovascular system with equal right and left ventricular outputs, the circulatory connections during the fetal period are complex. During fetal life, the right ventricle receives 65% of the venous return while the left ventricle receives about 35% of the total venous return.[10–12] Both ventricles provide systemic blood flow. In the fetus, around 30% to 45% of the combined cardiac output is directed to the placental circulation, while only 8% to 15% reaches the pulmonary circulation.[11,12] The fetal cardiovascular system is adapted to allow more oxygenated blood from placenta to be delivered preferentially to the brain and heart while right ventricular output is diverted away from the lungs. This complex parallel circulatory arrangement in a fetus is possible because of the following four fetal shunts (**Fig. 1**):

1. Placenta has a low vascular resistance, and hence, systemic vascular resistance (SVR) in the fetus is maintained low. It allows the fetus to receive oxygenated blood easily from the maternal circulation. The umbilical arteries receive around 30% to 45% of the fetal cardiac output to the placenta, and the oxygenated blood is returned to the fetus via umbilical vein[13];
2. Ductus venosus (DV) plays an important role in directing oxygenated blood from umbilical vein to inferior vena cava;
3. Foramen ovale: The shape of DV and eustachian ridge (at the junction of inferior vena cava with right atrium) helps in preferential shunting of oxygenated blood from inferior vena cava to left atrium via foramen ovale. Hence, more oxygenated blood is returned to the left ventricle allowing coronary arteries and upper part of the body (brain) to receive more oxygenated blood than the lower part of the body[13,14]; and
4. Ductus arteriosus (DA), channel connecting pulmonary artery to the descending aorta, allows diversion of most of the right ventricular cardiac output to the descending aorta. This is facilitated by the high pulmonary vascular resistance (PVR) and low SVR during the fetal period. The patency of DA is primarily maintained by the high prostaglandin levels synthesized in the placenta and within the ductal tissue and increased levels of nitric oxide and endothelin-1 during the fetal

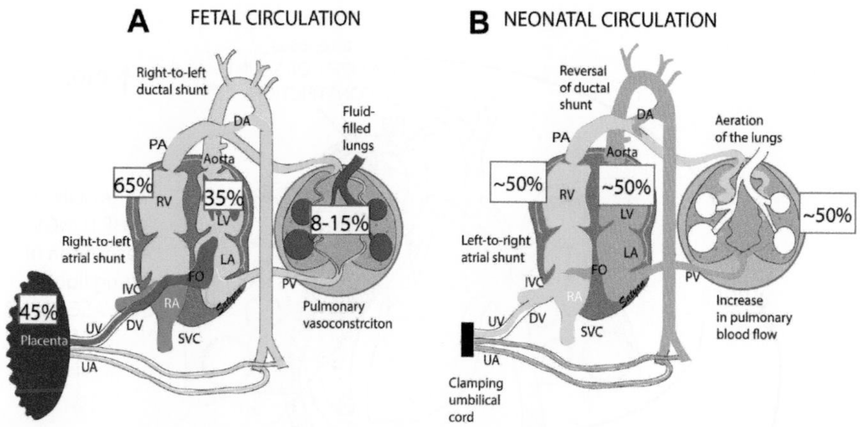
A FETAL CIRCULATION
Right-to-left ductal shunt
DA
Fluid-filled lungs
PA
Aorta
65%
RV
35%
LV
8-15%
Right-to-left atrial shunt
LA
FO
IVC
PV
45%
RA
Pulmonary vasoconstrciton
Placenta
UV
DV
SVC
UA
B NEONATAL CIRCULATION
Reversal of ductal shunt
DA
Aeration of the lungs
PA
Aorta
~50%
RV
~50%
LV
~50%
Left-to-right atrial shunt
LA
FO
IVC
PV
RA
Increase in pulmonary blood flow
UV
DV
SVC
UA
Clamping umbilical cord

Fig. 1. Schematic diagram showing fetal and neonatal circulation. (*A*) Fetal circulation with fetal shunts, and (*B*) neonatal circulation after transition. The percentages in large boxes indicates % combined ventricular output based on human and lamb studies. DA, ductus arteriosus; DV, ductus venosus; FO, oval foramen; IVC, inferior vena cava; LA, left atrium; LV, left ventricle; PA, pulmonary artery; PV, pulmonary vein; RA, right atrium; RV, right ventricle; SVC, superior vena cava; UV, umbilical vein; UA, umbilical artery. (*Courtesy of* Satyan Lakshminrusimha and Yogen Singh.)

period. The animal studies demonstrate that up to 90% of the right ventricular output is shunted away from unaerated lungs via ductus arteriosus, although, in a human fetus, this proportion is thought to be slightly lower.[14,15]

TRANSITION FROM FETAL TO NEONATAL CIRCULATION IN TERM INFANTS

The transition from fetal to neonatal circulation is accompanied by drastic physiologic changes in the cardiovascular system soon after birth. In a term infant, a successful cardiovascular transition is accomplished by rapid drop in PVR after expansion of the lungs and an increase in SVR after removal of the placenta.[13,15]

The drop in PVR is primarily from aeration of lungs, resorption of fetal lung liquid, and increased production of potent pulmonary arterial vasodilators such as nitric oxide, bradykinins, histamine, and prostaglandins.[16,17] In a term infant, there is a 5- to 10-fold drop in PVR soon after normal birth. PVR continues to drop over 4 to 6 weeks after birth. The SVR is increased primarily from removal of placenta (low vascular resistance shunt) and increase in vasoconstrictors such as thromboxane 2 and vasopressin. This rapid change in PVR and SVR soon after birth is the key to a successful and smooth transition, which results in reversal of shunt across DA to left-to-right increasing pulmonary blood flow (PBF), and hence pulmonary venous return (see **Fig. 1**B). This results in an increase in left atrial pressure and reversal of intra-atrial shunt across foramen ovale to left-to-right leading to its functional closure within first few days after birth. The ductus venosus closes soon after birth[2,8,15] (**Fig. 2**).

The mechanism for ductus arteriosus (DA) closure is multifactorial, primarily facilitated by the direct vasoconstriction of ductal smooth muscle in response to oxygenated blood from left-to-right shunt via DA and a drop in prostaglandins from decreased production (after removal of placenta) and increased degradation in the aerated lungs. In a term infant, the functional closure of DA occurs within 24 to 48 hours after birth while anatomic closure may take up to 10 to 14 days.[8,18] A patent DA maintains

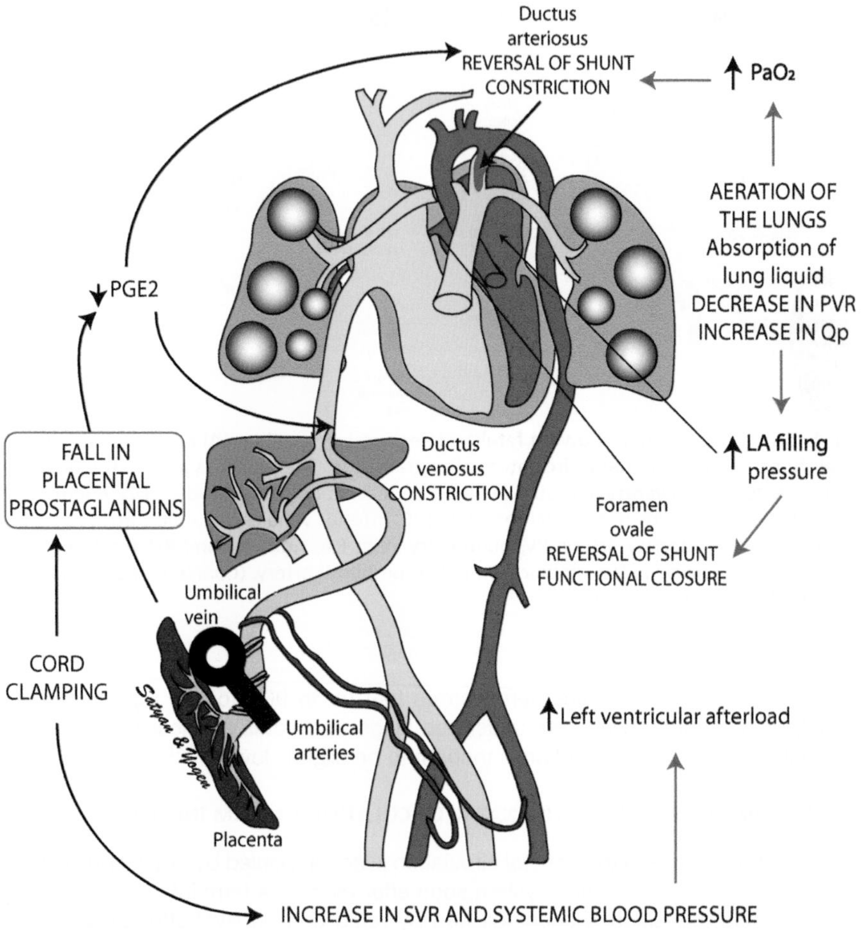
Ductus
arteriosus
REVERSAL OF SHUNT
CONSTRICTION
PaO2
AERATION OF
THE LUNGS
Absorption of
lung liquid
DECREASE IN PVR
INCREASE IN Qp
LA filling
pressure
PGE2
FALL IN
PLACENTAL
PROSTAGLANDINS
Ductus
venosus
CONSTRICTION
Foramen
ovale
REVERSAL OF SHUNT
FUNCTIONAL CLOSURE
Umbilical
vein
CORD
CLAMPING
Umbilical
arteries
Left ventricular afterload
Placenta
INCREASE IN SVR AND SYSTEMIC BLOOD PRESSURE

Fig. 2. Schematic diagram showing events during transition of circulation: fetal to neonatal circulation. DA, ductus arteriosus; FO, foramen ovale; L, left; $Pa{O_2}$, arterial partial pressure of oxygen; PBF, pulmonary blood flow; PG, prostaglandin; PVR, pulmonary vascular resistance; R, right. (*Adapted from* Singh Y and Tissot C (2018) Echocardiographic Evaluation of Transitional Circulation for the Neonatologists. Front. Pediatr. 6:140. https://doi.org/10.3389/fped.2018.00140.)

pulmonary and/or systemic circulation in several critical CHDs, and closure of the ductus compromises gas exchange and hemodynamics.

The removal of placenta and closure of fetal shunts (placenta, ductus arteriosus, ductus venosus, and foramen ovale) result in change of cardiovascular connections from parallel to series, and this accomplishes a successful adaptation to neonatal circulation with left and right ventricular outputs.

RESUSCITATION AND DELAYED CORD CLAMPING IN INFANTS WITH CONGENITAL HEART DEFECTS

Almost all infants with CHDs, including those with critical congenital heart defects, are usually born in a good condition and rarely need resuscitation because of their underlying heart condition. When required, resuscitation should be started in air (21% O_2), and oxygen therapy may be given if required like in other term infants without CHD. However, in infants with confirmed antenatal diagnosis of duct-dependent critical CHD, inadvertent use of oxygen therapy should be avoided.

Physiologically, delayed cord clamping (DCC) may provide better hemodynamic stability during transition, similar to term and preterm infants without any CHD. Backes and colleagues showed DCC in infants with critical CHD appears both safe and feasible.[19] Infants with DCC had deceased number of red cell transfusions as compared to those with early cord clamping.[19]

CLINICAL PRESENTATION OF INFANTS WITH CONGENITAL HEART DEFECTS

The signs and symptoms of CHD in the neonatal period are often nonspecific and may be absent during the transitional period while fetal shunts are still patent and/or when the PVR is still high. The signs and symptoms suggestive of CHD are summarized in **Table 1**.

CYANOTIC CHDs

Cyanotic CHDs constitute about 20% of congenital heart lesions. Most of the cyanotic CHDs presenting in the neonatal period start with 'T' as summarized in **Table 2**.

ACYANOTIC CONGENITAL HEART DEFECTS

Acyanotic CHDs are a spectrum of congenital heart lesions with variable presentation—completely asymptomatic presenting as heart murmur to sudden collapse. These include CHDs involving left-to-right shunts (who may present after days or weeks or even months after birth) and left heart obstructive lesions. Left heart obstructive CHDs may remain asymptomatic for week to years, but ductal dependent lesions may present with acute deterioration when ductus arteriosus closes.

Table 1
Signs and symptoms suggestive of underlying CHD

Signs and Symptoms	Comment
• Unwell infant, poor feeding • Feeble or absent pulses (brachial or femoral) • Persistent cyanosis in absence of respiratory distress or cyanotic episodes • Low oxygen saturation (<95% in air) or difference of >3% between preductal and postductal saturations • Heart murmur maybe present but often absent in critical CHDs • Presence of dysmorphic features or other congenital anomalies • Presence of arrhythmias • Heart failure • Collapse/sudden death	• Nonspecific • Suggestive of low cardiac output shock or critical CHD with LV outflow obstruction • Pulse oximetry helps in detecting cyanotic CHDs but can be normal in lesions with left-to-right shunt even when they are critical • Heart murmur often absent in critical CHDs especially during transitional circulation • May suggest underlying CHD • Signs of heart failure such as tachypnea, tachycardia, hepatomegaly • Rule out critical CHD in collapsed infants
Other risk factors • Suspicion of CHD on fetal anomaly screening (FAS) • Positive family history of CHD	• Around 50%–60% critical CHDs are detected on antenatal FAS

Abbreviations: LV, left ventricle.

Table 2
Cyanotic CHDs presenting in neonatal period

Type of CHD	Comment
• Transposition of great arteries (TGA) (**Fig. 3**) • Tetralogy of Fallot (TOF) and double outlet right ventricle (DORV) (**Fig. 4**) • Truncus arteriosus • Total anomalous pulmonary venous connection (TAPVC) • Tricuspid atresia • Pulmonary atresia with no VSD (severe spectrum of TOF) • Ebstein anomaly (rare with variable presentation)	TGA - most common CHD presenting in neonatal period TOF is the most common cyanotic CHD

There are many classifications of CHDs such as cyanotic versus acyanotic (as discussed previously) or duct-dependent versus non-duct-dependent (as summarized in **Table 3**).

While classifying CHDs into cyanotic and acyanotic is helpful, from the acute neonatologist/pediatrician's perspective, it is helpful to divide them into critical and noncritical types linking the lesions to its pathophysiology. This helps in recognizing critical CHDs during the neonatal period and initiating management while waiting for a confirmative diagnosis by echocardiography.[8] This article is focused on critical CHDs presenting as neonatal emergencies that may be faced by acute care physicians such as neonatologist, pediatrician, emergency room physician, pediatric cardiologist, or pediatric intensivist.

CLINICAL PRESENTATION OF INFANT WITH CRITICAL CHD

The timing of presentation and severity of the presentation depends on

1. Nature and severity of underlying defect
2. The alteration in cardiovascular physiology secondary to the effect of the transitional circulation as
   A. Closure of ductus arteriosus (DA)
   B. Restriction of patent foramen ovale (PFO)
   C. Fall in pulmonary vascular resistance (PVR)

The critical CHDs can broadly be divided into acyanotic and cyanotic type, and their presentation and underlying pathophysiology is briefly discussed below.[20]

Critical Acyanotic Congenital Heart Diseases

Patients with acyanotic heart diseases may present acutely in a critical condition either because of left-sided obstructive lesion or due to heart failure.

Critical acyanotic ductal-dependent heart diseases presenting with shock

In this category of CHDs, the normal flow from the left ventricle to systemic arterial circulation may be compromised because of either stenosis or complete interruption of flow. During the fetal and transitional circulation, PDA maintains the blood flow to systemic circulation bypassing the area of stenosis or interruption. When PDA closes, the flow to descending aorta, that depends on PDA in these situations, will be

Table 3
Classification of congenital heart defects based on postnatal adaptation

Types of CHDs		Examples of Pathologies
Duct-dependent CHDs	Duct-dependent pulmonary circulation (cyanotic CHDs)	Pulmonary atresia (PA) Tricuspid atresia with intact IVS Critical TOF Critical pulmonary stenosis (PS) Single ventricle with PS/PA Severe Ebstein anomaly
	Duct dependent systemic circulation (Acyanotic CHDs)	Hypoplastic left heart syndrome (HLHS) Critical aortic stenosis (AS) Severe coarctation of aorta CoA Interrupted aortic arch (IAA) Single ventricle (SV) with severe AS or CoA
	Poor central mixing (cyanotic CHD)	TGA with intact ventricular septum
Non-duct-dependent CHDs	Mild cyanotic CHDs	TAPVC TOF TAC with mild PS TGA with VSD Single ventricle
	Left-to-right shunt CHDs	Ventricular septal defect (VSD) Patent ductus arteriosus (PDA) Atrio-ventricular septal defect (AVSD) Aorto-pulmonary window (APW) Double outlet right ventricle (DORV) without or with mild PS Truncus arteriosus communis (TAC) with no PS Single ventricle

Abbreviations: APW, aorto-pulmonary window; AS, aortic stenosis; ASD, atrial septal defect; AVSD, atrio-ventricular septal defect; CHD, congenital heart disease; COA, coarctation of aorta; DORV, double outlet right ventricle; HLHS, hypoplastic left heart disease; IAA, interrupted aortic arch; IVS, intact ventricular septum; PA, pulmonary atresia; PDA, patent ductus arteriosus; PS, pulmonary stenosis; SV, single ventricle; TA, tricuspid atresia; TAC, truncus arteriosus communis; TAPVC, total anomalous pulmonary venous connection; TGA, transposition of great arteries; TOF, tetralogy of fallot; VSD, ventricular septal defect.

Adapted from Singh Y and Tissot C (2018) Echocardiographic Evaluation of Transitional Circulation for the Neonatologists. Front. Pediatr. 6:140. https://doi.org/10.3389/fped.2018.00140.

compromised, thus leading to tissue hypoperfusion and tissue hypoxia. This subsequently leads to lactic acidosis and shock.[1,20–22]

The most common acyanotic critical CHD is neonatal coarctation of the aorta (**Fig. 5**). In infants with critical or significant coarctation of aorta, the blood flow in post-ductal descending aorta depends on the patency of ductus arteriosus. When PDA closes, the infant may present with shock due to a significant decrease in blood flow to lower part of the body or with early heart failure due to increased left ventricle afterload from the narrowing. It is not unusual for the infants with a left-sided obstructive lesion to present in heart failure with poor cardiac function, increased left ventricle end-diastolic volume, and severe pulmonary edema. The pulmonary edema occurs from increased pressure in left atrium, due to poor left ventricular compliance and increased end-diastolic volume, leading to increased pulmonary wedge pressure. Without a timely and appropriate intervention, an infant with critical coarctation or severe left-sided obstruction may deteriorate rapidly with possible demise.[1,21,23]

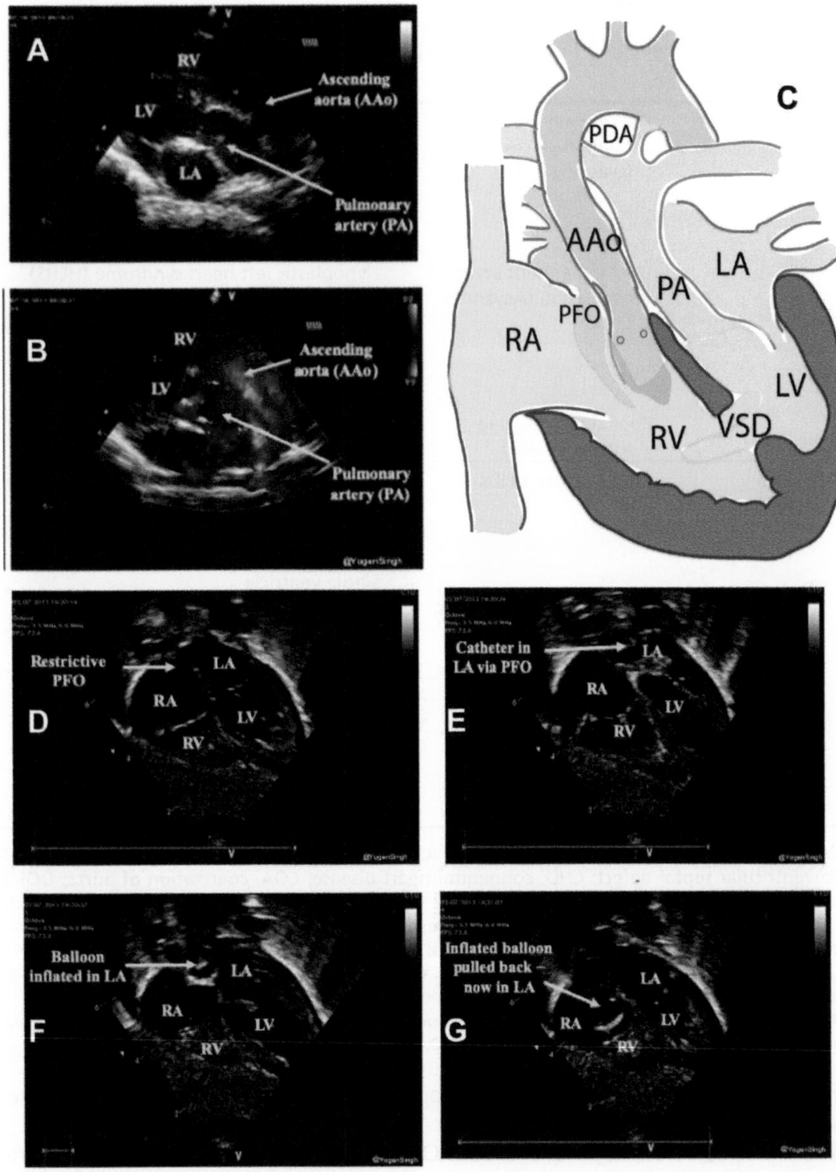
A
RV
LV
LA
Ascending aorta (AAo)
Pulmonary artery (PA)
B
RV
LV
Ascending aorta (AAo)
Pulmonary artery (PA)
C
PDA
AAo
LA
PA
PFO
RA
LV
RV
VSD
D
Restrictive PFO
LA
RA
LV
RV
E
Catheter in LA via PFO
LA
RA
LV
RV
F
Balloon inflated in LA
LA
RA
LV
RV
G
Inflated balloon pulled back - now in LA
LA
RA
LV
RV

Fig. 3. Transposition of great arteries (TGA), most common cyanotic congenital heart defect presenting in the neonatal period. (*A*) Anatomy in 2 D and (*B*) with color Doppler—pulmonary artery originating from posterior ventricle (left ventricle) and dividing soon after origin while ascending aorta originating from anterior (right) ventricle. (*C*) Flow pattern in TGA with two parallel circulations with admixture occurring at the level of PDA (patent ductus arteriosus), PFO (patent foramen ovale), and in this case, VSD (ventricular septal defect). (*D*) A restrictive PFO in a four-chamber view. (*E*) The balloon atrial septostomy catheter in the left atrium. The balloon is inflated in the left atrium in image (*F*) and pulled back to the right atrium in image (*G*). (*Courtesy of* Satyan Lakshminrusimha and Yogen Singh.)

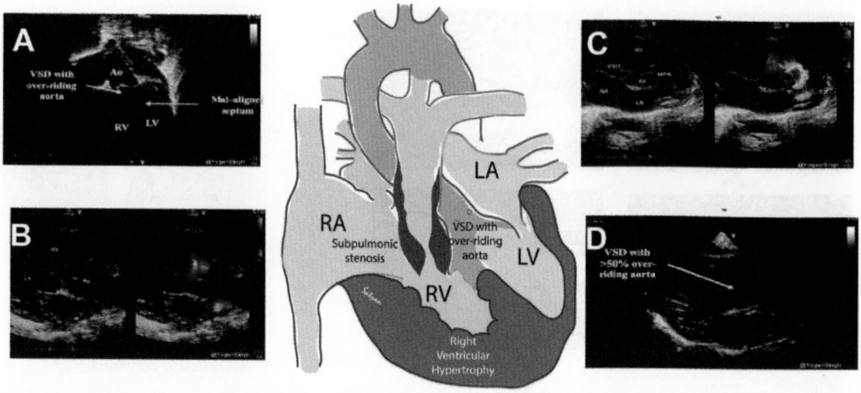
A
VSD with over-riding aorta
Ao
RV
LV
B
LA
RA
Subpulmonic stenosis
VSD with over-riding aorta
LV
RV
Right Ventricular Hypertrophy
C
D
VSD with >50% over-riding aorta

Fig. 4. Anatomy in tetralogy of Fallot tetralogy—the most common cyanotic congenital heart defect. (*A*) and (*B*) Bigger right side of the heart with caudally deviated interventricular septum, mal-aligned ventricular septal defect (VSD) leading to over-riding of aorta. (*C*) VSD position at 10 O'clock with right ventricular outflow obstruction in parasternal short axis view. (*D*) A similar anatomy but with greater than 50% over-riding of aorta, hence classified as double outlet right ventricle (DORV). The central image shows the flow pattern. Ao, aorta (ascending aorta); LV, left ventricle; RV, right ventricle. (*Courtesy of* Satyan Lakshminrusimha and Yogen Singh.)

Clinicians should have a low index of suspicion of critical acyanotic CHD in infants presenting with shock during the first couple of weeks after birth. These infants may mimic the clinical picture of septic or hypovolemic shock—with early nonspecific signs and symptoms and then sudden deterioration leading to shock. Coarctation of aorta, and less commonly other left-sided obstructive cardiac lesions such as interrupted aortic arch (IAA), critical aortic stenosis (AS), and aortic valve atresia, is the most common cause of cardiogenic shock and early congestive heart failure presenting during the neonatal period. Infants with critical AS or aortic atresia have weak systemic arterial pulses (both brachial and femoral pulses) while neonates with critical coarctation or IAA who have weak or absent femoral pulses as compared to brachial pulses. However, with the onset of shock, poor left-ventricle function, and low cardiac output, these infants often have all systemic pulses weak on palpation.[1,20]

Management of infants with suspected critical acyanotic CHD including ductal-dependent acyanotic heart lesion should include hemodynamic stabilization and initiation of appropriate dose of prostaglandin E1 infusion (discussed in the following section) as soon as possible, in addition to general approach to cardiorespiratory stabilization in a shocked infant (see **Fig. 5**). When there is a clinical suspicion of acyanotic critical CHD, there should not be any delay in starting prostaglandin E1 infusion and clinicians should not wait for a confirmatory echocardiography or cardiologist opinion to start the drug, although they should be sought urgently.[20,24] Appropriate dose of prostaglandin E1 to open ductus arteriosus can be lifesaving and once ductus arteriosus opens it improves the systemic blood flow and perfusion resulting in improvement in acidosis and shock. Once diagnosis is confirmed these infants need definitive intervention. Timing and type of such intervention is decided by the specialist pediatric cardiologist.[20,24]

Acyanotic heart diseases presenting with heart failure

This category of CHDs compromise infants with significant left to right shunt resulting in increased pulmonary blood flow and thus leading to heart failure. The common heart

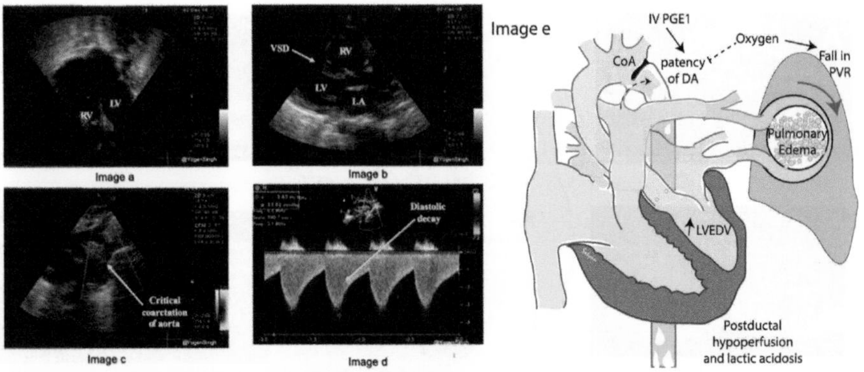
Image a
RV
LV
Image b
VSD
RV
LV
LA
Image c
Critical coarctation of aorta
Image d
Diastolic decay
Image e
IV PGE1
Oxygen
Fall in PVR
CoA
patency of DA
Pulmonary Edema
LVEDV
Postductal hypoperfusion and lactic acidosis

Fig. 5. Left-sided obstructive lesion with ductal dependent systemic circulation such as coarctation of aorta (CoA). CoA is the most common left ventricular outflow tract obstruction leading to collapse or hemodynamic compromise in an undiagnosed infant. Image a and b show dilated right side of the heart with right ventricle (RV) being big and rounded in image b. There is a muscular VSD seen in image b. Image c showing critical coarctation of aorta with severe narrowing at the isthmus, junction between transverse arch and descending aorta. Image d shows classical diastolic decay seen in infants with coarctation of aorta—there is increased velocity in systole which remains high during diastole and slows decreased but never reached back to baseline. The consequences of ductal closure are shown in image e. Oxygen constricts the ductus arteriosus (DA) and reduces pulmonary vascular resistance (PVR) leading to reduced right-to-left flow across the DA (dashed, curved *arrow*). Ductal closure leads to increased left ventricular end diastolic volume (LVEDV), increased left atrial pressure and pulmonary edema. Reduced perfusion of the postductal region causes lactic acidosis and oliguria. Infusion of prostaglandin E1 (IV PGE1) restores and maintains ductal patency. (*Courtesy of* Satyan Lakshminrusimha and Yogen Singh.)

lesions include ventricle septal defect (VSD), atrioventricular septal defect (AVSD), PDA, or combination of lesions.[20] The degree of the shunt across heart lesion is directly proportional to the pressure gradient between the two chambers or vessels where the shunt occurs, often left to right shunt because of high pressure on the left side. Hence, infants with isolated ASD do not present with signs of heart failure in infancy as there is minimal pressure gradient between the left and right atrium.[1,20]

In general, pulmonary vascular resistance (PVR) drops drastically soon after birth as a result of increasing Pa_{O_2} due to lungs expansion and aeration with air.[20,25] During the early neonatal stage, the PVR is relatively high, and it continues to drop during the first 6 weeks after birth. High PVR during the early neonatal period restricts the left to right shunt, and hence, infants with isolated left to right shunt do not present with heart failure during the first few weeks after birth, unless they have multiple lesions. As the PVR drops, there is increased left (systemic) to right (pulmonary) shunt leading to congestion of lungs from increased pulmonary blood flow. They often present with signs and symptoms of heart failure (breathlessness, tachypnoea, tachycardiac, poor feeding, hepatomegaly, and cardiomegaly) around 6 weeks after birth.[1,8,20]

Any infant presenting with heart failure during the first 1 to 2 weeks after should be suspected to have more serious critical CHD as discussed previously. On the other hand, an infant with acyanotic CHD (VSD, AVSD, or PDA) may present in an emergency or critical condition with decompensated heart failure or respiratory failure due to respiratory infection, which they are more prone to from the increased pulmonary congestion.[20]

Management of these cases requires initial stabilization, the use of positive pressure ventilation as indicated (It is important to avoid excess Fi_{O_2} as it may enhance pulmonary vasodilation and overcirculation.), diuretics, and may need reducing afterload with angiotensin-converting enzyme inhibitor or phosphodiesterase III inhibitor, which should be started after consultation with the cardiologist and establishing the definitive diagnosis. Later, these infants need definitive corrective surgery for the underlying heart defect. These infants often have poor weight gain and failure to thrive because of increased demand from breathlessness and increased work of breathing, and poor intake from feeding difficulties due to easily tiring and poor oral intake.[20] Some of these infants may need supplementation with fortified feeds either through a nasogastric (or gastrostomy) tube until their failure is under control or corrective surgery can be performed (**Fig. 6**).

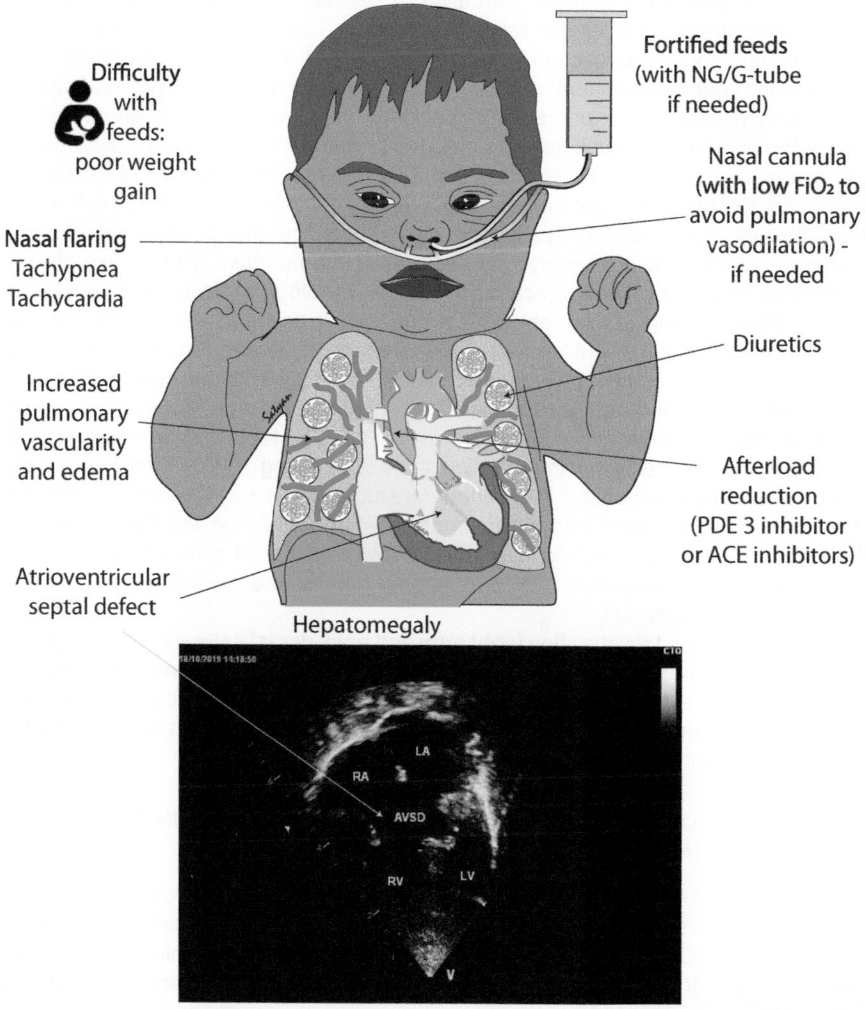
Difficulty with feeds: poor weight gain
Nasal flaring
Tachypnea
Tachycardia
Increased pulmonary vascularity and edema
Atrioventricular septal defect
Hepatomegaly
Fortified feeds (with NG/G-tube if needed)
Nasal cannula (with low FiO2 to avoid pulmonary vasodilation) - if needed
Diuretics
Afterload reduction (PDE 3 inhibitor or ACE inhibitors)
LA
RA
AVSD
RV
LV

Fig. 6. Atrioventricular septal defect (AVSD, endocardial cushion defect) in an infant with trisomy 21. The clinical features are shown on the left and therapies on the right. The inset shows an apical 4-chamber view of AVSD. ACE, angiotensin converting enzyme; G-tube, gastrostomy tube; NG, nasogastric; PDE 3, phosphodiesterase 3. (*Courtesy of* Satyan Lakshminrusimha and Yogen Singh.)

Critical Cyanotic Congenital Heart Diseases

The cyanosis results from the presence of deoxygenated hemoglobin more than 5 g/dL. The ability to recognize cyanosis is related to the level of hemoglobin. With higher hemoglobin concentration, cyanosis can be recognized more easily.[26]

In general, this may be due to one of four causes (**Fig. 7**)[1]: Incomplete oxygenation process of blood passing through the lung due to lung pathology leading to intrapulmonary shunt,[2] extrapulmonary right-to-left shunts at PDA or PFO in pulmonary hypertension,[3] due to shunting of deoxygenated blood from the right side of the heart to the left side systemic circulation leading to intracardiac shunt secondary to cyanotic CHD, or[4] due to having abnormal hemoglobin that cannot bind to oxygen. Examples of the first cause where the blood does not get fully oxygenated in the lungs include cases of collapsed lung or those with alveolar diseases such as pulmonary edema, respiratory distress syndrome, or severe pneumonia. This type of ventilation/perfusion (V/Q) mismatching is the result of intrapulmonary shunt. The oxygen saturation of patient with intrapulmonary shunt may improve with supplementing oxygen and positive pressure ventilation as it improves V/Q matching.[20] The second type of shunt that can lead to the presence of deoxygenated blood in systemic circulation is extrapulmonary and extracardiac (PDA) or intracardiac shunt that is, present when the blood coming from venous circulation (right side of heart) crosses to systemic circulation (left side of heart) through abnormal communication within heart chamber or great vessels. One example is persistent pulmonary hypertension of the newborn (PPHN; see chapter 9). Another example of this intracardiac shunt is Tetralogy of Fallot (TOF) where the venous blood coming to the right side of the heart crosses to the left side through VSD in association with right ventricle outflow obstruction (see **Fig. 4**). When deoxygenated blood is mixed with oxygenated blood, the resulted blood has a lower saturation than normal and may lead to significant central cyanosis. This type of shunt is called intracardiac shunt.[20,27] One of the clinical bedside tests that can help in differentiating intrapulmonary from intracardiac shunt is by giving 100% O_2 through oxygen hood to the affected neonate. The peripheral saturation usually improves in cases of lung diseases associated with intrapulmonary shunt; while on the other hand, the cyanosis, O_2 saturation, and Pao_2 do not improve in cases of intracardiac shunt due to congenital heart diseases (for hyperoxia test details, see the following section on approach to management).

Measuring preductal saturation (right arm) and post-ductal saturation (right leg) may show a significant difference between pre- and post-ductal Pao_2 indicating that the blood is shunted at the level of PDA from pulmonary to systemic circulation as it happens in cases of severe PPHN or CHDs with right to left ductal shunt (such as in interrupted arch of aorta).[20,28]

AN APPROACH TO UNDERSTAND CARDIOVASCULAR PHYSIOLOGY IN INFANTS PRESENTING AS NEONATAL EMERGENCY

As discussed previously, both acyanotic and cyanotic CHDs can present as neonatal emergencies. These cardiac emergencies can be broadly divided into 3 categories: (A) duct-dependent CHDs, (B) circulation dependent upon mixing of blood centrally via foramen ovale, and (C) obstructed total anomalous pulmonary venous connection (TAPVC).[8,20]

Ductal Dependent CHDs

As discussed previously, in a normal term neonate, ductus arteriosus closes smoothly in the first few days of life without causing any hemodynamic compromise. In neonates

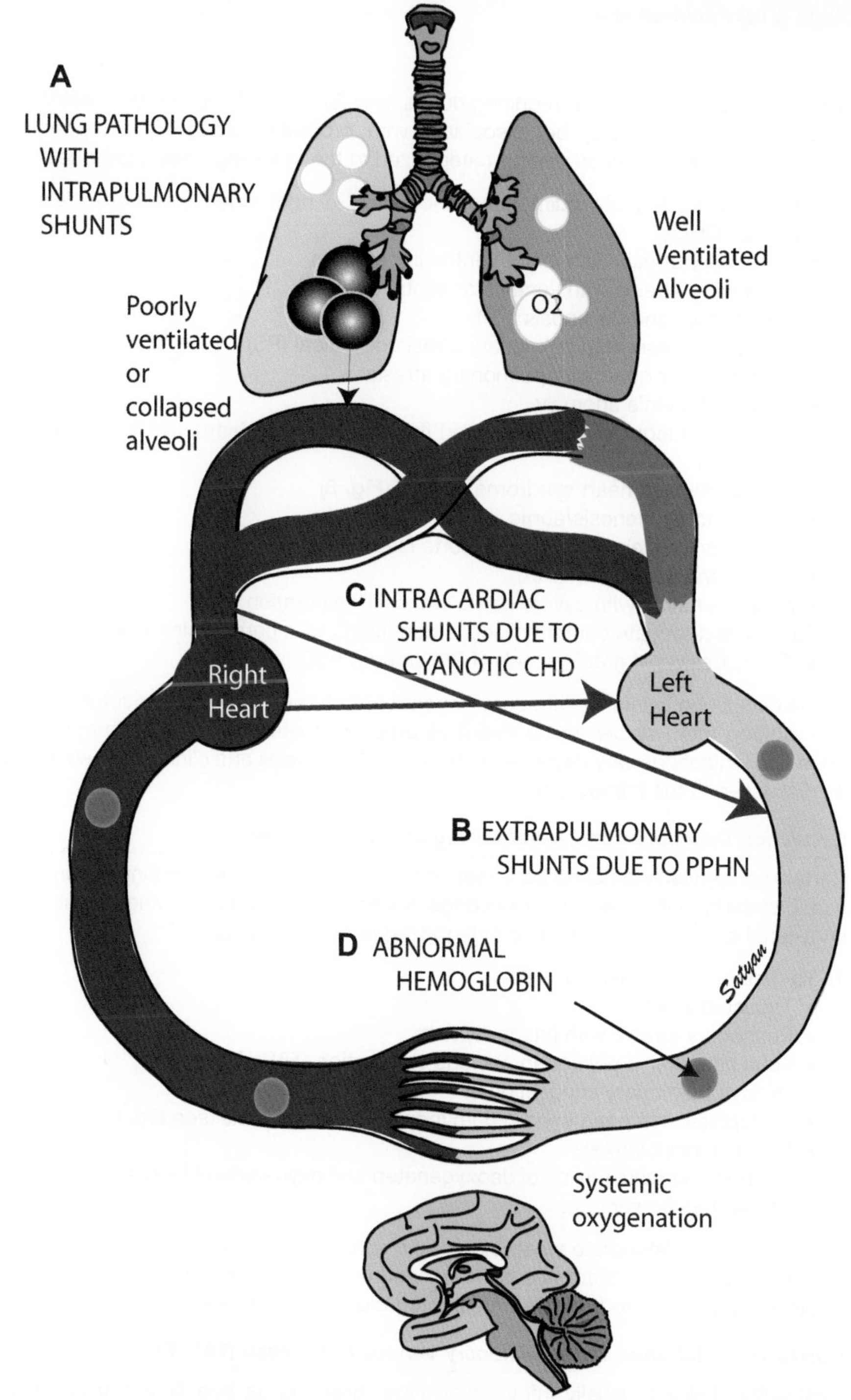
A
LUNG PATHOLOGY WITH INTRAPULMONARY SHUNTS
Well Ventilated Alveoli
O2
Poorly ventilated or collapsed alveoli
C INTRACARDIAC SHUNTS DUE TO CYANOTIC CHD
Right Heart
Left Heart
B EXTRAPULMONARY SHUNTS DUE TO PPHN
D ABNORMAL HEMOGLOBIN
Satyan
Systemic oxygenation

Fig. 7. Causes of neonatal cyanosis. Lung pathology such as meconium aspiration syndrome, respiratory distress syndrome and atelectasis cause intrapulmonary shunting (A). Elevated pulmonary arterial pressure leads to right-to-left shunts at patent ductus arteriosus and patent foramen ovale in persistent pulmonary hypertension of the newborn (PPHN; B). In cyanotic CHD, intracardiac shunting of deoxygenated blood to the left heart is common (C). Finally, abnormal hemoglobins such as methemoglobin do not bind to oxygen and contribute to hypoxia and cyanosis (D). (*Courtesy of* Satyan Lakshminrusimha and Yogen Singh.)

with duct-dependent CHDs, requiring ductal flow for survival, closure or constriction of ductus arteriosus may be associated with profound circulatory compromise. Duct-dependent circulation can be categorized in the following three categories[8,20]:

1. To maintain adequate pulmonary blood flow in right sided obstructive lesions (cyanotic CHDs)
   - Pulmonary atresia with intact ventricular septum
   - Pulmonary atresia with ventricular septal defect
   - Critical pulmonary stenosis (PS)
   - Tricuspid atresia with pulmonary atresia or critical (PS)
   - Univentricular heart with pulmonary atresia
   - Severe Ebstein's anomaly
2. To maintain adequate systemic blood flow in left sided obstructive lesions (Acyanotic CHDs)
   - Hypoplastic left heart syndrome (HLHS) (**Fig. 8**)
   - Critical aortic stenosis/aortic atresia
   - Severe or critical coarctation of aorta (see **Fig. 5**)
   - Interrupted aortic arch (IAA)
   - Single ventricle with severe aortic stenosis/coarctation
3. To ensure adequate central mixing in conditions with parallel circulation
   - Transposition of great vessels (TGA) without VSD (see **Fig. 3**)

The circulation in infants with duct-dependent CHDs require patent ductus arteriosus to keep them stable until a definitive procedure/intervention is performed. The dose and indications vary depending on timing of diagnosis and clinical presentations as discussed in the following section.

Circulation Dependent on Central Mixing at Foramen Ovale

Certain congenital heart conditions require patent foramen ovale to maintain hemodynamic stability in the newborn. The congenital heart conditions requiring unrestricted intra-atrial communication can be categorized in two sub-groups[8,20]:

1. To maintain systemic blood flow
   - Tricuspid atresia
   - Pulmonary atresia with intact septum
   - Total anomalous pulmonary venous connection (TAPVC)
2. To relieve pulmonary congestion in
   - Hypoplastic left heart syndrome/hypoplastic left ventricle (see **Fig. 8**E, F)
   - Mitral stenosis/atresia
3. To permit adequate mixing of deoxygenated and oxygenated blood as in TGA with intact ventricular septum.

These infants deteriorate when blood flow across the foramen ovale is restricted, despite a patent ductus arteriosus. They need urgent intervention (atrial septostomy or atrial septectomy) to facilitate unrestricted blood flow via foramen ovale.

Obstructed Total Anomalous Pulmonary Venous Connection (TAPVC)

Obstructed TAPVC, usually infracardiac type, presents as true time critical emergency, and clinical picture mimics severe PPHN (**Fig. 9**). However, these infants get worse with fall in PVR as compared to persistent pulmonary hypertension of the newborn (PPHN), and they often deteriorate after starting nitric oxide to manage PPHN-like clinical picture. Drop in PVR leads to increased pulmonary blood flow, but it increases pulmonary congestion because drainage in obstructed TAPVC is

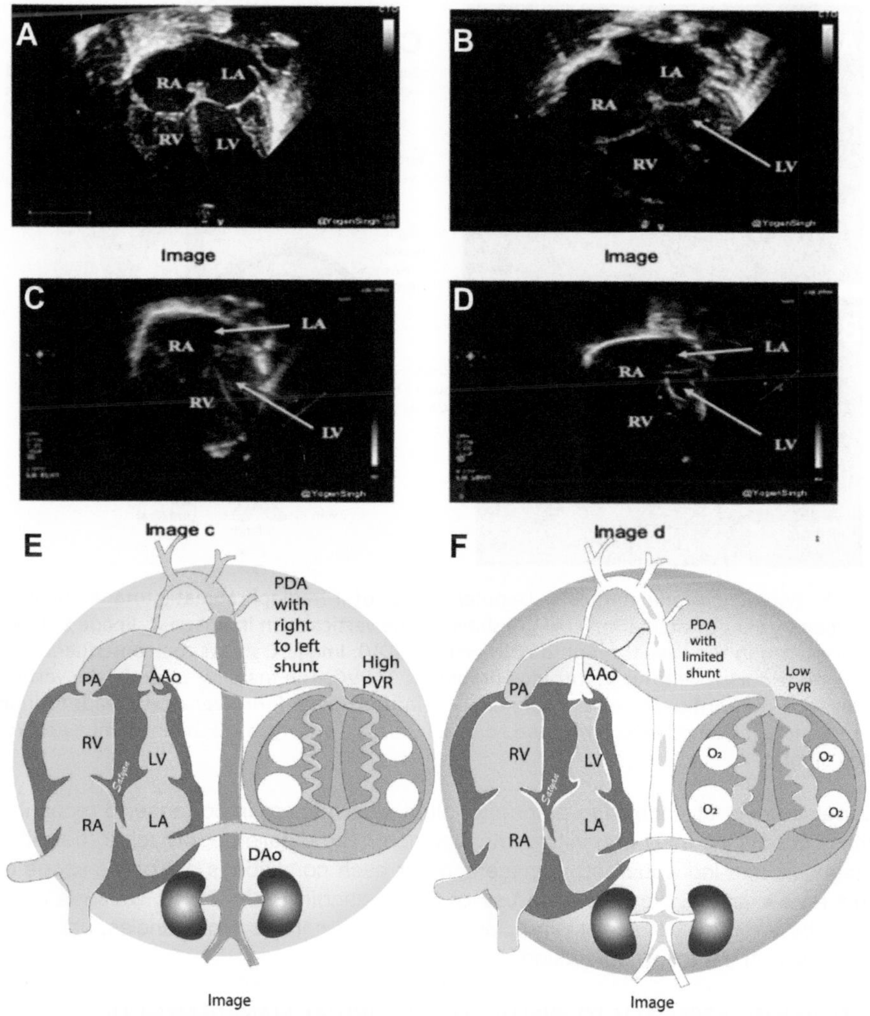
A
RA
LA
RV
LV
Image
B
LA
RA
RV
LV
Image
C
LA
RA
RV
LV
Image c
D
LA
RA
RV
LV
Image d
E
PDA with right to left shunt
High PVR
PA
AAo
RV
LV
RA
LA
DAo
Image
F
PDA with limited shunt
Low PVR
PA
AAo
RV
LV
LA
RA
Image

Fig. 8. Left ventricle in hypoplastic left heart syndrome (HLHS). Image a showing normal left ventricle (LV) with normal cardiac symmetry. Image b showing borderline left ventricle while Image c shoes hypoplastic left ventricle. Image d shows severely hypoplastic left ventricle with tiny left ventricle and mitral atresia. Image e shows pathophysiology of HLHS with atrial and ductal communication and high pulmonary vascular resistance (PVR). Image f shows decreased PVR and ductal closure from oxygen therapy leading to systemic hypoperfusion. AAo, ascending aorta; DAo, descending aorta; LA, left atrium; RA, right atrium; RV, right ventricle. (*Courtesy of* Satyan Lakshminrusimha and Yogen Singh.)

blocked. Maintaining ductal patency or wide open intra-atrial communication does not help in this situation. The only definitive and lifesaving intervention is urgent cardiac surgery to relieve the obstruction.

An urgent pediatric cardiology consultation is warranted when a critical CHD is suspected, and a comprehensive echocardiography would provide a definitive diagnosis. The neonatologist, pediatrician, or emergency room physician may encounter any of the aforementioned situations with an undiagnosed critical CHD. Therefore,

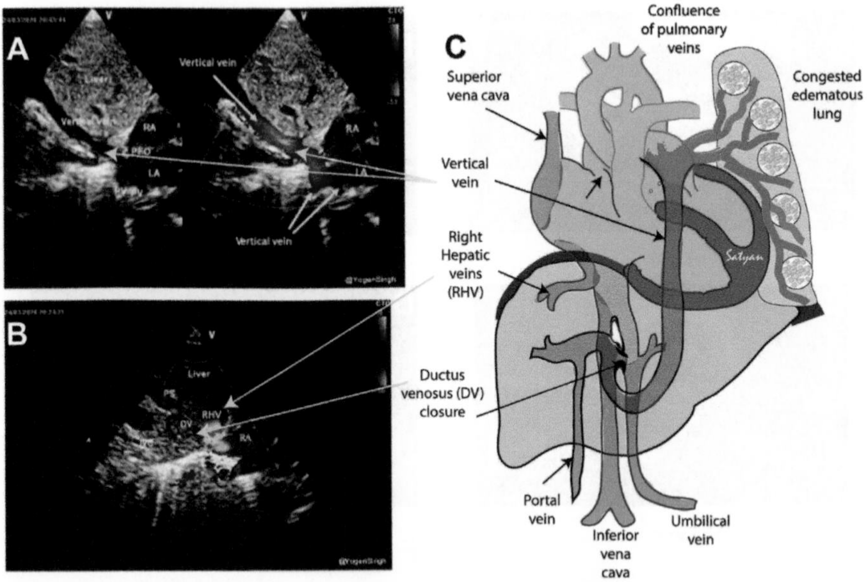
A
Vertical vein
Vertical vein
RA
LA
B
Liver
RHV
DV
RA
C
Confluence of pulmonary veins
Superior vena cava
Congested edematous lung
Vertical vein
Right Hepatic veins (RHV)
Ductus venosus (DV) closure
Portal vein
Inferior vena cava
Umbilical vein

Fig. 9. Two-dimensional and color Doppler images of infradiaphragmatic total anomalous pulmonary venous circulation (TAPVC) showing the vertical vein in image A. Image B shows connections in the liver through ductus venosus (DV). Image C shows the consequences of closure of ductus venosus in infradiaphragmatic TAPVC. The inability to drain the vertical vein from the confluence of the pulmonary veins into the inferior vena cava leads to lung congestion, increased vascularity, and edema. (*Courtesy of* Satyan Lakshminrusimha and Yogen Singh.)

understanding of underlying pathophysiology is of utmost importance to recognize these conditions early and initiate management. The detailed approach to definitive diagnosis and individualized management for each condition is out of the scope of this review article. However, the use of prostaglandin E1 in CHDs, which is often used by the noncardiologist physicians in neonatal cardiac emergencies, has been discussed in the following section.

A SIMPLIFIED APPROACH TO EVALUATION AND INITIAL MANAGEMENT OF INFANTS WITH SUSPECTED CONGENITAL HEART DISEASE

The clinical presentation of CHD in the neonatal period can be nonspecific mimicking other more common conditions in infancy such as sepsis, respiratory, hypovolemia, or metabolic condition. Therefore, having a high index of suspicion and a systematic approach is vitally important for the timely diagnosis and management.

The initial evaluation of an infant with suspected CHD should include a detailed history including obstetric history and family history, meticulous physical examination including palpation of peripheral pulses and measuring preductal and postductal saturations, and hyperoxia test. The presence of dysmorphic features and other congenital anomalies may help in suspecting underlying CHD.

During the fetal period the shunt direction across ductus arteriosus is right-to-left shunt (from pulmonary artery to aorta) because of high PVR and low SVR. This leads to higher preductal saturation than postductal saturation, which is often seen soon after birth during early transitional circulation and infants with persistently high PVR (such in infants with severe Persistent Pulmonary Hypertension of Newborn). Right to left shunt can also be seen in certain critical CHDs such as interrupted arch of aorta and critical aortic stenosis/aortic atresia. Persistently reversed differential cyanosis (higher postductal saturation than the preductal saturation) is rare. It is sometimes seen in TGA with PPHN or coarctation. It can be noted transiently in PPHN or even in otherwise well infants soon after birth.

As discussed previously, hyperoxia test can be useful in differentiating between the cardiac and respiratory causes of cyanosis in newborns infants. It works on the assumption that in infants with cyanotic CHDs or those with right to left shunt, regardless of the level of alveolar oxygenation, the desaturating effect of the lesion/shunt will not alter. Oxygen is administered through a plastic hood for at least 10 minutes to fill the alveolar spaces completely with oxygen and arterial partial pressure of oxygen (Pao_2) is measured before and after delivering 100% oxygen to assess the response to inhaled oxygen (hyperoxia test). In infants with cyanotic CHD, the rise in Pao_2 is usually no more than 10 to 30 mm Hg and rarely exceeds 100 mm Hg. In comparison, in infants with pulmonary diseases, Pao_2 often rises to over 100 mm Hg. However, infants with massive intrapulmonary shunt from a respiratory disease may not show a rise in Pao_2 to greater than 100 mm Hg. Conversely, some infants with cyanotic defects with a large pulmonary blood flow, such as TAPVC, may demonstrate a rise in Pao_2 of 100 mm Hg or higher. Therefore, hyperoxia test should be interpreted in the light of clinical picture and the degree of pulmonary pathology seen on radiographs.[1,27] In NICUs with easy access to echocardiography, it may be better to skip hyperoxia test to minimize adverse effects of 100% oxygen including free radical injury, ductal closure and rapid drop in PVR (see **Figs. 5** and **8**). In addition, echocardiography provides additional hemodynamic information that is, beneficial to management of an infant with CHD.

Four limb blood pressures are of limited value in neonates but can be helpful in older children. If the systolic pressure in right arm exceeds 10 mm Hg difference as measured in the leg, an aortic arch anomaly is likely. PDA may not allow this gradient to manifest. Therefore, the absence of a systolic pressure gradient alone does not rule out aortic arch anomaly in neonates.[27]

Chest X-ray is important in excluding respiratory pathology, although its role is limited in diagnosing CHDs. The presence of cardiomegaly or pulmonary vascular markings (plethoric or oligemic lung fields) may help in suspecting underlying CHD. ECG may be diagnostic in certain categories of CHD such as superior axis deviation seen in infants with tricuspid atresia, atrioventricular septal defect (AVSD) and congenitally corrected TGA (ccTGA).[27]

Echocardiogram remains the gold standard in diagnosing CHDs and delineating the underlying anatomy. It may be available immediately in the emergency room or when acute neonatologist/pediatrician encounters an undiagnosed CHD. As discussed previously, management should not be delayed in infants with suspected duct-dependent CHDs while waiting for an echocardiography or cardiology consultation.

Infants presenting with cardiorespiratory failure should first be stabilized as per Advanced Pediatric Life Support guidelines, and infants with cardiorespiratory failure will often need endotracheal intubation and mechanical ventilation, and infants with suspected duct-dependent CHD should be started on prostaglandin E1 as soon as possible.[20,24,27]

USE OF PROSTAGLANDIN E1 INFANTS WITH CRITICAL CHDs

In infants with suspected duct-dependent critical CHDs maintaining ductal patency can be lifesaving, and there should not be a delay in starting prostaglandin E1 while waiting for echocardiography or specialist advice (**Fig. 10**).

Infants with an 'open duct' (those with antenatal diagnosis or early presentation) need a small dose (0.005–0.01 μg/kg/min or 5–10 ng/kg/minute) to maintain ductal patency while collapsed infants with weak or absent femoral pulses will need a much higher dose, up to 0.1 μg/kg/min or 100 ng/kg/min. The expected desired response would be an improvement in acidosis, lactate or femoral pulses in collapsed acyanotic infant and an improvement in oxygen saturation in the cyanotic CHD (**Table 4**). The dose can be doubled if response is inadequate, and progress should be reassessed every 20 to 30 minutes. These infants should be discussed with pediatric cardiologists as soon as possible.[24]

Infants on a low dose of prostaglandin E1 (less than 15 ng/kg/min) are unlikely to have adverse effects such as apnea and they do not routinely need mechanical ventilation. A 10-year retrospective population-based audit conducted by the New South Wales transport service in Australia and a UK study reported safe transfer of infants with low dose prostaglandin E1 without mechanical ventilation. As prostaglandin

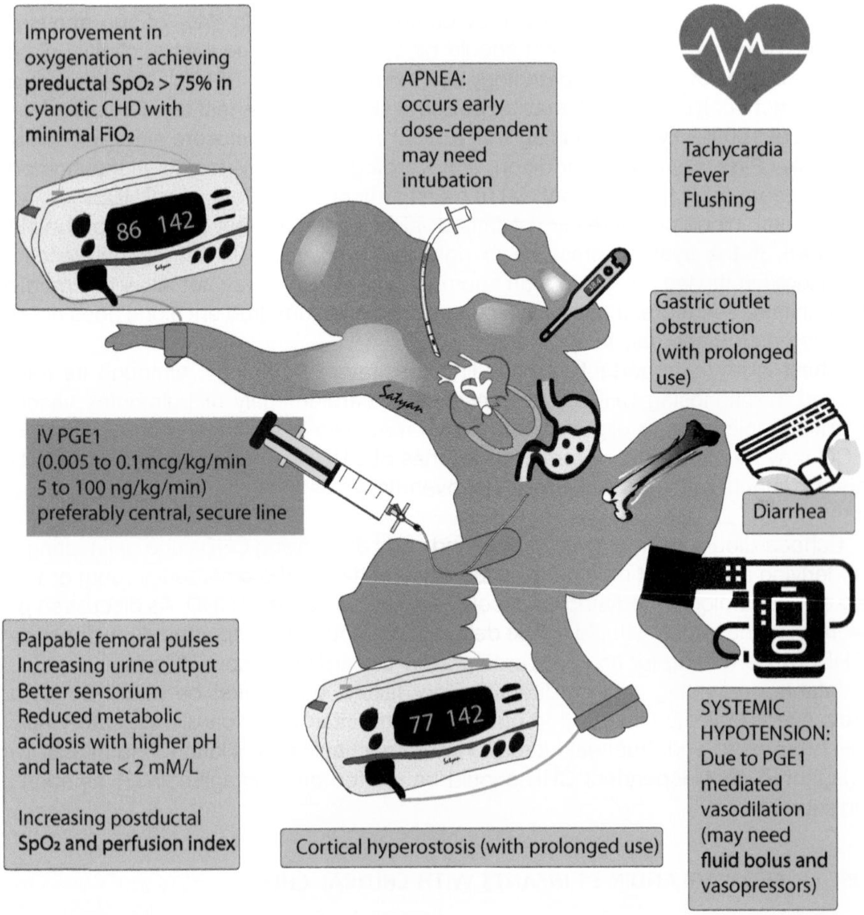
Improvement in oxygenation - achieving preductal SpO2 > 75% in cyanotic CHD with minimal FiO2
86 142
APNEA:
occurs early
dose-dependent
may need intubation
Tachycardia
Fever
Flushing
Gastric outlet obstruction (with prolonged use)
IV PGE1
(0.005 to 0.1mcg/kg/min
5 to 100 ng/kg/min)
preferably central, secure line
Diarrhea
Palpable femoral pulses
Increasing urine output
Better sensorium
Reduced metabolic acidosis with higher pH and lactate < 2 mM/L
Increasing postductal SpO2 and perfusion index
77 142
Cortical hyperostosis (with prolonged use)
SYSTEMIC HYPOTENSION:
Due to PGE1 mediated vasodilation
(may need fluid bolus and vasopressors)

Fig. 10. The dose (*green box*), benefits (*pink boxes*), and adverse effects (*blue boxes*) associated with intravenous PGE1 therapy in newborn infants. (*Courtesy of* Satyan Lakshminrusimha and Yogen Singh.)

infusion can cause apnea and hypotension, continuous cardiorespiratory monitoring is indicated.[24] The adverse effects of prostaglandin E1 are summarized in **Table 5**.

Failure to respond to prostaglandin E1 infusion could be because of incorrect diagnosis, insufficient central mixing despite ductal patency (such as in transposition great arteries (TGA) with restrictive atrial septum, HLHS with restrictive atrial septum, etc.) or a lack of ductal response to prostaglandin E1. These infants may deteriorate rapidly without atrial septostomy irrespective of maintaining ductal patency and this a time critical emergency needing urgent discussion with a pediatric cardiologist.[26,28]

ESTABLISHING A DEFINITIVE DIAGNOSIS OF CHD

The definitive diagnosis of CHD is made by diagnostic echocardiography which should be performed by a pediatric cardiologist or clinician trained in performing echocardiography for congenital heart defects. If a CHD is suspected on neonatologist performed echocardiography (NPE) or targeted neonatal echocardiography (TNE), even when NPE/TNE trained clinician, the infant should be referred to the pediatric cardiologist.[29–31] The infants with suspected critical CHDs should be discussed urgently with the pediatric cardiologist.[30,31] The diagnosis of congenital heart disease can be challenging, even in expert hands, during transitional circulation (such as coarctation in presence of an open ductus arteriosus) or in very sick infants (such as TAPVC in infants with PPHN).[29–31]

Point-of-care ultrasound (POCUS) is increasingly being adopted by the acute care physicians (neonatologists, pediatricians, intensivists and emergency room physicians) to gain anatomic and physiologic information which can help in making timely diagnosis in sick infants and provide targeted specific intervention. However, POCUS should not be used as screening tool to diagnose or rule out CHDs, although underlying pathology may be seen or suspected while performing POCUS. Those infants with suspected CHDs on POCUS assessment should be discussed with the pediatric cardiologist and they will need formal echocardiography to establish the diagnosis.[32]

Table 4
Dose of prostaglandin E1 infusion and desired response in infants with critical congenital heart defects[24]

Dose of prostaglandin E1 in different clinical scenarios of critical CHDs	
Antenatal diagnosis of Duct-dependent CHD	5–10 ng/Kg/min or 0.005–0.01 μg/kg/min
Cyanotic infant, well and not acidotic	5–10 ng/Kg/min or 0.005–0.01 μg/kg/min
Infant with absent femoral pulses, well and not acidotic	10–15 ng/Kg/min or 0.01–0.015 μg/kg/min
Unwell or acidotic infant with suspected duct-dependent CHD	50–100 ng/Kg/min or 0.05–0.1 μg/kg/min
Desired response to prostaglandin E1 infusion in infants with critical CHDs	
Suspected or known left-heart obstruction	Palpable femorals, normal pH and lactate <2 mmols/L
Suspected or known right-heart obstruction	Oxygen saturations 75%–85% with normal lactate <2 mmols/L
Transposition of Great Arteries (TGA)	Oxygen saturations >75% with normal lactate <2 mmols/L

Table 5
Adverse effects of prostaglandin E1 infusion in neonates

Common Adverse Effects	Less Common and Rare Adverse Effects	Adverse Effects due to Prolonged Use
• Apnea (usually occurs within 1st hour and with increasing dosing) • Hypotension (due to vasodilatation consider fluid bolus) • Fever • Tachycardia • Flushing	• Hypothermia • Bradycardia • Convulsions • Diarrhoea • Cardiac arrest • Disseminated intravascular coagulation (DIC)	• Gastric outlet obstruction syndrome • Cortical hyperostosis

SUMMARY

The hemodynamic changes during after birth are probably the most significant and dramatic that will ever occur during life. The cardiovascular transition physiology is complex and it is affected by multiple factors. Infants with CHDs, even those with critical CHDs, may remain completely asymptomatic during the transitional period when fetal shunts are open. The clinical diagnosis of CHD during transitional circulation may be difficult and in certain situations it can be challenging even on echocardiography. There should be low a low index of suspicion of critical CHDs in infants presenting with shock during the neonatal period. Acute care physicians (neonatologists, pediatricians, intensivists and emergency room physicians) need understanding of cardiovascular physiology and the varied presentations of undiagnosed critical CHDs. Timely and the appropriate dose of prostaglandin E1 infusion can be lifesaving in ductal-dependent CHDs. Providers should not be any delay in starting prostaglandin E1 infusion in infants with suspected critical CHD while waiting for the echocardiography or cardiology consultation.

CLINICS CARE POINTS

- A high degree of suspicion is warranted in diagnosing critical CHDs in infants presenting with shock, hypoxia or unexplained deterioration.
- The understanding perinatal cardiovascular physiology is essential for timely diagnosis and management of congenital heart defects.
- The signs and symptoms of critical congenital heart defects are often non-specific soon after birth.
- Appropriate dose of prostaglandin E1 should be started as soon as possible in infants suspected to have duct dependent CHD.

Best Practices

- Infants with suspected critical congenital heart defects should be discussed with the pediatric cardiologists as soon as possible.
- Timely recognition and therapy with prostaglandin E1 infusion can be lifesaving in neonatal cardiac emergencies.

- Infants with obstructive TAPVD and those with restrictive central mixing atrial septum (such as TGA and HLHS with restrictive atrial septum) are time critical emergencies and may continue to deteriorate despite starting prostaglandin E1.

REFERENCES

1. Singh Y. Evaluation of a child with suspected congenital heart disease. Paediatrics Child Health 2018;28(12):556–61.
2. Plana MN, Zamora J, Suresh G, et al. Pulse oximetry screening for critical congenital heart defects. Cochrane Database Syst Rev 2018;3(3):CD011912.
3. Levey A, Glickstein JS, Kleinman CS, et al. The impact of prenatal diagnosis of complex congenital heart disease on neonatal outcomes. Pediatr Cardiol 2010; 31:587–97.
4. Connor JA, Thiagarajan R. Hypoplastic left heart syndrome. Orphanet J Rare Dis 2007;2:23.
5. Franklin O, Burch M, Manning N, et al. Prenatal diagnosis of coarctation of the aorta improves survival and reduces morbidity. Heart 2002;87:67–9.
6. Bonnet D, Coltri A, Butera G, et al. [Prenatal diagnosis of transposition of great vessels reduces neonatal morbidity and mortality]. Arch Mal Coeur Vaiss 1999; 92:637–40.
7. Oster ME, Kim CH, Kusano AS, et al. A population-based study of the association of prenatal diagnosis with survival rate for infants with congenital heart defects. Am J Cardiol 2014;113:1036–40.
8. Singh Y, Tissot C. Echocardiographic evaluation of transitional circulation for the neonatologists. Front Pediatr 2018;6:140.
9. Singh Y. Echocardiographic evaluation of hemodynamics in neonates and children. Front Pediatr 2017;5:201.
10. Kiserud T. Physiology of the fetal circulation. Semin Fetal Neonatal Med 2005;10: 493–503.
11. Rudolph AM, Heymann MA. The circulation of the fetus in utero. Methods for studying distribution of blood flow, cardiac output and organ blood flow. Circ Res 1967;21:163–84.
12. Mielke G, Benda N. Cardiac output and central distribution of blood flow in the human fetus. Circulation 2001;103:1662–8.
13. Rudolph AM. Fetal and neonatal pulmonary circulation. Ann Rev Physiol 1979;41: 383–95.
14. Rasanen J, Wood DC, Weiner S, et al. Role of the pulmonary circulation in the distribution of human fetal cardiac output during the second half of pregnancy. Circulation 1996;94:1068–73.
15. Hooper SB, Te Pas AB, Lang J, et al. Cardiovascular transition at birth: a physiological sequence. Pediatr Res 2015;77:608–14.
16. Lang JA, Pearson JT, te Pas AB, et al. Ventilation/perfusion mismatch during lung aeration at birth. J Appl Physiol 1985;117(5):535–43.
17. van Vonderen JJ, Roest AA, Siew ML, et al. Measuring physiological changes during the transition to life after birth. Neonatology 2014;105:230–42.
18. Bökenkamp R, DeRuiter MC, van Munsteren C, et al. Insights into the pathogenesis and genetic background of patency of the ductus arteriosus. Neonatology 2010;98:6–17.
19. Backes CH, Huang H, Cua CL, et al. Early versus delayed umbilical cord clamping in infants with congenital heart disease: a pilot, randomized, controlled trial. J Perinatol 2015;35(10):826–31.

20. Park MK. Paediatric cardiology for practitioners. Philadelphia: Mosby Elsevier; 2008. p. 151e2.
21. Watson T, Kakar P, Srivastava S, et al. Eustachian valve remnant. Cardiol J 2007; 14:508–9.
22. Rosenthal E. Coarctation of the aorta from fetus to adult: Curable condition or life-long disease process? Heart 2005;91:1495–502.
23. Ward KE, Pryor RW, Matson JR, et al. Delayed detection of coarctation in infancy: Implications for timing of newborn follow-up. Pediatrics 1990;86:972–6.
24. Singh Y, Mikrou P. Use of prostaglandins in duct-dependent congenital heart conditions. Arch Dis Child Educ Pract Ed 2017;103:137–40.
25. Rudolph AM. High pulmonary vascular resistance after birth: I. Pathophysiologic considerations and etiologic classification. Clin Pediatr (Phila) 1980;19:585–90.
26. Martin L, Khalil H. How much reduced hemoglobin is necessary to generate central cyanosis? Chest 1990;97:182–5.
27. Singh Y, Gahlaut R, Chee Y. Evaluation of a child with suspected congenital heart disease. Paediatrics Child Health 2015;25(1):7–12.
28. Gardner TH. Cardiac emergencies in the newborn period. Radiol clinic North America 1971;9:385–97.
29. Mertens L, Seri I, Marek J, et al. Targeted neonatal echocardiography in the neonatal intensive care unit: practice guidelines and recommendations for training. J Am Soc Echocardiogr 2011;24:1057–78.
30. Singh Y, Gupta S, Groves AM, et al. Expert consensus statement 'neonatologist-performed echocardiography (NoPE)'—training and accreditation in UK. Eur J Pediatr 2016;175:281–7.
31. de Boode WP, Singh Y, Gupta S, et al. Recommendations for neonatologist performed echocardiography in Europe: consensus statement endorsed by European Society for Paediatric Research (ESPR) and European Society for Neonatology (ESN). Pediatr Res 2016;80:465–71.
32. Singh Y, Tissot C, Fraga MV, et al. International evidence-based guidelines on Point of care ultrasound (POCUS) for critically ill neonates and children issued by the POCUS working group of the European Society of Paediatric and neonatal intensive care (ESPNIC). Crit Care 2020;24:65.

Pathophysiology and Management of Persistent Pulmonary Hypertension of the Newborn

Yogen Singh, MD, MA (Cantab)[a,b], Satyan Lakshminrusimha, MD[c,*]

KEYWORDS

- Persistent pulmonary hypertension of the newborn (PPHN) • Inhaled nitric oxide
- Oxygen • Echocardiography • Term infant

KEY POINTS

- Understanding the pathophysiology is of paramount importance in diagnosis and management of persistent pulmonary hypertension of the newborn (PPHN).
- Echocardiography is diagnostic in PPHN for confirming diagnosis, assessing the severity, understanding pathophysiology, guiding targeted specific therapy, and monitoring response to therapy.
- Inhaled nitric oxide (iNO) is the pulmonary vasodilator of choice. However, alternative therapy (such as, sildenafil, milrinone, or iloprost) should be considered in iNO-resistant cases.
- Hypoxia and hyperoxia both should be avoided in managing PPHN.
- Alkalosis and hyperventilation should be avoided and gentle lung recruitment strategy should be preferred in conjunction with early iNO, surfactant, and a "cardiocentric" approach to manage hemodynamic instability.

INTRODUCTION

Persistent pulmonary hypertension of the newborn (PPHN), previously referred to as persistent fetal circulation, is a syndrome of impaired circulatory adaptation at birth.[1] The hallmark of PPHN physiology is sustained elevation of pulmonary vascular

Funding: NICHD – 5 R01 HD072929-10 (S. Lakshminrusimha).
[a] Department of Pediatrics - Neonatology and Pediatric Cardiology, Cambridge University Hospitals NHS Foundation Trust and University of Cambridge School of Clinical Medicine, Cambridge, UK; [b] Department of Pediatrics - Division of Neonatology, Loma Linda University Children's Hospital and Loma Linda University School of Medicine, 11175 Coleman Pavillion, Loma Linda, CA 92374, USA; [c] Department of Pediatrics, UC Davis Children's Hospital, UC Davis Health, Sacramento, CA 95817, USA
* Corresponding author.
E-mail address: slakshmi@ucdavis.edu

Clin Perinatol 48 (2021) 595–618
https://doi.org/10.1016/j.clp.2021.05.009 perinatology.theclinics.com

resistance (PVR) and persistent hypoxemia after birth.[2] Despite advances in understanding of perinatal pathophysiology and neonatal management strategies, its prevalence (2 per 1000 live births) has not changed significantly.[2] The vast majority of infants with PPHN are born at term or near term, although approximately 2% of cases are born prematurely.[3] Mortality has not changed (5%–10%) and PPHN remains one of the leading causes of critical illness in the neonatal intensive care unit.[4]

PPHN is secondary to impaired or delayed relaxation of the pulmonary vasculature associated with a diverse group of cardiopulmonary pathologies such as meconium aspiration syndrome (MAS), congenital diaphragmatic hernia (CDH), congenital pneumonia, hypoxic ischemic encephalopathy (HIE/perinatal asphyxia), premature prolonged rupture of membranes (pPROM), respiratory distress syndrome (RDS), and underlying or associated congenital heart disease (CHD).[5,6] It is critical to understand the etiopathogenesis, altered physiology, and impact of the interventions on the pathophysiology to manage these patients effectively. A physiology-based approach toward PPHN is essential to decrease morbidity and mortality.

This article reviews the pathophysiology and hemodynamic changes that occur in PPHN. We also review a cardiocentric echo-based approach in the management of PPHN in late preterm, term, and post-term infants.

CLASSIFICATION OF PERSISTENT PULMONARY HYPERTENSION OF THE NEWBORN

During the sixth World Symposium of Pulmonary Arterial Hypertension (PAH) held in 2018 in Nice, France, the classification of PAH was updated.[7] Because of its particular anatomic and physiologic nature, PPHN has been moved to a separate subcategory. Although this classification of pediatric pulmonary hypertension is useful, a more commonly used classification of PPHN is based on etiology: primary (idiopathic) and secondary PPHN (**Table 1**).

Primary or idiopathic PPHN refers to the absence of parenchymal lung disease to explain elevated pulmonary arterial pressure and implies intrauterine pulmonary vascular remodeling. Compared with pediatric pulmonary hypertension, only approximately 10% to 20% of cases of PPHN are idiopathic and a vast majority of PPHN cases, from abnormally constricted pulmonary vasculature, are due to other acute

Table 1
Etiology of persistent pulmonary hypertension of the newborn (PPHN)

A). Secondary PPHN (80%–90% of all PPHN cases)	
Lung parenchymal diseases (abnormal constriction of pulmonary vasculature)	Meconium aspiration syndrome (MAS) Pneumonia/sepsis Respiratory distress syndrome (RDS)
Abnormal or delayed transition at birth (impaired pulmonary vasculature vasodilation)	Transient tachypnea of the newborn (TTN) Perinatal stress/asphyxia Alveolar capillary dysplasia (ACD) Syndromic – Trisomy 21 Associated congenital heart disease (CHD)
Lung hypoplasia Hypoplastic pulmonary vasculature	Congenital diaphragmatic hernia (CDH) Oligohydramnios/Premature prolonged rupture of membranes Syndromic – Trisomy 21
B. Idiopathic PPHN (10%–20% of all PPHN cases)	
Normal pulmonary parenchyma with abnormally remodeled pulmonary vasculature	

respiratory disease processes, such as MAS, RDS, pneumonia, or CDH; this is referred to as secondary PPHN.[6] Recent data from California suggest that infection (30%), MAS (24%), idiopathic (20%), RDS (7%), and CDH (6%) are the 5 leading causes of PPHN.[8] In these cases, it can be difficult to separate chronic intrauterine remodeling from acute pulmonary vasoconstriction due to parenchymal lung disease. A practical list of congenital and acquired causes of PPHN with mnemonics is shown in **Fig. 1**.

PATHOPHYSIOLOGY OF PERSISTENT PULMONARY HYPERTENSION OF THE NEWBORN

The pathophysiology of PPHN is complex, multifactorial, and dynamic; it evolves with time and is significantly affected by the intervention and disease process (**Fig. 2**). The hallmark of the PPHN pathophysiology is increased PVR resulting in decreased pulmonary blood flow (PBF) and hence, decreased amount of oxygenated blood returning to left side of the heart leading to hypoxia, decreased end-organ perfusion, acidosis and cyanosis.[9] Hypoxemia and acidosis are potent vasoconstrictors leading to increase in PVR and worsening of PPHN. Persistently elevated PVR results in hypertrophy of right ventricle (RV) from pumping of blood against high vascular resistance. If elevated PVR persists or worsens, it may lead to impaired RV function and RV dilatation, and in severe cases it can lead to in RV failure, which may further decrease PBF and worsen hypoxemia. In severe cases of PPHN, this becomes a vicious cycle until altered pathophysiology is changed.[9]

RV dysfunction may impair left ventricle (LV) function because of interventricular functional independence. Poor LV function may decrease LV cardiac output and

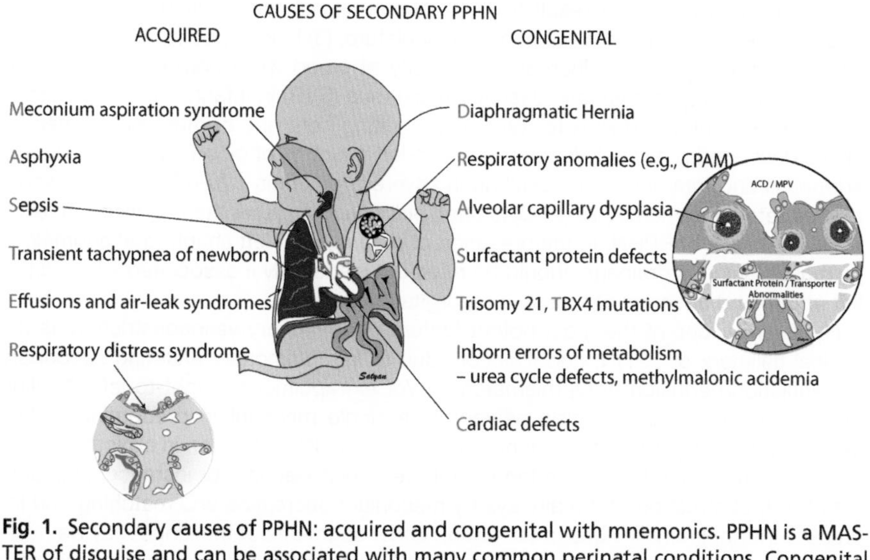
CAUSES OF SECONDARY PPHN
ACQUIRED
CONGENITAL
Meconium aspiration syndrome
Asphyxia
Sepsis
Transient tachypnea of newborn
Effusions and air-leak syndromes
Respiratory distress syndrome
Diaphragmatic Hernia
Respiratory anomalies (e.g., CPAM)
Alveolar capillary dysplasia
Surfactant protein defects
Trisomy 21, TBX4 mutations
Inborn errors of metabolism
– urea cycle defects, methylmalonic acidemia
Cardiac defects
ACD / MPV
Surfactant Protein / Transporter Abnormalities

Fig. 1. Secondary causes of PPHN: acquired and congenital with mnemonics. PPHN is a MASTER of disguise and can be associated with many common perinatal conditions. Congenital causes of PPHN, if not recognized early, can be associated with DRASTIC consequences. ACD, alveolar capillary dysplasia; CPAM, congenital pulmonary adenomatoid malformation; MPV, malalignment of pulmonary veins; TBX4 – T-box transcription factor 4 gene mutations. (*Modified from* PK R, Lakshminrusimha S, Vidyasagar D. Essentials of Neonatal Ventilation, 1st Edition: Elsevier India; 2019;with permission.)

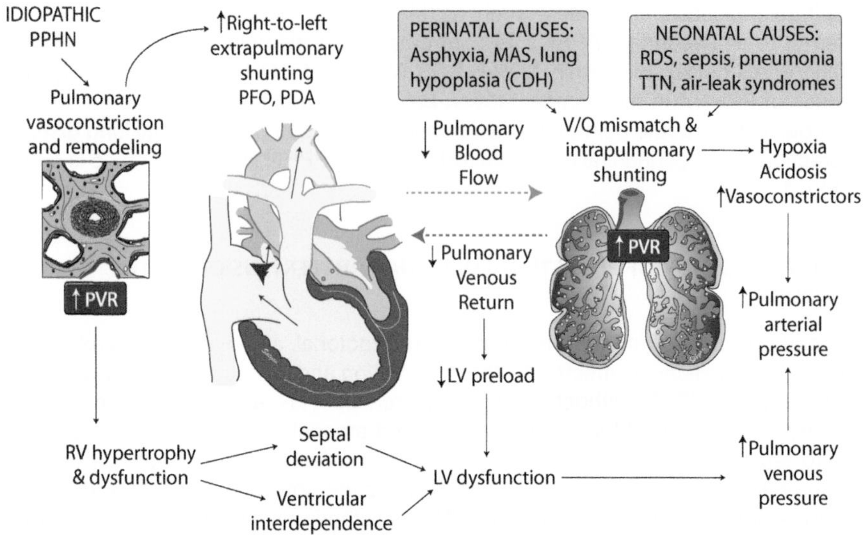
IDIOPATHIC PPHN
↑Right-to-left extrapulmonary shunting PFO, PDA
PERINATAL CAUSES: Asphyxia, MAS, lung hypoplasia (CDH)
NEONATAL CAUSES: RDS, sepsis, pneumonia TTN, air-leak syndromes
Pulmonary vasoconstriction and remodeling
↓Pulmonary Blood Flow
V/Q mismatch & intrapulmonary shunting
Hypoxia Acidosis ↑Vasoconstrictors
↑PVR
↑PVR
↓Pulmonary Venous Return
↑Pulmonary arterial pressure
↓LV preload
RV hypertrophy & dysfunction
Septal deviation
Ventricular interdependence
LV dysfunction
↑Pulmonary venous pressure

Fig. 2. Pathophysiology of extrapulmonary shunts, ventricular dysfunction, and interventricular function interdependence in PPHN.[10] TTN, transient tachypnea of newborn. (*Courtesy of* Satyan Lakshminrusimha and Yogen Singh.)

systemic blood flow, leading to poor end-organ perfusion and acidosis, and hence worsening of PPHN. Severe LV dysfunction may also impair LV filling due to poor compliance, which can lead to increased left atrial and pulmonary wedge pressure resulting in pulmonary venous hypertension.[5]

The elevated PVR may result from (1) abnormal pulmonary vasoconstriction, (2) structural remodeling of the pulmonary vasculature, (3) lung hypoplasia, and (4) intravascular obstruction from increased viscosity of blood as in polycythemia. PVR is often higher than the systemic vascular resistance (SVR) in infants with moderate to severe PPHN. Elevated PVR to SVR ratio resulting from one or more of the mechanisms described previously leads to right-to-left shunting of blood across the ductus arteriosus and foramen ovale resulting in severe hypoxemia[11] (see **Fig. 2**). The shunt across patent foramen ovale (PFO) is often bidirectional, rather than right-to-left, even in severe cases of PPHN. In the presence of pure right-to-left shunt, total anomalous pulmonary venous drainage should be ruled out (especially if associated with a small left atrium and absence of tricuspid regurgitation).

Hypoxemia, one of the most potent factors of pulmonary vasoconstriction, is the clinical hallmark of PPHN, and it occurs due to intrapulmonary shunting secondary to ventilation/perfusion (V/Q) mismatch and/or extrapulmonary right-to-left shunting of blood (see **Fig. 2**). In some newborns, a single mechanism predominates (eg, extrapulmonary right-to-left shunting in idiopathic PPHN). However, in clinical practice several of these mechanisms often contribute to hypoxemia. For instance, in infants with MAS, obstruction of the airways by meconium decreases V/Q matching and increases intrapulmonary right-to-left shunt. Other segments of the lungs may be overventilated relative to perfusion resulting in V/Q mismatch and increase in physiologic dead space. The same patient may also exhibit severe hypoxemia due to extrapulmonary right-to-left shunting at the ductus arteriosus and foramen ovale.[9,12,13] Similarly, pathophysiological changes may be seen infants with severe congenital pneumonia. On the other hand, PPHN in infants with MAS and congenital pneumonia may result from alveolar hypoxia, from inflammatory mediators, metabolic acidosis, and from abnormal pulmonary vascular muscularization. Similar mechanisms may play a significant role in infants with sepsis. Infants with severe HIE may have associated PPHN both from altered or delayed transition leading to persistent high PVR, which could also be worsened by the therapeutic hypothermia. Perinatal asphyxia can also lead to myocardial ischemia leading to poor cardiac function, acidosis, and low cardiac output, which may contribute to PPHN.[13]

On the other hand, lung hypoplasia resulting from impaired in utero lung development or anatomic causes may be the primary cause of increased PVR and PPHN in infants with pPROM or anatomic abnormalities such as CDH.[12]

Infants with CDH have abnormal cardiopulmonary vascular development leading to in utero LV hypoplasia, lung hypoplasia, and increased PVR.[14] In infants with PPHN, previously the primary focus was on lowering of PVR. However, now with better understanding of altered pathophysiology, the focus is shifting to managing PPHN with gentle ventilation to improve V/Q mismatch and supporting the LV (such as with early introduction of a low dose of epinephrine and milrinone) to stabilize the cardiovascular hemodynamics.[5,14] The article is primarily focused on PPHN and a detailed description of impaired pathophysiology and management of CDH is out of the scope of this article.

Other causes of PPHN include constriction of the fetal ductus arteriosus in utero, which can occur after exposure of fetus to nonsteroidal anti-inflammatory drugs or selective serotonin reuptake inhibitors during late gestation.[15–17] There is a sixfold increase in the prevalence of PPHN after exposure to these medications during the third trimester.[17] These findings have been confirmed in animal models: ductal constriction or surgical ligation in lambs produces a rapid antenatal remodeling of pulmonary vasculature resulting in increased fetal pulmonary artery pressure and profound hypoxemia after birth, similar to human infants.[15,18] Similarly, in utero exposure to fluoxetine resulted in pulmonary vasculature remodeling and hypoxemia in newborn rats after birth.[18]

MECHANISM OF PULMONARY VASCULATURE REMODELING AND BASIS OF THERAPEUTIC INTERVENTION IN PERSISTENT PULMONARY HYPERTENSION OF THE NEWBORN

From animal studies there is good evidence that remodeling of the pulmonary vasculature occurs as a result of the disruption of the following 1 or more pathways: (1) nitric oxide (NO)–cyclic guanosine monophosphate (cGMP) pathway, (2) prostacyclin–cyclic adenosine monophosphate (cAMP) pathway, (3) endothelin signaling pathway, and (4) oxidant stress pathway[5,6] (**Fig. 3**).

The NO-cGMP pathway is the best studied mechanism of PPHN and has been the basis of NO therapeutic trials in treatment of PPHN.[4,5] NO produced by the endothelium stimulates soluble guanylyl cyclase (sGC) in the pulmonary arterial smooth muscle cell (PASMC) to produce cGMP. Both NO and cGMP produce pulmonary vasodilation. Abnormal vasodilator responses to NO secondary to impaired sGC activity are well described in animal models of neonatal pulmonary hypertension and CDH.[19,20] In fetal lambs, disruption of the NO-cGMP pathway by chronic in utero inhibition of endothelial nitric oxide synthase (eNOS) resulted in the physiologic characteristics of PPHN.[21] Decreased expression of eNOS has also been reported in the umbilical venous endothelial cultures and reduced levels of NO metabolites in urine have been noted in human infants with MAS and PPHN.[22–24] Because NO and cGMP both vasodilate and inhibit vascular smooth muscle growth, it is possible that

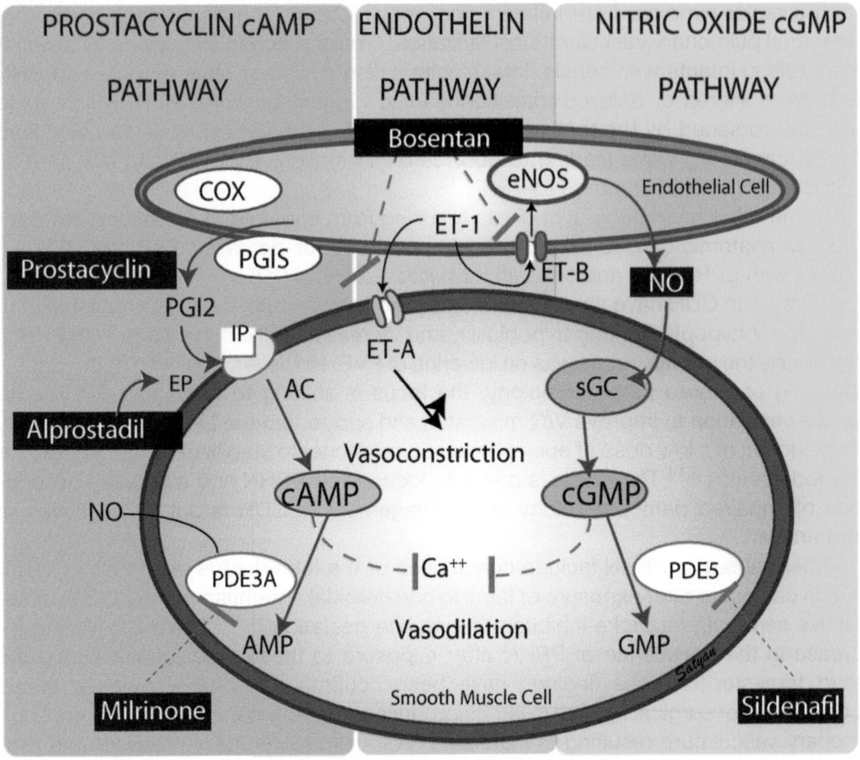
PROSTACYCLIN cAMP
PATHWAY
ENDOTHELIN
PATHWAY
NITRIC OXIDE cGMP
PATHWAY
Bosentan
COX
eNOS
Endothelial Cell
ET-1
PGIS
Prostacyclin
ET-B
NO
PGI2
IP
ET-A
EP
AC
sGC
Alprostadil
Vasoconstriction
cAMP
cGMP
NO
Ca++
PDE3A
PDE5
Vasodilation
AMP
GMP
Milrinone
Smooth Muscle Cell
Sildenafil

Fig. 3. Pathways of vasoactive agents in the pulmonary circulation and agents used for therapy of PPHN including endothelium-derived vasodilators: prostacyclin (PGI_2) and NO and blockers of vasoconstrictors (endothelin, ET-1). The enzymes, cyclooxygenase (COX) and prostacyclin synthase (PGIS) are involved in the production of prostacyclin. Prostacyclin acts on its receptor (IP) in the smooth muscle cell and stimulates adenylate cyclase (AC) to produce cAMP. Similarly, alprostadil acts on the EP receptor to stimulate cAMP production. Cyclic AMP is broken down by phosphodiesterase 3A (PDE 3A) in the smooth muscle cell. Milrinone inhibits PDE 3A and increases cAMP levels in pulmonary arterial smooth muscle cells and cardiac myocytes resulting in pulmonary (and systemic) vasodilation and inotropy. Endothelin is a powerful vasoconstrictor and acts on ET-A receptors in the smooth muscle cell and increases ionic calcium concentration. A second endothelin receptor (ET-B) on the endothelial cell stimulates NO release and vasodilation. Endothelin receptor blockers such as Bosentan are beneficial in intractable PPHN. eNOS produces NO, which diffuses from the endothelium to the smooth muscle cell and stimulates soluble guanylate cyclase (sGC) enzyme to produce cGMP. Cyclic GMP is broken down by PDE 5 enzyme in the smooth muscle cell. Sildenafil inhibits PDE5 and increases cGMP levels in pulmonary arterial smooth muscle cells. Cyclic AMP and cGMP reduce cytosolic ionic calcium concentrations and induce smooth muscle cell relaxation and pulmonary vasodilation. (*Modified from* PK R, Lakshminrusimha S, Vidyasagar D. Essentials of Neonatal Ventilation, 1st Edition: Elsevier India; 2019;with permission.)

the combination of diminished eNOS expression, inactivation of sGC, and reduced cGMP levels contribute to both abnormal vasoreactivity and excessive muscularization of pulmonary vessels in PPHN. Inhaled NO (iNO) therapy, exogenous nitric oxide, stimulates PASMC to produce cGMP resulting in pulmonary vasodilation.

Increased phosphodiesterase 5 (PDE5) activity results in catabolism of cGMP and limitation of NO-induced vasodilation.[25] Hence, inhibition of PDE5 with the use of sildenafil is a promising strategy in the treatment of PPHN.[5] Sildenafil may also augment the effect of iNO in patients with partial or poorly sustained responses to iNO. It may be particularly effective in patients following prolonged hyperoxic ventilation, which increases production of superoxide anions and stimulates PDE5 activity.[25–27] Oral sildenafil has been used in infants with prolonged pulmonary hypertension associated with BPD and it is the mainstay of treatment in children with chronic pulmonary hypertension.[28]

The disruption of the prostacyclin pathway can also play an important role in PPHN. Prostacyclin I_2 (PGI_2) mediates vasodilation by activating adenylate cyclase and increasing cAMP in the PASMC.[29] Prostacyclin I_2 (PGI_2) analogs administered by the intravenous route are the mainstay of pulmonary vasodilator therapy in adults with PAH. Inhaled PGI_2 (epoprostenol) acts synergistically with iNO; it improves oxygenation in PPHN and prevents rebound hypertension when iNO is weaned off.[30,31] Use of inhaled iloprost has also been reported in combination with iNO for intractable PPHN.[32] However, as there are no randomized controlled trials evaluating the effect of prostaglandin vasodilators, their use remains limited.

cAMP levels can be enhanced through inhibition of its metabolism by phosphodiesterase 3 (PDE3A) modulation. Milrinone inhibits PDE3A activity in pulmonary arterial smooth muscle and increases cAMP, resulting in pulmonary vasodilation.[33] The pulmonary vasodilatory response to milrinone is proportional to PDE3A activity in PASMCs.[34] Animal studies suggest that exposure to iNO increases PDE3A activity, and that milrinone may be especially effective in promoting pulmonary vasodilation and improving oxygenation in iNO-resistant PPHN.[34,35] Milrinone also enhances the heart's inotropic effect through inhibition of cardiac PDE3A and is considered an inodilator.[36] In some infants with PPHN, especially those with LV dysfunction or hypoplasia (due to CDH, asphyxia, or sepsis), milrinone can help in augmenting LV function and induce pulmonary vasodilation. It can also be particularly helpful in infants with pulmonary venous hypertension from raised left atrial pressure secondary to impaired LV dysfunction or mitral regurgitation. Administration of iNO to infants with pulmonary venous hypertension may flood the pulmonary capillary bed and worsen pulmonary edema, resulting in clinical deterioration.[5] Three case series have demonstrated the effectiveness of milrinone in improving oxygenation in iNO-resistant PPHN,[33–35] and currently multicentric randomized controlled trials are under way to study the effects of milrinone in infants with CDH and pulmonary hypertension.

The disruption of the endothelial signaling pathway can also play an important role in infants with PPHN. Endothelin-1 (ET-1) synthesized by vascular endothelial cells is a potent vasoconstrictor and acts through 2 receptors: ET_A and ET_B. The ET_A receptor plays a critical role in vasoconstriction, whereas the endothelin-B receptor (ET_B) receptor promotes vasodilation mediated by endothelium-derived NO.[37,38] Selective blockade of the ET_A receptor causes fetal pulmonary vasodilation.[39] Chronic intrauterine ET_A receptor blockade following ductal ligation decreases pulmonary arterial pressure and distal muscularization of small pulmonary arteries in utero, decreases RV hypertrophy, and increases the fall in PVR at delivery in newborn lambs with PPHN.[40] Thus, ET-1 acting through the ET_A receptor might contribute to the pathogenesis and pathophysiology of PPHN. Bosentan, a nonspecific ET-1 receptor blocker, has mainly been used to treat PH in adults. Two recent trials show that bosentan is well tolerated in neonates with PPHN, although its efficacy is variable, possibly due to inconsistent intestinal absorption.[41,42]

Last, there is mounting evidence for the role of oxidant stress in the pathogenesis of PPHN. Reactive oxygen species (ROS), such as hydrogen peroxide, superoxide, and peroxynitrite, cause pulmonary vasoconstriction. In animal studies, lamb PPHN model, an increase in superoxide and hydrogen peroxide in the smooth muscle and adventitia of pulmonary arteries has been demonstrated.[43,44] In addition to direct inactivation of NO, ROS can decrease eNOS and sGC activity and increase PDE5 activity, resulting in decreased cGMP levels.[45] Increased ROS can be secondary to (1) exposure to high concentrations of oxygen; (2) reduced levels of antioxidant enzymes such as superoxide dismutase, catalase, and glutathione peroxidase; and (3) increased activity of prooxidant enzymes such as NADPH oxidase.[43] Oxidative stress can be minimized by judicious use of inspired oxygen or possibly by the use of targeted antioxidants.

Oxygen is one of the most potent pulmonary vasodilators and increased oxygenation is the primary mediator of the reduction in PVR at birth. Alveolar hypoxia and hypoxemia increase PVR and contribute to the pathophysiology of PPHN. Avoiding hypoxemia by mechanical ventilation and high concentrations of oxygen is the mainstay of PPHN management.[5,12] Furthermore, animal studies demonstrate exaggerated hypoxic pulmonary vasoconstriction with pH less than 7.25, suggesting that acidosis should be avoided.[46] However, exposure to extreme hyperoxia promotes formation of ROS and may lead to lung injury. The animal studies demonstrated that even brief exposure to 100% oxygen in newborn lambs increased the contractility responses of pulmonary arteries and resulted in formation of superoxide anions and reduced response to iNO.[47,48]

DIAGNOSIS OF PERSISTENT PULMONARY HYPERTENSION OF THE NEWBORN

Hypoxic respiratory failure is a hallmark feature of PPHN, but differentiating cyanotic CHD from PPHN is critical in a hypoxemic infant.[5] The initial evaluation should include a thorough history of risk factors for PPHN, a meticulous physical examination, simultaneous measurement of preductal (right upper limb) and post-ductal (lower limb) oxygen saturation to check the difference between them, chest radiography, and arterial blood gas analysis. Pre- and post-ductal oxygen saturation and Pa_{O_2} measurements can help in differentiating PPHN from cyanotic CHD. Saturation differences of greater than 5% to 10% or Pa_{O_2} differences of 10 to 20 mm Hg between right upper limb and lower limbs, with preductal levels being higher than post-ductal levels, are considered significant. Hypoxemia is often labile in PPHN, unlike fixed hypoxemia seen in cyanotic CHD.[4–6]

The chest radiograph is particularly helpful in diagnosing respiratory pathology (**Fig. 4**). It may help in differentiating etiology of PPHN (such as MAS, pneumonia, RDS, or CDH) and differentiating types of CHD.[49] Hypoxemia disproportionate to the severity of parenchymal disease on chest radiography suggests idiopathic PPHN (or cyanotic heart disease). Pulmonary oligemia is seen in tetralogy of Fallot, Ebstein anomaly, critical pulmonary stenosis, and pulmonary atresia due to decreased pulmonary flow. Pulmonary plethora is seen in transposition of the great arteries with intact interventricular septum, truncus arteriosus, tricuspid atresia, total anomalous pulmonary venous connection (TAPVC), and single ventricle.[9,50,51]

The hyperoxia test may be useful in differentiating the cardiac causes from respiratory causes in cyanotic newborns. On confirmation of central cyanosis by measuring the arterial partial pressure of oxygen (Pa_{O_2}), response of Pa_{O_2} to 100% oxygen inhalation is tested (hyperoxia test). Oxygen should be administered through a plastic hood for at least 10 minutes to fill the alveolar spaces completely with oxygen. In a cyanotic

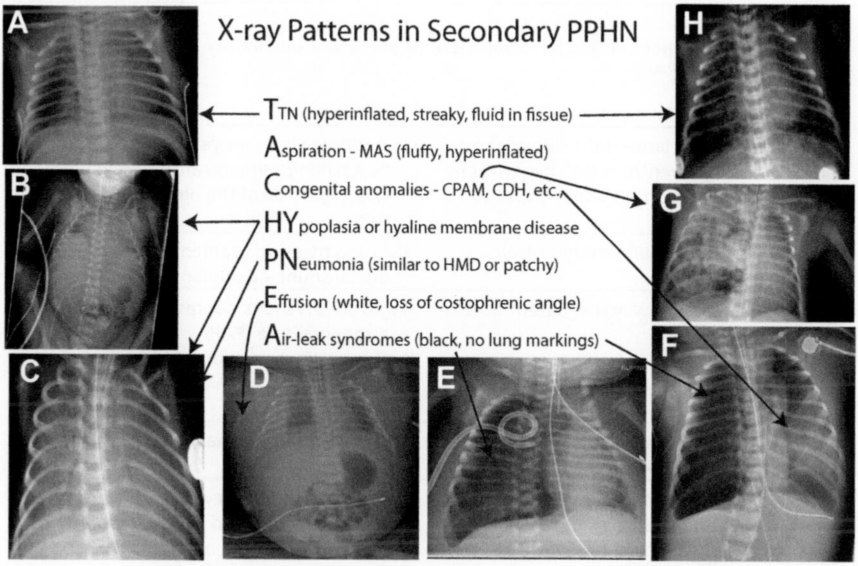
A
X-ray Patterns in Secondary PPHN
H
TTN (hyperinflated, streaky, fluid in fissue)
Aspiration - MAS (fluffy, hyperinflated)
B
Congenital anomalies - CPAM, CDH, etc.
G
HYpoplasia or hyaline membrane disease
PNeumonia (similar to HMD or patchy)
Effusion (white, loss of costophrenic angle)
Air-leak syndromes (black, no lung markings)
F
C
D
E

Fig. 4. X-ray patterns in secondary PPHN in term infants. (*A*) Transient tachypnea of the newborn (TTN). (*B*) Severe lung hypoplasia secondary to prolonged oligohydramnios. (*C*) Hyaline membrane disease (HMD) or RDS with ground glass appearance with air bronchograms. (*D*) Hydrops with pleural effusions and ascites. (*E*) Airleak with pneumothorax with chest tube in place. (*F*) CDH on the left and pneumothorax on the right. (*G*) Congenital cystic pulmonary adenomatoid malformation (CPAM). (*H*) MAS with fluffy infiltrates and hyperexpanded lung fields. (*Modified from* Alhassen Z, Vali P, Guglani L, Lakshminrusimha S, Ryan RM. Recent advances in pathophysiology and management of transient tachypnea of newborn. Journal of Perinatology. 2020 Aug 4:1-1.)

CHD case, the rise in Pao_2 is usually no more than 10 to 30 mm Hg and hardly ever exceeds 100 mm Hg. With pulmonary diseases, Pao_2 often rises more than 100 mm Hg; however, infants with massive intrapulmonary shunt from a respiratory disease may not show a rise in Pao_2 to 100 mm Hg. Conversely, some infants with cyanotic defects with a large PBF, such as TAPVC, may demonstrate a rise in Pao_2 of 100 mm Hg or higher. A hyperoxia test should be interpreted in the context of the clinical picture and the degree of pulmonary pathology seen on radiograph.[49–51] With the availability of bedside echocardiography, the hyperoxia test is seldom performed but can be helpful when echocardiography is not available.

Echocardiography is the gold standard to confirm the diagnosis of PPHN, monitor the response to the therapeutic interventions, and rule out underlying cyanotic or critical CHD. It can help in assessing the severity of PPHN. Pulmonary artery systolic pressure (PASP) can be estimated using tricuspid regurgitation velocity or ductus arteriosus shunt when present. Serial echocardiographic assessment can help in understanding evolving pathophysiology and response to the therapeutic intervention. Echocardiographic assessment and hemodynamic evaluation can help in targeting specific intervention and they can guide the choice of appropriate pulmonary vasodilator and vasoactive therapy.[9,10,52–54] Detailed description of echocardiographic technique used for assessment of PPHN is out of the scope of this article, a summary of echocardiography parameters commonly used in clinical practice have been summarized in **Figs. 3** and **4**, and **Table 2**. We recommend serial echocardiography (**Fig. 5**)

Table 2
Echocardiographic parameters for assessment of persistent pulmonary hypertension of the newborn (PPHN)[9,10,52–54]

Echocardiographic Parameter	Comment
Disproportionately large right side of the heart with right ventricle (RV) hypertrophy and/or RV dilatation on visual inspection	In multiple views on visual inspection "eyeballing" shows cardiac asymmetry with right ride of the heart bigger than left side
Estimation of pulmonary artery systolic pressure (PASP)	By using tricuspid gradient (when present) or ductal shunt – Doppler assessment
Direction of blood flow across patent ductus arteriosus (PDA)	Right-to-left shunt: suprasystemic pulmonary artery pressure (PAP) Left-to-right shunt: sub-systemic PAP Bidirectional shunt: PAP equal to systemic blood pressure
Direction of blood flow across patent foramen ovale (PFO)	Often it is bidirectional and seldom purely right-to-left
Flattening of interventricular septum (due to sustained high pressure in the RV and flattening proportional to severity of PPHN)	Helps in estimating severity of PPHN in absence of tricuspid regurgitation or PDA; can be categorized as mild, moderate, and severe flattening
Assessment of RV function	On visual inspection Tricuspid annular pan systolic excursion (TAPSE) Tei index using Tissue Doppler Imaging (TDI)
Assessment of left ventricle function	On visual inspection Tei index using TDI (note fraction shortening may be unreliable in presence of RV hypertrophy and dysfunction)
Assessment of cardiac filling (preload)	Inferior vena cava size and collapsibility
Advanced echocardiography and hemodynamic evaluation	RV fractional area change Pulmonary arterial acceleration time (PAAT) and PAAT/RV ejection time ratio Speckle tracking and strain rate Estimation of left and right cardiac output and serial assessment to see the response to therapy

assessment to monitor the disease progress, changing pathophysiology and response to treatment in PPHN, especially in infants with moderate to severe PPHN with hemodynamic instability (**Fig. 6**).

GENERAL SUPPORTIVE MANAGEMENT

The severity of PPHN can range from mild hypoxemia with minimal respiratory distress to severe hypoxemic respiratory failure and cardiopulmonary instability. General management principles for the newborn with PPHN include maintenance of normal temperature, electrolytes (particularly calcium and magnesium), glucose, nutritional support, avoidance of stress, maintaining good hemostasis (Hb >140 g/L), and handling with sedation and analgesia as needed. Paralysis should be avoided if possible because it has been associated with increased mortality.[5] As sepsis is

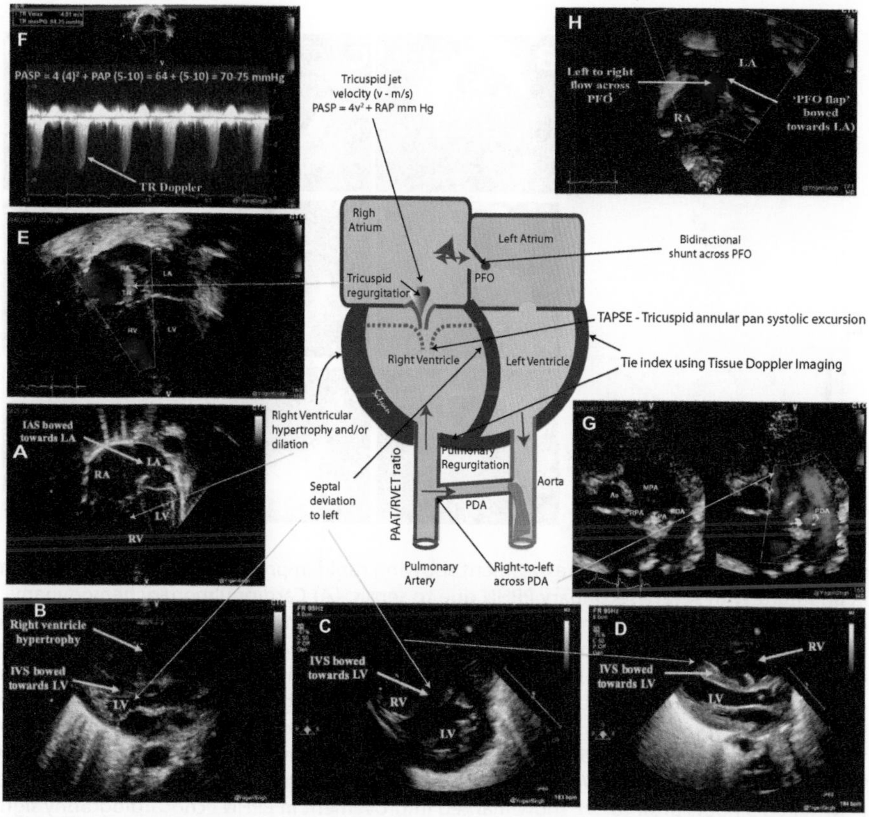
F
PASP = 4 (4)² + PAP (5-10) = 64 + (5-10) = 70-75 mmHg
TR Doppler
Tricuspid jet
velocity (v - m/s)
PASP = 4v² + RAP mm Hg
H
Left to right
flow across
PFO
LA
RA
'PFO flap'
bowed
towards LA)
E
LA
RV
LV
Righ
Atrium
Left Atrium
Bidirectional
shunt across PFO
Tricuspid
regurgitatior
PFO
TAPSE - Tricuspid annular pan systolic excursion
Right Ventricle
Left Ventricle
Tie index using Tissue Doppler Imaging
IAS bowed
towards LA
A
RA
LA
LV
RV
Right Ventricular
hypertrophy and/or
dilation
Septal
deviation
to left
PAAT/RVET ratio
Regurgitation
Aorta
PDA
Pulmonary
Artery
Right-to-left
across PDA
G
MPA
PDA
B
Right ventricle
hypertrophy
IVS bowed
towards LV
LV
C
IVS bowed
towards LV
RV
LV
D
RV
IVS bowed
towards LV
LV

Fig. 5. Echocardiography images showing features on PPHN on 2D images. (*A*) Apical 4-chamber view (A4C) showing RV hypertrophy, interventricular septum (IVS) bowed toward LV and interatrial septum bowed toward LA. (*B*) Parasternal long axis view (PLAX) showing RV and IVS hypertrophy with bowing of IVS toward LV. (*C*) Parasternal short axis showing significant bowing of IVS toward LV due to suprasystemic pulmonary artery pressure. (*D*) PLAX view showing RV dilatation and hypertrophy with paradoxic septal movements in an infant with PPHN and RV failure. Echocardiography images showing estimation of PASP and shunts in PPHN are shown in (*E–H*). (*E*) Apical 4 chamber showing tricuspid regurgitation (TR) jet on color flow mapping. (*F*) Doppler assessment of TR velocity (Vmax 4 m/s), which equates to an estimated PASP of approximately 70 to 75 mm Hg. (*H*) PSAX view showing right-to-left shunt across PDA suggesting suprasystemic PASP. (*H*) Subcostal view showing bidirectional transatrial shunt across PFO (left-to-right blood flow direction seen on frozen image and "flap of PFO" bowed toward left atrium). Tricuspid annular pan systolic excursion (TAPSE) can assess RV function. Tei index using tissue Doppler imaging can be used to assess both right and left ventricular function. PAAT, pulmonary arterial acceleration time; RVET, right ventricular ejection time. (*Courtesy of* Satyan Lakshminrusimha and Yogen Singh.)

difficult to rule out in critically unwell infants, empirical antibiotic therapy for pneumonia or sepsis is required. Hyperventilation and infusion of alkali were used in the past but should be avoided because of adverse effects on cerebral perfusion and increased risk of sensorineural deafness.[55,56] Alkali infusion was associated with increased use of extracorporeal membrane oxygenation (ECMO) and need for oxygen

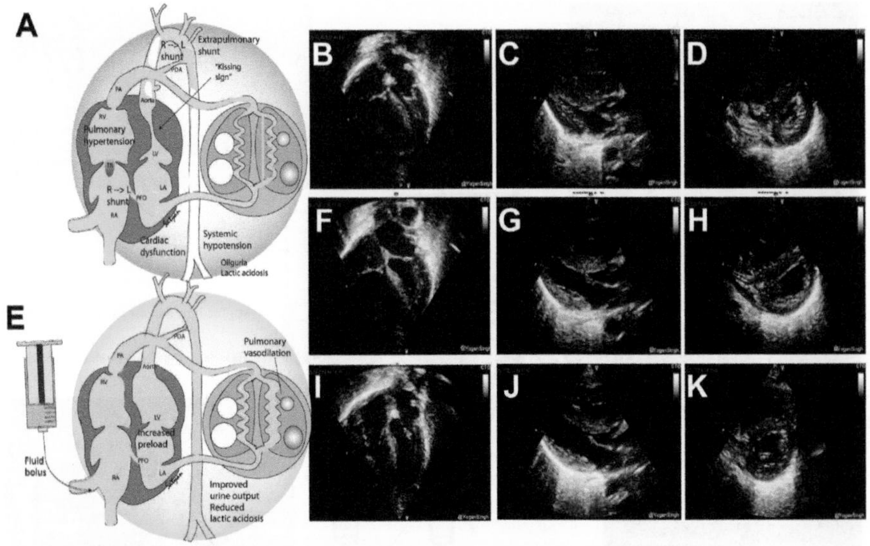
A
Extrapulmonary shunt
"Kissing sign"
Systemic hypotension
Oliguria
Lactic acidosis
E
Pulmonary vasodilation
preload
Fluid bolus
Improved urine output
Reduced lactic acidosis
B
C
D
F
G
H
I
J
K

Fig. 6. Serial echocardiography assessment showing rapid improvement in clinical condition in an infant with severe secondary PPHN due to sepsis. (*A*) Cardiopulmonary hemodynamics in an infant with high PVR and low SVR with intravascular hypovolemia. (*B–D*) Echocardiographic signs of PPHN and hypovolemia: RV hypertrophy, bowing of interventricular septum (IVS) toward LV, and "kissing sign" of hypovolemia in (*C*) with IVS touching LV free wall in parasternal long axis view (PLAX); when infant was needing maximum intensive care support showing hypovolemia. Image E shows effect of a fluid bolus and pulmonary vasodilator therapy. (*F–H*) Significant improvement in signs within 35 minutes after echocardiography targeted intervention (30 mL/kg fluid bolus) and optimizing "cardiocentric" management. (*I–K*) Taken 5 hours after (*B–D*), show marked improvement in PPHN echocardiography signs and hypovolemia, which was reflected in dramatic clinical improvement. (*Courtesy of* Satyan Lakshminrusimha and Yogen Singh.)

at 28 days.[2] Most centers continue to avoid acidosis based on animal studies that found exaggerated hypoxic pulmonary vasoconstriction with pH less than 7.25.[2,5] Maintaining pH greater than 7.25, preferably 7.30 to 7.40, during the acute phase of PPHN is recommended.

OXYGEN SATURATION TARGETS IN MANAGING INFANTS WITH PERSISTENT PULMONARY HYPERTENSION OF THE NEWBORN

The optimal Pao_2 in the management of PPHN is not clear. Wung and colleagues[57] have suggested that gentle ventilation with avoidance of hyperoxia and hyperventilation results in good outcomes for neonates with respiratory failure. In lamb studies with PPHN model, decreasing Pao_2 below 45 to 50 mm Hg results in increased PVR in newborn calves and lambs, and maintaining Pao_2 above 80 mm Hg does not result in any additional decrease in PVR.[46,47] Maintaining preductal oxygen saturations in the mid-90s appears to maximize the drop in PVR in the ductal ligation model of PPHN and meconium aspiration model of PPHN (**Fig. 7**). In summary, animal studies show that hypoxemia results in pulmonary vasoconstriction and normoxemia reduces PVR, but hyperoxemia does not enhance pulmonary vasodilation. Furthermore, ventilation with 100% oxygen in lambs with PPHN prevents the normal postnatal increase in eNOS expression in pulmonary arteries and increases PDE5 activity.[58] Randomized

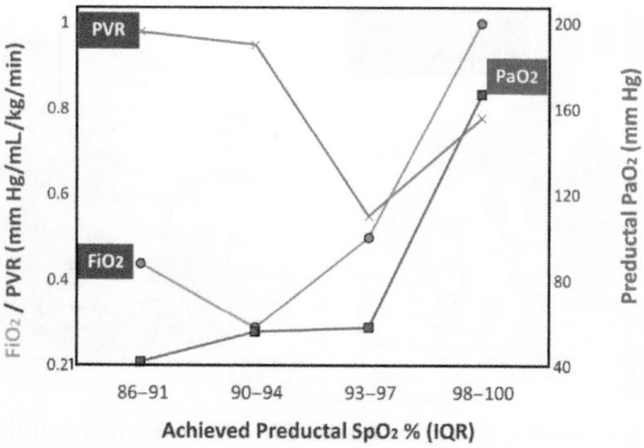
PVR
PaO2
FiO2
FiO2 / PVR (mm Hg/mL/kg/min)
Preductal PaO2 (mm Hg)
1
0.8
0.6
0.4
0.21
200
160
120
80
40
86–91
90–94
93–97
98–100
Achieved Preductal SpO2 % (IQR)

Fig. 7. Preductal oxygen saturation and PVR in lambs with meconium aspiration and pulmonary hypertension based on Rawat and colleagues[73] Term lambs with asphyxia, meconium aspiration, and pulmonary hypertension were randomized to preductal SpO_2 target of 85% to 89%, 90% to 94%, 95% to 99%, and fixed inspired oxygen at 100%. The achieved SpO_2, PVR in the left pulmonary circuit (in mm Hg/mL/kg/min), preductal Pao_2 (mm Hg), and Fio_2 are shown. Achieved SpO_2 interquartile range (IQR) are shown on the horizonal axis. Achieving preductal 93% to 97% SpO_2 resulted in lowest PVR; however, 90% to 94% SpO_2 was associated with lowest Fio_2 requirement. Targeting 85% to 89% SpO_2 was associated with high PVR. Fixed inspired Fio_2 of 1.0 resulted in median SpO_2 of 100% (IQR 96%–100%) with supraphysiological Pao_2 (mean 167 mm Hg). However, despite high Fio_2 and Pao_2, no further reduction in PVR was observed compared with 93% to 97% achieved SpO_2. (*Modified from* Rawat M, Chandrasekharan P, Gugino SF, Koenigsknecht C, Nielsen L, Wedgwood S, Mathew B, Nair J, Steinhorn R, Lakshminrusimha S. Optimal oxygen targets in term lambs with meconium aspiration syndrome and pulmonary hypertension. American Journal of Respiratory Cell and Molecular Biology. 2020 Oct;63(4):510-8.)

studies comparing different Pao_2 targets have not been conducted in infants with PPHN. Based on the current evidence from translational studies, it appears that avoiding both hyperoxia and hypoxia is critical.

MECHANICAL VENTILATION

Underinflation and overinflation of the lung will lead to elevation of PVR (**Fig. 8**A). Optimal lung recruitment (8–9 posterior-rib expansion on an inspiratory chest radiograph) decreases PVR. Gentle ventilation strategies with optimal positive end expiratory pressure, relatively low peak inflation pressure or tidal volume, and a degree of permissive hypercapnia are recommended to ensure adequate lung expansion while limiting barotrauma and volutrauma.[57] In newborns with severe lung disease, high-frequency (jet or oscillator) ventilation is frequently used to optimize lung inflation and minimize lung injury.[59] In clinical studies, the combination of high-frequency ventilation and iNO resulted in the greatest improvement in oxygenation in PPHN associated with diffuse parenchymal lung disease, such as RDS, MAS, and pneumonia, but had no benefit in idiopathic PPHN.[60]

SURFACTANT THERAPY

In patients with PPHN secondary to parenchymal lung disease, early administration of surfactant and lung recruitment is associated with better outcomes and reduced risk of ECMO or death (**Fig. 8**B).[61,62] A recent randomized trial of surfactant + iNO compared with iNO alone in PPHN showed less progression of hypoxemia and

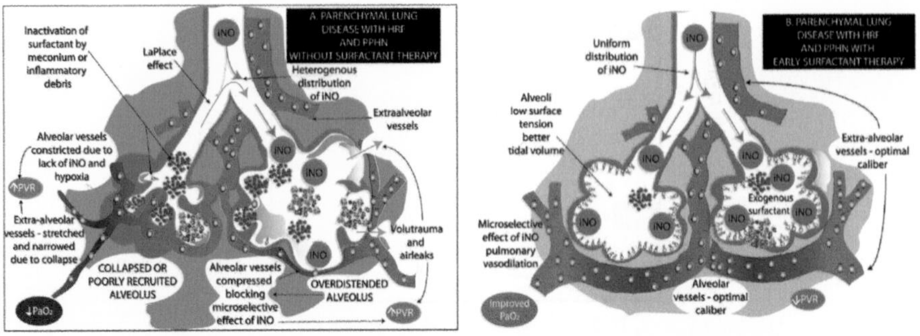
A. PARENCHYMAL LUNG DISEASE WITH HRF AND PPHN WITHOUT SURFACTANT THERAPY
Inactivation of surfactant by meconium or inflammatory debris
LaPlace effect
iNO
Heterogenous distribution of iNO
Extraalveolar vessels
Alveolar vessels constricted due to lack of iNO and hypoxia
↑PVR
Extra-alveolar vessels - stretched and narrowed due to collapse
COLLAPSED OR POORLY RECRUITED ALVEOLUS
Alveolar vessels compressed blocking microselective effect of iNO
OVERDISTENDED ALVEOLUS
Volutrauma and airleaks
↓PaO₂
B. PARENCHYMAL LUNG DISEASE WITH HRF AND PPHN WITH EARLY SURFACTANT THERAPY
Uniform distribution of iNO
Alveoli low surface tension better tidal volume
Extra-alveolar vessels - optimal caliber
Exogenous surfactant
Microselective effect of iNO pulmonary vasodilation
Alveolar vessels - optimal caliber
↓PVR
Improved PaO₂

Fig. 8. Effect of lung inflation, surfactant, and iNO on PVR. In conditions such as MAS and pneumonia, heterogeneous lung disease with surfactant deficiency leads to collapsed and overdistended alveoli (*A*). Underinflation or collapse compresses extraalveolar pulmonary vessels and prevents their access to oxygen and iNO causing high PVR (left-sided alveolus in [*A*]). Overdistended alveoli compress alveolar pulmonary vessels and prevent them from dilating in response to iNO and oxygen; overdistension increases the risk of airleak (right-sided alveolus in [*A*]). Following optimal lung recruitment and surfactant use, uniform distension of alveoli and optimal recruitment will allow oxygen and iNO to reach pulmonary vessels decreasing PVR and improving Pa_{O_2} (*B*). (*Modified from* Konduri GG, Lakshminrusimha S. Surf early to higher tides: surfactant therapy to optimize tidal volume, lung recruitment, and iNO response. Journal of Perinatology: Official Journal of the California Perinatal Association. 2020 Aug 13;with permission.)

reduced incidence of death/ECMO with surfactant use (**Fig. 9**). Surfactant inactivation and deficiency are observed in many neonatal respiratory disorders, such as MAS, pneumonia, and RDS. In infants with PPHN secondary to parenchymal lung disease, a dose of surfactant rich in surfactant protein B (such as calfactant or poractant alfa) is recommended.[5]

PULMONARY VASODILATOR THERAPY

Inhaled Nitric Oxide

iNO is a potent and selective pulmonary vasodilator; it is considered as the first-line therapy to decrease PVR in infants with PPHN needing mechanical ventilation. It is preferentially distributed to the ventilated segments of the lung, resulting in increased perfusion of the ventilated segments, optimizing ventilation-perfusion match (microselective effect of iNO) and a marked improvement in oxygenation in term newborns with PPHN.[61–63] Multicenter randomized clinical studies demonstrated that iNO therapy reduced the need for ECMO in term neonates with hypoxemic respiratory failure.[61,64,65] iNO is the only therapy approved by the US Food and Drug Administration for clinical use in term or near-term newborn infants (>34 weeks' gestation) with hypoxemic respiratory failure with clinical or echocardiographic evidence of PPHN.[5]

A dose of 20 ppm results in improved oxygenation and the most optimal decrease in pulmonary to systemic arterial pressure ratio[66] and is the typical starting dose. Higher doses are not recommended because they are associated with increased levels of nitrogen dioxide and methemoglobin.[63] iNO should be initiated early in the disease process to break the vicious cycle of PPHN; it should be commenced at a dose of 20 ppm if oxygenation index is approximately 20. An optimal response to iNO is defined as an increase in Pa_{O_2}/Fi_{O_2} ratio of 20 mm Hg or more (20–20–20 rule for initiation of iNO). However, in the presence of echocardiographic evidence of pulmonary hypertension,

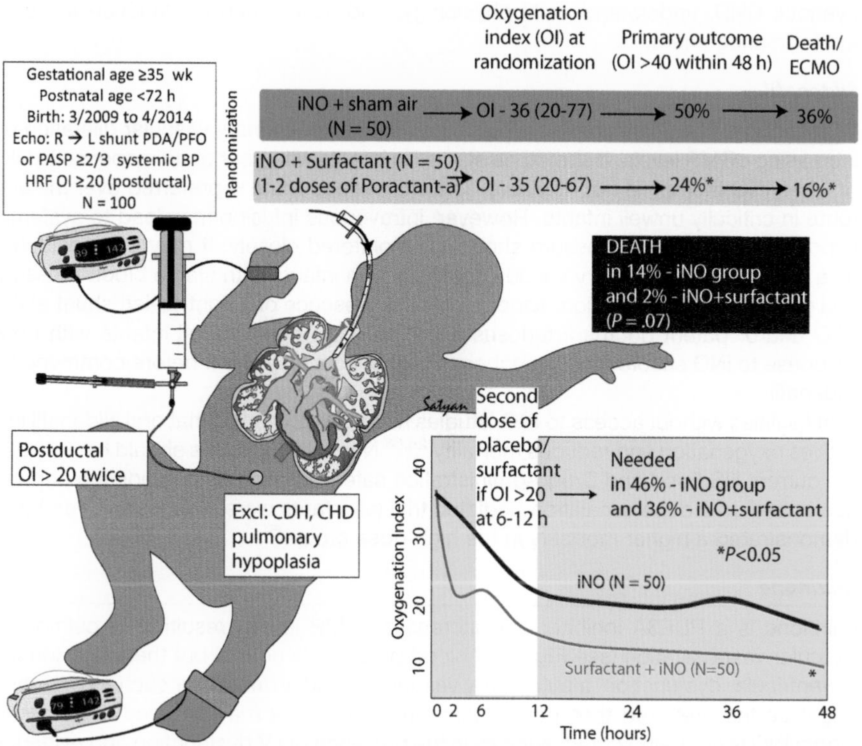
Oxygenation index (OI) at randomization
Primary outcome (OI >40 within 48 h)
Death/ ECMO
Gestational age ≥35 wk
Postnatal age <72 h
Birth: 3/2009 to 4/2014
Echo: R → L shunt PDA/PFO or PASP ≥2/3 systemic BP
HRF OI ≥20 (postductal)
N = 100
Randomization
iNO + sham air (N = 50)
OI - 36 (20-77)
50%
36%
iNO + Surfactant (N = 50)
(1-2 doses of Poractant-a)
OI - 35 (20-67)
24%*
16%*
DEATH
in 14% - iNO group
and 2% - iNO+surfactant
(P = .07)
Postductal
OI > 20 twice
Excl: CDH, CHD pulmonary hypoplasia
Second dose of placebo/ surfactant if OI >20 at 6-12 h
Needed
in 46% - iNO group
and 36% - iNO+surfactant
*P<0.05
iNO (N = 50)
Surfactant + iNO (N=50)
Oxygenation Index
Time (hours)

Fig. 9. Graphic abstract of randomized controlled trial of surfactant + iNO versus iNO only in infants with PPHN by González and colleagues.[74] Addition of surfactant to iNO resulted in reduced progression of hypoxemic respiratory failure (HRF), decreased incidence of ECMO/death, and more rapid reduction in oxygenation index (OI). (*Courtesy of* Satyan Lakshminrusimha.)

it should be commenced early without any delay. Methemoglobin levels should be monitored regularly, at 2 hours, 8 hours after initiation of iNO, and then once a day for the duration of iNO therapy,[5] although with most modern blood gas analyses it is almost always available.

Weaning iNO is a gradual process to minimize the risk of rebound vasoconstriction and resultant pulmonary hypertension associated with abrupt withdrawal. If there is good response to iNO, weaning should start 30 minutes after initiation, if inspired oxygen concentration is less than 60%, and then iNO is weaned only if Pa_{O_2} can be maintained at 60 mm Hg or higher (or preductal oxygen saturation as measured by pulse oximetry >90%) (30–60–90 rule of weaning iNO).[5] The authors' practice is to wean iNO by 5 ppm every 4 hours, and once iNO dose is 5 ppm, gradual weaning by 1 ppm every 2 to 4 hours is performed. Continuing iNO in infants unresponsive to iNO or failure to wean iNO can potentially lead to prolonged dependence on iNO due to suppression of endogenous eNOS.[67]

Ideally, all infants with PPHN should have an echocardiographic assessment before or soon after starting PPHN when available, but it should definitely be performed in iNO nonresponders or infants who deteriorate after starting iNO to rule out underlying cyanotic CHD, understand pathophysiology, and assess cardiac function to guide further management.

Sildenafil

Sildenafil is a PDE5 inhibitor (see **Fig. 3**) and causes pulmonary vascular dilatation by increasing cGMP levels. It should be started in infants with poor or no response to iNO or when iNO therapy is not available. The intravenous route is preferred over the oral route in critically unwell infants. However, intravenous infusion may lead to systemic hypotension, so blood pressure should be monitored closely. It may be considered as a second-line pulmonary vasodilator therapy in infants with stable blood pressure and good ventricular function, especially in the presence of a right-to-left shunt at the PFO and/or patent ductus arteriosus (PDA) levels.[5] Therefore, all infants with poor response to iNO should have an echocardiographic assessment before commencing sildenafil.

In facilities without access to iNO, studies have demonstrated that oral sildenafil improves oxygenation and reduces mortality.[26,68] Neonatal clinicians should be aware of the current US Food and Drug Administration safety warning in the pediatric population based on a dose escalation pediatric trial (all infants were older than 1 year) that demonstrated a higher mortality in the high-dose group.[69]

Milrinone

Milrinone is a PDE3A inhibitor and increases cAMP levels, resulting in pulmonary vascular vasodilatation (see **Fig. 3**). If blood pressure is normal but there is evidence of ventricular dysfunction, a pulmonary vasodilator and an inodilator such as milrinone might be the preferred therapeutic agent in PPHN.[5,36] It may be used in infants in whom iNO is contraindicated, such as in the presence of LV dysfunction and evidence

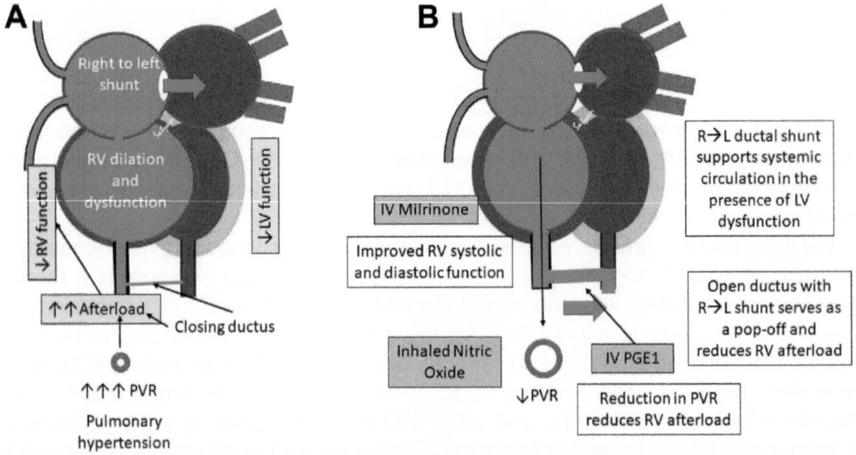
A
Right to left shunt
RV dilation and dysfunction
↓RV function
↓LV function
↑↑Afterload
Closing ductus
↑↑↑ PVR
Pulmonary hypertension
B
R→L ductal shunt supports systemic circulation in the presence of LV dysfunction
IV Milrinone
Improved RV systolic and diastolic function
Open ductus with R→L shunt serves as a pop-off and reduces RV afterload
Inhaled Nitric Oxide
IV PGE1
↓PVR
Reduction in PVR reduces RV afterload

Fig. 10. Cardiac pathophysiology in PPHN. (*A*) In severe PPHN, the PFO and PDA shunt right-to-left with IVS bulging to the left decreasing LV preload. Extremely high RV afterload leads to uncoupling of RV function leading to RV dilation. An open PDA might benefit the RV by providing a pop-off mechanism to reduce RV afterload. (*B*) iNO reduces PVR and reduces RV afterload and milrinone can improve RV function leading to synergy with ductal patency maintained by intravenous prostaglandin E1 (PGE1). (*Courtesy* of Satyan Lakshminrusimha.)

pulmonary venous hypertension from raised left atrial pressure or in iNO nonresponders.[33,36] It can be used as an adjunct therapy (**Fig. 10**). We recommend using intravenous infusion without loading dose in neonates because of the risk of systemic hypotension. Optimal cardiac filling may help in reducing the risk of hypotension and a 10 mL/kg fluid bolus may be given before commencing milrinone infusion, especially if decreased preload is suspected,[5] or stabilizing blood pressure with low dose of epinephrine before commencing milrinone infusion.

Prostacyclin

Alternate agents (not approved by the US Food and Drug Administration) for iNO-resistant PPHN include aerosolized prostaglandin E1 and inhaled prostaglandin I_2 (PGI_2).[30,70] The intravenous formulation epoprostenol carries a significant risk of systemic hypotension and is often avoided in critically unwell infants with PPHN. Iloprost is a synthetic prostacyclin that can also be delivered by aerosolization or by intravenous route, and it improves oxygenation in PPHN.[71]

ROLE OF PROSTAGLANDIN E1 IN MANAGEMENT OF PERSISTENT PULMONARY HYPERTENSION OF THE NEWBORN

Critically unwell infants with failing RV may benefit from a PDA, which can work as a "pop-off" valve in cases with severely elated PVR. In infants with a constricting PDA, prostaglandin E1 will open the ductus arteriosus and keep in patent. This will decrease the RV afterload by allowing right-to-left shunt[5] (see **Fig. 10**). In the authors' experience, prostaglandin E1 use should be guided by the echocardiography, and it would be specifically useful in infants with failing RV and a constricting ductus arteriosus.

SUPPORTING SYSTEMIC BLOOD PRESSURE

Hypotension in critically unwell infants with PPHN should be treated promptly and most clinicians, including the authors, would support systemic blood pressure with vasoactive medications such as epinephrine, norepinephrine, dobutamine, low-dose dopamine, or vasopressin.[5,13,72] Maintaining systemic pressure at a reasonable level (for example approximately 50 mm Hg in a term infant) may help in reversing shunt direction across ductus arteriosus, from right-to-left to left-to-right. This will increase PBF (and hence oxygenation and systemic end-organ perfusion) by increasing LV cardiac output. However, the authors do not recommend using a very high dose of vasoactive medications because all of these vasoactive medications have significant adverse effects profiles, especially at higher doses. Risks versus benefits should always be assessed. These medications should be weaned off as soon as possible and this can be guided by functional echocardiography. A detailed description of all the vasoactive medications is out of the scope of this article but their mechanisms and important hemodynamic effects are summarized in **Table 3**, along with an algorithm for PPHN management that is shown in **Fig. 11**.

ROLE OF EXTRACORPOREAL MEMBRANE OXYGENATION

Hypotension associated with cardiac dysfunction and rapid deterioration with hemodynamic instability should precipitate cannulation for ECMO. We recommend considering commencing ECMO or discussion with the ECMO center early in iNO nonresponders or those who continue to deteriorate despite the conventional therapy described previously.

Table 3
Commonly used vasoactive medications and pulmonary vasodilators in PPHN

Name of Drug	Dose	Site of Action	Hemodynamic Effects
Epinephrine	0.02–0.3 μg/kg/min 0.3–1 μg/kg/min	β1 and β2 receptors α1 receptors	Inotropic effects; Decrease SVR Vasopressor effects; Increase SVR
Norepinephrine	0.1–1 μg/kg/min	α1 and α2 receptors	Vasopressor effects; Increase SVR
Milrinone	0.25–0.75 μg/kg/min	Phosphodiesterase III inhibitor and effects at β1 and β2 receptors	Inodilator effects; Lusitropic effects; Increase contractility; Decrease SVR
Dobutamine	5–20 μg/kg/min	β1 and β2 receptors, some effect on α receptors	Inotropic effects; Decrease SVR; Increase cardiac output
Dopamine	1–4 μg/kg/min 4–10 μg/kg/min 11–20 μg/kg/min	Dopaminergic receptors 1 and 2 α receptors β receptors	Renal and mesenteric dilatation Inotropic effects Vasopressor, increase SVR and increase PVR
Hydrocortisone	1–2.5 mg/kg; 4–6 hourly		Uncertain - enhance sensitivity to catecholamines
Vasopressin	0.018–0.12 units/kg/h	Vasopressin 1 receptors	Increase SVR; No inotropic effect
Pulmonary vasodilators			
Inhaled nitric oxide	1–20 ppm	Selective pulmonary vasodilator	Decrease PVR
Sildenafil	IV: load of 0.42 mg/kg for 3 h followed by 1.6 mg/kg per day as a continuous maintenance infusion Oral: 1–2 mg/kg every 6 h	Phosphodiesterase (PDE) 5 inhibitor	Pulmonary and systemic vasodilator; Decreases PVR, decreases SVR
Synthetic prostacyclin (Iloprost)	Aerosolized: 1–2.5 mg/kg every 2–4 h IV 0.5–3 ng/kg per minute and titrated to 1–10 ng/kg per minute	Pulmonary vasodilator acting locally Pulmonary and systemic vasodilator	Decreases PVR Decreases SVR and hypotension
Prostacyclin I_2 (PGI_2)	Inhaled prostaglandin I2 at a dose of 50 ng/kg per minute	Pulmonary vasodilator acting locally	Decreases SVR

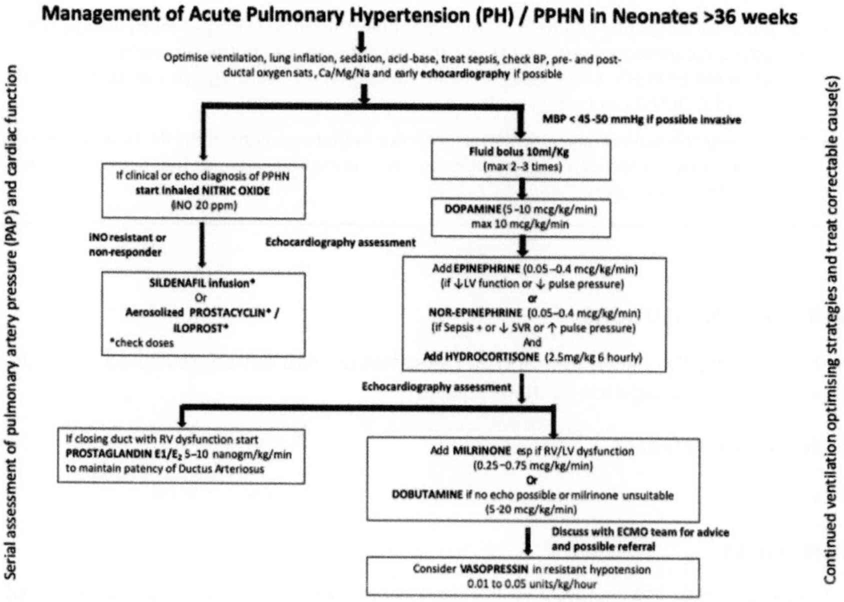
Management of Acute Pulmonary Hypertension (PH) / PPHN in Neonates >36 weeks
Optimise ventilation, lung inflation, sedation, acid-base, treat sepsis, check BP, pre- and post-ductal oxygen sats, Ca/Mg/Na and early echocardiography if possible
MBP < 45-50 mmHg if possible invasive
If clinical or echo diagnosis of PPHN start Inhaled NITRIC OXIDE (iNO 20 ppm)
Fluid bolus 10ml/Kg (max 2-3 times)
DOPAMINE (5-10 mcg/kg/min) max 10 mcg/kg/min
iNO resistant or non-responder
Echocardiography assessment
SILDENAFIL infusion* Or Aerosolized PROSTACYCLIN* / ILOPROST* *check doses
Add EPINEPHRINE (0.05–0.4 mcg/kg/min) (if ↓LV function or ↓ pulse pressure) or NOR-EPINEPHRINE (0.05–0.4 mcg/kg/min) (if Sepsis + or ↓ SVR or ↑ pulse pressure) And Add HYDROCORTISONE (2.5mg/kg 6 hourly)
Echocardiography assessment
If closing duct with RV dysfunction start PROSTAGLANDIN E1/E2 5–10 nanogm/kg/min to maintain patency of Ductus Arteriosus
Add MILRINONE esp if RV/LV dysfunction (0.25–0.75 mcg/kg/min) Or DOBUTAMINE if no echo possible or milrinone unsuitable (5-20 mcg/kg/min)
Discuss with ECMO team for advice and possible referral
Consider VASOPRESSIN in resistant hypotension 0.01 to 0.05 units/kg/hour
Serial assessment of pulmonary artery pressure (PAP) and cardiac function
Continued ventilation optimising strategies and treat correctable cause(s)

Fig. 11. An approach to management of PPHN in term or near-term infants. (*Courtesy of* Yogen Singh.)

SUMMARY

There has been a substantial gain in understanding of pathophysiology of PPHN over the past 2 decades, and biochemical pathways responsible for abnormal vasoconstriction of pulmonary vasculature are now better understood. Availability of bedside echocardiography establishes early diagnosis, provides an understanding of the pathophysiology and hemodynamic abnormalities, and allows for monitoring of the disease process and response to the therapeutic intervention in PPHN. There have been significant advances in the management of PPHN targeting biochemical pathways and hemodynamic instability. When available, iNO is the pulmonary vasodilator of choice. Clinical practice has shifted from hyperoxygenation-hyperventilation-alkalosis to improved gentle ventilation strategies to optimize lung recruitment and allow permissive hypercapnia, early use of iNO and surfactant therapy, and avoid hypoxia-hyperoxia. These changes have led to a substantial decrease in the number of infants with PPHN requiring ECMO for respiratory disorders. Newer pulmonary vasodilators, such as antioxidants (superoxide dismutase), soluble guanylate cyclase activators, and rho-kinase inhibitors, are promising but still under investigation and currently their use is limited to research studies. They may play an important role in targeting specific therapy in PPHN, especially in infants resistant to iNO.

CLINICS CARE POINTS

- In the management of PPHN, clinical practice has shifted from hyperoxygenation-hyperventilation-alkalosis to improved gentle ventilation strategies to optimize lung recruitment, allow permissive hypercarbia, early use of iNO and avoid hypoxia.

- Early echocardiography can help in understanding the underlying pathophysiology, detect hemodynamic abnormalities, and target specific therapy, key to the successful management of PPHN. Serial assessment on functional echocardiography or point of care ultrasound (POCUS) can help in evaluating response to therapy.
- iNO remains the pulmonary vasodilator of choice in management of PPHN. However, newer pulmonary vasodilators can play an important role in management of these cases, especially in the iNO resistant cases.

AUTHOR CONTRIBUTIONS

Y. Singh wrote the initial draft and S. Lakshminrusimha edited, reviewed, and added figures and figure legends to the article.

CONFLICT OF INTEREST

None.

REFERENCES

1. Gersony WM. Persistence of the fetal circulation: a commentary. J Pediatr 1972; 82(6):1103–6.
2. Walsh-Sukys MC, Tyson JE, Wright LL, et al. Persistent pulmonary hypertension of the newborn in the era before nitric oxide: practice variation and outcomes. Pediatrics 2000;105:14–20.
3. Kumar VH, Hutchison AA, Lakshminrusimha S, et al. Characteristics of pulmonary hypertension in preterm neonates. J Perinatol 2007;27(4):214–9.
4. Steinhorn RH. Neonatal pulmonary hypertension. Pediatr Crit Care Med 2010; 11(2):S79–84.
5. Lakshminrusimha S. Persistent pulmonary hypertension of the newborn. Neoreviews 2015;16(12):e680.
6. Martinho S, Adão R, Leite-Moreira AF, et al. Persistent pulmonary hypertension of the newborn: pathophysiological mechanisms and novel therapeutic approaches. Front Pediatr 2020;8:342.
7. Simonneau G, Gatzoulis MA, Adatia I, et al. Updated clinical classification of pulmonary hypertension. J Am Coll Cardiol 2013;62(25 Suppl):D34–41.
8. Steurer MA, Jelliffe-Pawlowski LL, Baer RJ, et al. Persistent pulmonary hypertension of the newborn in late preterm and term infants in California. Pediatrics 2017; 139(1):e20161165.
9. Singh Y, Tissot C. Echocardiographic evaluation of transitional circulation for the neonatologists. Front Pediatr 2018;6:140.
10. Singh Y. Echocardiographic evaluation of hemodynamics in neonates and children. Front Pediatr 2017;5:201.
11. Abman SH, Hansmann G, Archer SL, et al. Pediatric pulmonary hypertension: guidelines from the American Heart Association and American Thoracic Society. Circulation 2015;132(21):2037–99.
12. Nair J, Lakshminrusimha S. Update on PPHN: mechanisms and treatment. Semin Perinatol 2014;38(2):78–91.
13. Gupta S, Singh Y. Hemodynamic assessment in hypoxic-ischaemic encephalopathy. In: Seri I, Martin K, editors. Hemodynamics and cardiology: neonatology questions and controversies. 3rd edition. Philadelphia: Elsevier; 2018.

14. Kinsella JP, Steinhorn RH, Mullen MP, et al, Pediatric Pulmonary Hypertension Network (PPHNet). The left ventricle in congenital diaphragmatic hernia: implications for the management of pulmonary hypertension. J Pediatr 2018;197:17–22.
15. Alano MA, Ngougmna E, Ostrea EM Jr, et al. Analysis of nonsteroidal antiinflammatory drugs in meconium and its relation to persistent pulmonary hypertension of the newborn. Pediatrics 2001;107:519–23.
16. Levin DL, Mills LJ, Parkey M, et al. Constriction of the fetal ductus arteriosus after administration of indomethacin to the pregnant ewe. J Pediatr 1979;94:647–50.
17. Chambers CD, Hernandez-Diaz S, Van Marter LJ, et al. Selective serotonin-reuptake inhibitors and risk of persistent pulmonary hypertension of the newborn. N Engl J Med 2006;354:579–87.
18. Fornaro E, Li D, Pan J, et al. Prenatal exposure to fluoxetine induces fetal pulmonary hypertension in the rat. Am J Respir Crit Care Med 2007;176:1035–40.
19. Steinhorn RH, Russell JA, Morin FC. Disruption of cGMP production in pulmonary arteries isolated from fetal lambs with pulmonary hypertension. Am J Physiol 1995;268:H1483–9.
20. de Buys Roessingh A, Fouquet V, Aigrain Y, et al. Nitric oxide activity through guanylate cyclase and phosphodiesterase modulation is impaired in fetal lambs with congenital diaphragmatic hernia. J Pediatr Surg 2011;46(8):1516–22.
21. Fineman JR, Wong J, Morin FC III, et al. Chronic nitric oxide inhibition in utero produces persistent pulmonary hypertension in newborn lambs. J Clin Invest 1994; 93(6):2675–83.
22. Villanueva ME, Zaher FM, Svinarich DM, et al. Decreased gene expression of endothelial nitric oxide synthase in newborns with persistent pulmonary hypertension. Pediatr Res 1998;44(3):338–43.
23. Pearson DL, Dawling S, Walsh WF, et al. Neonatal pulmonary hypertension—urea-cycle intermediates, nitric oxide production, and carbamoyl-phosphate synthetase function. N Engl J Med 2001;344(24):1832–8.
24. Steinhorn RH, Morin FC III, Fineman JR. Models of persistent pulmonary hypertension of the newborn (PPHN) and the role of cyclic guanosine monophosphate (GMP) in pulmonary vasorelaxation. Semin Perinatol 1997;21(5):393–408.
25. Farrow KN, Groh BS, Schumacker PT, et al. Hyperoxia increases phosphodiesterase 5 expression and activity in ovine fetal pulmonary artery smooth muscle cells. Circ Res 2008;102(2):226–33.
26. Baquero H, Soliz A, Neira F, et al. Oral sildenafil in infants with persistent pulmonary hypertension of the newborn: a pilot randomized blinded study. Pediatrics 2006;117(4):1077–83.
27. Steinhorn RH, Kinsella JP, Pierce C, et al. Intravenous sildenafil in the treatment of neonates with persistent pulmonary hypertension. J Pediatr 2009;155(6):841–7.
28. Mourani PM, Sontag MK, Ivy DD, et al. Effects of long-term sildenafil treatment for pulmonary hypertension in infants with chronic lung disease. J Pediatr 2009; 154(3):379–84, 384.e1-2.
29. Lakshminrusimha S, Porta NF, Farrow KN, et al. Milrinone enhances relaxation to prostacyclin and iloprost in pulmonary arteries isolated from lambs with persistent pulmonary hypertension of the newborn. Pediatr Crit Care Med 2009;10(1): 106–12.
30. Kelly LK, Porta NF, Goodman DM, et al. Inhaled prostacyclin for term infants with persistent pulmonary hypertension refractory to inhaled nitric oxide. J Pediatr 2002;141(6):830–2.

31. Soditt V, Aring C, Groneck P. Improvement of oxygenation induced by aerosolized prostacyclin in a preterm infant with persistent pulmonary hypertension of the newborn. Intensive Care Med 1997;23(12):1275–8.
32. Ehlen M, Wiebe B. Iloprost in persistent pulmonary hypertension of the newborn. Cardiol Young 2003;13(4):361–3.
33. McNamara PJ, Shivananda SP, Sahni M, et al. Pharmacology of milrinone in neonates with persistent pulmonary hypertension of the newborn and suboptimal response to inhaled nitric oxide. Pediatr Crit Care Med 2013;14(1):74–84.
34. Busch CJ, Graveline AR, Jiramongkolchai K, et al. Phosphodiesterase 3A expression is modulated by nitric oxide in rat pulmonary artery smooth muscle cells. J Physiol Pharmacol 2010;61(6):663–9.
35. Bassler D, Choong K, McNamara P, et al. Neonatal persistent pulmonary hypertension treated with milrinone: four case reports. Biol Neonate 2006;89(1):1–5.
36. Lakshminrusimha S, Steinhorn RH. Inodilators in nitric oxide resistant persistent pulmonary hypertension of the newborn. Pediatr Crit Care Med 2013;14(1):107–9.
37. Perreault T, Coceani F. Endothelin in the perinatal circulation. Can J Physiol Pharmacol 2003;81(6):644–53.
38. Mann J, Farrukh IS, Michael JR. Mechanisms by which endothelin 1 induces pulmonary vasoconstriction in the rabbit. J Appl Physiol (1985) 1991;71(2):410–6.
39. Ivy DD, Kinsella JP, Abman SH. Physiologic characterization of endothelin A and B receptor activity in the ovine fetal pulmonary circulation. J Clin Invest 1994;93(5):2141–8.
40. Ivy DD, Parker TA, Ziegler JW, et al. Prolonged endothelin A receptor blockade attenuates chronic pulmonary hypertension in the ovine fetus. J Clin Invest 1997;99(6):1179–86.
41. Mohamed WA, Ismail M. A randomized, double-blind, placebo-controlled, prospective study of bosentan for the treatment of persistent pulmonary hypertension of the newborn. J Perinatol 2012;32(8):608–11.
42. Steinhorn RH, Fineman J, Kusic-Pajic A, et al. Bosentan as adjunctive therapy for persistent pulmonary hypertension of the newborn: results of the FUTURE-4 study. Circulation 2014;130:A13503.
43. Brennan LA, Steinhorn RH, Wedgwood S, et al. Increased superoxide generation is associated with pulmonary hypertension in fetal lambs: a role for NADPH oxidase. Circ Res 2003;92(6):683–91.
44. Konduri GG, Bakhutashvili I, Eis A, et al. Oxidant stress from uncoupled nitric oxide synthase impairs vasodilation in fetal lambs with persistent pulmonary hypertension. Am J Physiol Heart Circ Physiol 2007;292(4):H1812–20.
45. Farrow KN, Wedgwood S, Lee KJ, et al. Mitochondrial oxidant stress increases PDE5 activity in persistent pulmonary hypertension of the newborn. Respir Physiolo Neurobiol 2010;174(3):272–81.
46. Rudolph AM, Yuan S. Response of the pulmonary vasculature to hypoxia and H+ ion concentration changes. J Clin Invest 1996;45(3):399–411.
47. Lakshminrusimha S, Swartz DD, Gugino SF, et al. Oxygen concentration and pulmonary hemodynamics in newborn lambs with pulmonary hypertension. Pediatr Res 2009;66(5):539–44.
48. Lakshminrusimha S, Steinhorn RH, Wedgwood S, et al. Pulmonary hemodynamics and vascular reactivity in asphyxiated term lambs resuscitated with 21 and 100% oxygen. J Appl Physiol (1985) 2011;111(5):1441–7.
49. Singh Y, Chee YH, Gahlaut R. Evaluation of suspected congenital heart disease. Paediatr Child Health 2014;25(1):7–12.

50. Singh Y. Evaluation of a child with suspected congenital heart disease. Paediatrics Child Health 2018;28(12):556–61.
51. Park MK. Paediatric cardiology for practitioners. Philadelphia: Mosby Elsevier; 2008. p. 151e2.
52. Lang RM, Bierig M, Devereux RB, et al. Recommendations for chamber quantification: a report from the American Society of Echocardiography's guidelines and standards committee and the chamber quantification writing group, developed in conjunction with the European Association of Echocardiography, a branch of the European Society of Cardiology. J Am Soc Echocardiogr 2005;18:1440–63.
53. Singh Y, Tissot C, Fraga M, et al. International evidence-based guidelines on Point of Care Ultrasound (POCUS) for critically ill neonates and children issued by the POCUS Working Group of the European Society of Paediatric and Neonatal Intensive Care (ESPNIC). Crit Care 2020;24:65.
54. de Boode WP, Singh Y, Molnar Z, et al, European Special Interest Group 'Neonatologist Performed Echocardiography' (NPE). Application of neonatologist performed echocardiography in the assessment and management of persistent pulmonary hypertension of the newborn. Pediatr Res 2018;84(Suppl 1):68–77.
55. Bifano EM, Pfannenstiel A. Duration of hyperventilation and outcome in infants with persistent pulmonary hypertension. Pediatrics 1988;81(5):657–61.
56. Hendricks-Muñoz KD, Walton JP. Hearing loss in infants with persistent fetal circulation. Pediatrics 1988;81(5):650–6.
57. Wung JT, James LS, Kilchevsky E, et al. Management of infants with severe respiratory failure and persistence of the fetal circulation, without hyperventilation. Pediatrics 1985;76(4):488–94.
58. Farrow KN, Lakshminrusimha S, Reda WJ, et al. Superoxide dismutase restores eNOS expression and function in resistance pulmonary arteries from neonatal lambs with persistent pulmonary hypertension. Am J Physiol Lung Cell Mol Physiol 2008;295(6):L979–87.
59. Kinsella JP, Abman SH. Clinical approaches to the use of high- frequency oscillatory ventilation in neonatal respiratory failure. J Perinatol 1996;16(2):S52–5.
60. Kinsella JP, Truog WE, Walsh WF, et al. Randomized, multicenter trial of inhaled nitric oxide and high-frequency oscillatory ventilation in severe, persistent pulmonary hypertension of the newborn. J Pediatr 1997;131(1):55–62.
61. Konduri GG, Sokol GM, Van Meurs KP, et al. Impact of early surfactant and inhaled nitric oxide therapies on outcomes in term/late preterm neonates with moderate hypoxic respiratory failure. J Perinatol 2013;33(12):944–9.
62. Lotze A, Mitchell BR, Bulas DI, et al, Survanta in Term Infants Study Group. Multicenter study of surfactant (Beractant) use in the treatment of term infants with severe respiratory failure. J Pediatr 1998;132(1):40–7.
63. Davidson D, Barefield ES, Kattwinkel J, et al, The I-NO/PPHN Study Group. Inhaled nitric oxide for the early treatment of persistent pulmonary hypertension of the term newborn: a random- ized, double-masked, placebo-controlled, dose-response, multicenter study. Pediatrics 1998;101(3):325–34.
64. Clark RH, Kueser TJ, Walker MW, et al, Clinical Inhaled Nitric Oxide Research Group. Low-dose nitric oxide therapy for persistent pulmonary hypertension of the newborn. N Engl J Med 2000;342(7):469–74.
65. Roberts JD Jr, Fineman JR, Morin FC III, et al, The Inhaled Nitric Oxide Study Group. Inhaled nitric oxide and persistent pulmonary hypertension of the newborn. N Engl J Med 1997;336(9):605–10.
66. Tworetzky W, Bristow J, Moore P, et al. Inhaled nitric oxide in neonates with persistent pulmonary hypertension. Lancet 2001;357(9250):118–20.

67. Sokol GM, Fineberg NS, Wright LL, et al. Changes in arterial oxygen tension when weaning neonates from inhaled nitric oxide. Pediatr Pulmonol 2001;32(1):14–9.
68. Vargas-Origel A, Gomez-Rodriguez G, Aldana-Valenzuela C, et al. The use of sildenafil in persistent pulmonary hypertension of the newborn. Am J Perinatol 2009;27(3):225–30.
69. Abman SH, Kinsella JP, Rosenzweig EB, et al, Pediatric Pulmonary Hypertension Network (PPHNet). Implications of the U.S. Food and Drug Administration warning against the use of sildenafil for the treatment of pediatric pulmonary hypertension. Am J Respir Crit Care Med 2013;187(6):572–5.
70. Kahveci H, Yilmaz O, Avsar UZ, et al. Oral sildenafil and inhaled iloprost in the treatment of pulmonary hypertension of the newborn. Pediatr Pulmonol 2014; 49(12):1205–13.
71. Janjindamai W, Thatrimontrichai A, Maneenil G, et al. Effectiveness and safety of intravenous iloprost for severe persistent pulmonary hypertension of the newborn. Indian Pediatr 2013;50(10):934–8.
72. Singh Y, Katheria AC, Vora F. Advances in diagnosis and management of hemodynamic instability in neonatal shock. Front Pediatr 2018;6:2.
73. Rawat M, Chandrasekharan P, Gugino SF, et al. Optimal oxygen targets in term lambs with meconium aspiration syndrome and pulmonary hypertension. Am J Respir Cell Mol Biol 2020;63(4):510–8.
74. González A, Bancalari A, Osorio W, et al. Early use of combined exogenous surfactant and inhaled nitric oxide reduces treatment failure in persistent pulmonary hypertension of the newborn: a randomized controlled trial. J Perinatol 2021; 41:32–8.

Sudden Unexpected Infant Death

Keeping the Newborn Safe in Hospital and at Home

Ann Kellams, MD, IBCLC[a,*], Lori Feldman-Winter, MD, MPH[b]

KEYWORDS

• Safe sleep • Breastfeeding • SUID • SIDS • Prevention • Quality improvement

KEY POINTS

- Safe sleep practices and breastfeeding decrease the risk of sudden unexpected infant death.
- Counseling and support for these practices begins prenatally and continues through at least the first 6 months.
- Maternity care practices must include modeling safe sleep strategies while optimally supporting the initiation of breastfeeding.
- A conversational approach to counseling and educating can help tailor advice using trusted relationships and troubleshoot barriers in order to improve adherence.

INTRODUCTION

Definition and Prevalence of Sudden Unexpected Infant Death

Sudden unexpected infant death (SUID), defined in 2006, is the combination of primarily sleep-related deaths during infancy that are due to (1) sudden infant death syndrome (SIDS), (2) accidental suffocation or strangulation in bed (or any other location) (ASSB), and (3) ill-defined or other unknown causes.[1,2]

Key points

These sleep-related deaths are the most common reason for postneonatal mortality and contribute to about 3500 deaths annually in the United States, as tracked by the Centers for Disease Control and Prevention (CDC).[3]

In 2018, there were about 1300 deaths due to SIDS, about 1300 deaths due to unknown causes, and about 800 deaths due to accidental suffocation and strangulation in bed in the United States. SUID rates in the United States have plateaued over the

[a] Department of Pediatrics, University of Virginia, PO Box 800386, Charlottesville, VA 22908, USA; [b] Children's Regional Hospital at Cooper University Healthcare, Cooper Medical School of Rowan University, Three Cooper Plaza Suite 200, Camden, NJ 08103, USA

* Corresponding author.

E-mail address: Alk9c@virginia.edu

Clin Perinatol 48 (2021) 619–630

https://doi.org/10.1016/j.clp.2021.05.010

perinatology.theclinics.com

past few decades, after a steep decline that followed the "Back to Sleep campaign. Although SIDS rates may seem to be declining over the past several decades, SUID rates are stagnant because many SIDS deaths in recent years have been reclassified as ASSB and unknown causes, a trend known as a diagnostic shift.[1,3] Given that the United States has the highest rate of SUID among developed countries around the world, it is important to identify risk factors and special populations that provide opportunities to save infant lives.

Risk Factors for Sudden Unexpected Infant Death

One of the most impactful interventions to decrease SIDS and SUID in the United States, beginning around the 1990s,[4] has been supine sleep. This practice was widely promoted in the "Back to Sleep" campaign initiated in 1994 by a collaboration between the National Institute of Child Health and Development, the American Academy of Pediatrics (AAP), the Maternal and Child Health Bureau of the Health Resources and Services Administration, and SIDS prevention advocacy groups. The success of the campaign led to a subsequent decline in SIDS/SUID in the United States. Despite this success, there continue to be opportunities to increase adherence and decrease disparities in this practice.

In addition to nonsupine sleeping, several risk factors have been identified as being associated with SUID. Smoking is one of the most impactful risk factors for SUID. This risk is most significant for maternal smoking while pregnant, but maternal smoking after birth and more general tobacco exposure also increase the risk of SUID.[5,6] Some estimate that up to one-third of infant mortality due to SIDS can be prevented by eliminating maternal smoking during pregnancy alone. Soft bedding, loose blankets, or bumper pads, as well as other objects in the crib and sleep surfaces other than an approved crib or bassinet have been associated with SUID. Sleeping on a sofa or arm chair may be the most hazardous location for infant sleep.[7] The crib or bassinet should be one that is approved by the Consumer Product Safety Commission and used in a manner consistent with safe sleep recommendations.[3] One alternative to a detached crib or bassinet that may facilitate breastfeeding is a bassinet that attaches to the side of the adult bed, making access to the infant easier for nighttime nursing.

Bedsharing is another risk factor for SUID and may be especially important from 1 to 4 months of age, the time frame with the highest risk of SUID. This risk factor is often confounded by the evidence that breastfeeding, a protective factor for SIDS, is often practiced with bedsharing. Others have argued that smoking, low socioeconomic status, and even sleep position confound the risk of bedsharing, particularly among nonbreastfeeding infants. There are conflicting studies examining the risk of bedsharing in the breastfeeding, nonsmoking, and "no other risk" population; however, the evidence suggests this risk cannot be eliminated.[8,9] Therefore, the AAP recommends room sharing without bedsharing for all infants and the use of counseling strategies to achieve both practices.[10]

Key points

- Risk Factors for SUID Include
  - Nonsupine sleep
  - Not breastfeeding
  - Maternal smoking during pregnancy
  - Newborn passive smoke exposure
  - Soft bedding, loose blankets, or bumper pads, as well as other objects in the crib
  - Sleep location other than an approved infant crib or bassinette

Sleep location on a couch, sofa, or padded armchair
Sharing a sleep surface with an adult, child, or pet
Infant aged 1 to 4 months
Overheating or overbundling

Breastfeeding is Protective Against Sudden Infant Death Syndrome

Breastfeeding is associated with as much as a 60% reduced risk of SIDS if breastfeeding continues for 6 months or more.[11] Therefore, strategies to integrate breastfeeding promotion and support, along with safe infant sleep, have been adopted to further decrease the rate of SUID.

Many Do Not Adhere to Safe Sleep and Breastfeeding Recommendations

Not all mothers successfully achieve all of the safe sleep and breastfeeding recommendations. In a nationally representative sample, fewer than half reported that they were exclusively placing their infants on their back to sleep, and only 43.7% of mothers both intended to and then actually placed their infants exclusively in a supine position for sleep.[12] In addition, the same study revealed that only 45.4% of mothers both intended to and then practiced room sharing without bedsharing.[13]

Breastfeeding rates are also suboptimal. The CDC publishes an annual Breastfeeding Report Card, which demonstrates for those infants born in 2017 that although 84% initiate breastfeeding, less than half are breastfeeding exclusively at 3 months, and only one-quarter are exclusively breastfeeding at 6 months. Notably, almost 20% of breastfed infants in the United States have already received infant formula by 2 days of age.[14] It is essential that any interventions that target at helping mothers intend and achieve adherence to both safe sleep and breastfeeding recommendations in order to reduce the risk of SUID for their infants.

There are many opportunities to improve safe sleep and increase rates of breastfeeding. In a national study of 32 hospitals and more than 3000 mothers, published in 2017, only 77.3% usually used the supine position for sleep; however, merely 49.2% used the supine position all of the time.[12] Furthermore, mothers with lower levels of education and African American mothers were least likely to use the supine sleep position. Practice patterns were strongly correlated with maternal attitudes, subjective norms, and mostly with perceived control, all stemming from the theory of planned behavior. Moreover, African Americans are more likely than ever to practice bedsharing, even if not breastfeeding.[15] In addition to African Americans, more Native American/Alaskan Natives and younger mothers choose bedsharing over other sleep arrangements.[16]

Breastfeeding must persist for at least 2 months for it to be protective against SIDS, yet in the United States the rates of breastfeeding among all groups fall precipitously during the first few months after birth. Factors such as avoidance of in-hospital supplementation[17]; the Baby-Friendly Hospital initiative[18]; peer-support in hospital, in the community, or on-line[18–20]; and workplace support[21] may help women achieve their breastfeeding goals and offset the risk of SIDS for their infants. Longer breastfeeding and exclusive breastfeeding provide additional protection.[11,22]

Racial and Ethnic Disparities in Sudden Unexpected Infant Death and Breastfeeding

Racial and ethnic disparities in SUID have been apparent because the United States has been tracking these data. SUID rates per 100,000 live births for American Indian/Alaska Native (215.8) and non-Hispanic black infants (186.5) were more than twice those of non-Hispanic white infants (85.4), whereas SUID rates per 100,000 live births were lowest among Hispanic (53.8) and Asian/Pacific Islander infants (33.5). It is unclear what underpins these disparities; however, risk factors such as prone sleeping and exposure to tobacco and protective factors such as breastfeeding may be at least partly responsible.

Non-Hispanic black women have the lowest rates of breastfeeding in the United States.[14] Compared with white infants, black infants were 15 percentage points lower for any breastfeeding at age 3 months (58.0% vs 72.7%), 17 percentage points lower for any breastfeeding at 6 months (44.7% vs 62.9%), and 12 percentage points lower for exclusive breastfeeding at 6 months (17.2% vs 29.5%).[23]

Key points

- To decrease SUID, programs must be inclusive and equitable for all race/ethnicities.
- To increase breastfeeding mothers must have access to optimal maternity care and newborn practices, peer and community support, and workplace accommodations including paid leave.
- Mothers can achieve both their personal breastfeeding goals and practice safe sleep.

Timing of Sudden Unexpected Infant Death

About 90% of SUID occurs in the first 6 months, 72% between 1 and 4 months,[24,25] and most of those deaths occur between 2 and 3 months. Although a minority of SUID occur in the neonatal period, merely 3.3% during the first week after birth,[25] practices and policies in the birth hospital can contribute to offsetting postneonatal SUID. Infant deaths during the first week, and more commonly in the first few days, are commonly referred to as sudden unexpected postnatal collapse (SUPC); however, there is no International Classification of Diseases, 10th Revision (ICD-10) code for SUPC or SUID. SUID combines codes for SIDS (R95), deaths from other ill-defined or unknown causes (R99), and accidental suffocation and strangulation in bed (W75). SUPC deaths are often coded within SUID deaths, even though the causes may be distinct from SUID and include conditions related to pregnancy and delivery.[25] Researchers have attempted to distinguish these early neonatal deaths by adding another term "sudden unexpected early neonatal death" (SUEND), yet there is no ICD-10 code for SUEND either.

Most of the SUID cases during the first week are classified as ill-defined or unknown (67%) compared with postperinatal SUID (7 days to 1 year) when most of the deaths are due to SIDS (55%).[25] Further evidence shows that there may be different causes of SUID among younger infants who die: prenatal smoking and being economically disadvantaged. Older infants who succumb are more likely to have been low birth weight, born prematurely, and spent time in the neonatal intensive care unit. Thus, opportunities to offset SUID risk begins before delivery and spans the prenatal period, as well as potentially into the preconception period.

Prenatal Preventive Strategies

Prenatal discussions such as smoking cessation and avoidance, preparing for safe infant sleep, and breastfeeding initiation as well as achieving one's own personal goals for breastfeeding continuation are enhanced when the maternal care provider, such as the obstetrician, either initiates or at least validates these important messages. Advice from health care providers has been shown to positively influence adherence to both safe sleep and breastfeeding recommendations[26]; however, only about one-third of mothers reported that their doctors discussed these topics with them as part of their routine care.[12]

Attitudes and social norms have been shown to play an extremely important role in changing infant care practices.[13,27] Innovative interventions that highlight both the recommendations as well as the reasoning behind them have also been shown to be helpful, such as one study using a mobile health intervention improved adherence to safe sleep infant care practices, namely supine sleep, room sharing without bed-sharing, and no soft bedding use.[28]

Expectant parents also need evidence-based advice about how to prepare for a newborn and what products are safe and/or recommended. Unfortunately, overadvertised products such as bumper pads, thick, fluffy receiving blankets, infant sleep positioners, large stuffed animals pictured with newborns cuddling them on the package, and images of baby bottles versus images of breastfeeding remain common, available in stores, and in the media. A simple list of useful items that are considered safe may help families avoid unsafe or questionable products and save their money for essential items such as diapers and clothing.

Key points

- Many infant products are purchased before the baby is born; prenatal conversations about breastfeeding and safe infant sleep are paramount during this time frame.
  - List of RECOMMENDED infant care products:
    - Crib and/or bassinette with firm mattress
    - Bassinet that attaches to adult bed
    - Thin, cotton receiving blankets for swaddling and/or one-piece sleepers or sleep sacks
    - Pacifiers
    - Tightly-fitted crib sheets
    - Diapers
    - Disposable wipes or washable cloths for diaper area
    - Onesies or shirts/pants for layering
  - List of infant care products to AVOID
    - Fluffy, thick, or nonbreathable receiving blankets
    - Pillows
    - Stuffed animals
    - Infant sleep positioners
    - Infant sleeping products other than cribs or bassinettes*
    - Bumper pads
    - Crib comforters or quilts

*Note: infant sleep spaces should always be flat and firm and items such as bouncy seats, car seats, swings, sheep skins, or breastfeeding pillows should not be used for infant sleeping. Sleeping infants should always be flat and on their backs.

In-Hospital Preventive Strategies

The birth hospital provides multiple opportunities to model a safe sleep environment and at the same time may pose challenges that can compromise safety. Because experiences while at the birth hospital can affect breastfeeding, and because breastfeeding has the potential to mitigate against the risk of SUID, hospital practices supportive of breastfeeding are paramount. Accordingly the AAP has endorsed the World Health Organization's (WHO) Ten Steps to Successful Breastfeeding as a bundle of care practices that increases the likelihood of breastfeeding initiation and duration. The CDC, since 2007, monitors implementation of the Ten Steps with a universal hospital survey, entitled Maternity Practices in Infant Nutrition and Care.

Practices such as immediate and uninterrupted skin-to-skin care (SSC) after delivery, and rooming-in throughout the birth hospital stay, increase overall and exclusive breastfeeding initiation.[18,29] However, these practices have also raised concerns about safe infant sleep.[30,31]

Key points

WHO Ten Steps to Successful Breastfeeding[32]

Critical management procedures

1a. Comply fully with the International Code of Marketing of Breast-milk Substitutes and relevant World Health Assembly resolutions.
1b. Have a written infant feeding policy that is routinely communicated to staff and parents.
1c. Establish ongoing monitoring and data management systems.
2. Ensure that staff have sufficient knowledge, competence, and skills to support breastfeeding.

Key clinical practices

3. Discuss the importance and management of breastfeeding with pregnant women and their families.
4. Facilitate immediate and uninterrupted skin-to-skin contact and support mothers to initiate breastfeeding as soon as possible after birth.
5. Support mothers to initiate and maintain breastfeeding and manage common difficulties.
6. Do not provide breastfed newborns any food or fluids other than breast milk, unless medically indicated.
7. Enable mothers and their infants to remain together and to practice rooming-in 24 hours a day.
8. Support mothers to recognize and respond to their infants' cues for feeding.
9. Counsel mothers on the use and risks of feeding bottles, teats, and pacifiers.
10. Coordinate discharge so that parents and their infants have timely access to ongoing support and care.

Nevertheless, despite a nationwide increase in hospitals adopting SSC as a safe and optimal standard of care, there has not been an increase in neonatal SUID or SUPC as discussed earlier. The AAP provides guidance on best practices for SSC, such as continuous observational monitoring during the period immediately following delivery, as well as safety standards for rooming-in to avoid bedsharing and infant falls. These guidelines have been further disseminated through the guidelines and evaluation criteria developed by the institution responsible for designating hospital compliance with the Ten Steps, Baby-Friendly USA, as part of the US Baby-Friendly Hospital Initiative.[33]

Key points

AAP Best Practices for Skin-to-Skin Care[34]

Components of safe positioning for the newborn while in skin-to-skin contact:

- Infant's face can be seen
- Infant's head is in "sniffing" position
- Infant's nose and mouth are not covered
- Infant's head is turned to one side
- Infant's neck is straight, not bent
- Infant's shoulders and chest face mother
- Infant's legs are flexed

- Infant's back is covered with blankets
- Mother-infant dyad is monitored continuously by staff in the delivery environment and regularly on the postpartum unit
- When mother wants to sleep, infant is placed in bassinet or with another support person who is awake and alert

ACHIEVING BOTH SAFE SLEEP AND BREASTFEEDING

The National Action Partnership for the Promotion of Safe Sleep-Improvement and Innovation Network (NAPPSS-IIN) strives to make safe infant sleep and breastfeeding a national norm. This quality improvement initiative involves numerous stakeholders uniting safe sleep and breastfeeding advocates working together to adopt ideal practices in multiple settings. The stakeholders meet regularly as part of a national coalition and are working on tangible products as teams focused on aligning messages within national, state, and local organizations, adopting the Georgetown Conversation Modules,[35] supporting early child care and education, and using public media and media relations to provide consistent and accurate information.

Hospital Quality Improvement

Hospital improvements were introduced by NAPPSS-IIN as safety bundles with goals to increase adoption and modeling of safe sleep practices, increase breastfeeding initiation, and increase breastfeeding duration to at least 6 months.[36] Safety bundles are a structured way of grouping about 3 to 5 evidence-based practices together to improve outcomes and decrease harm. In the NAPPSS-IIN project, these bundles were developed for modeling safe infant sleep, discharge readiness, and prenatal education. In-hospital modeling includes practices such as hospital staff always placing an infant supine, on a flat surface, and in a bassinet that is free from any other objects such as blankets, toys, or medical equipment and developing mechanisms to support breastfeeding while rooming-in, while at the same time avoiding mothers or other caregivers falling asleep while holding their baby. Pareto charts are useful in identifying the most common practices that need to be changed among hospital staff.

Risky Newborn Care Practices in the Hospital to Avoid

Common risky practices include elevating the head of the bed in the newborn bassinet, placing objects in the bassinet such as a suction bulb, and use of loose bedding. Additional practices include placing an infant on their sides to sleep and use of swaddling with blankets to prop the newborn either on the side or with the head elevated. Improvement strategies include education, reminders, and incentives for staff to follow AAP policies. Ongoing improvements require continuous measurement using strategies and regular reporting of run charts. Data that are stratified by race ethnicity, and other variables where disparities may exist, help to identify opportunities for change. Stratified data also help to identify implicit bias and inequitable care. As shown in breastfeeding care, quality improvement strategies used in maternity care practices can be an effective method of decreasing racial disparities.[37]

Key points

- Common Risky Newborn Sleep Practices in the Hospital to AVOID:
  - Elevating the head of the bed in the newborn bassinet
  - Placing objects in the bassinet such as a suction bulb
  - Use of loose bedding
  - Placing an infant on their side to sleep

Use of blankets to prop the newborn either on the side or with the head elevated

Teachable Moments in the Hospital

Among the potential interventions to decrease SUID within the birth hospital, crucial conversations can occur during "teachable moments." One of the advantages of rooming-in is the opportunity to observe the mother and other support persons caring for the newborn. Instead of the hospital staff providing all of the care in a separate location, such as an infant nursery, the hospital staff and providers can assist new mothers in the care of their newborn while providing anticipatory guidance about how to room share without bedsharing and how to breastfeed safely. Staff can also explore health beliefs and social norms as a method to offset high-risk behaviors such as placing a baby prone to sleep, bedsharing, or using loose or fluffy blankets and soft bedding.[13] In-hospital counseling strategies should include individuals who are part of the mother's support system and provide trusted advice. Using a conversations approach, staff can explore the beliefs and norms for the most trusted caregivers and identify opportunities to enhance learning and adoption of breastfeeding along with safe infant sleep.

Feeding and Holding When the Mother Is at Risk of Falling Asleep

New parents are exhausted and at risk of falling asleep while holding and feeding their baby. The AAP recommends that mothers feed their infant in an adult bed with a flat, firm mattress free of loose bedding and soft objects and then place the infant in a crib or bassinette after the feeding or when the mother awakens (**Fig. 1**). Feeding on a couch, sofa, or padded armchair is not recommended, as these are particularly unsafe surfaces for sleeping with an infant due to the risk of accidental suffocation or entrapment. New parents need guidance to plan ahead for where they will feed their baby when they are at risk of falling asleep[3].

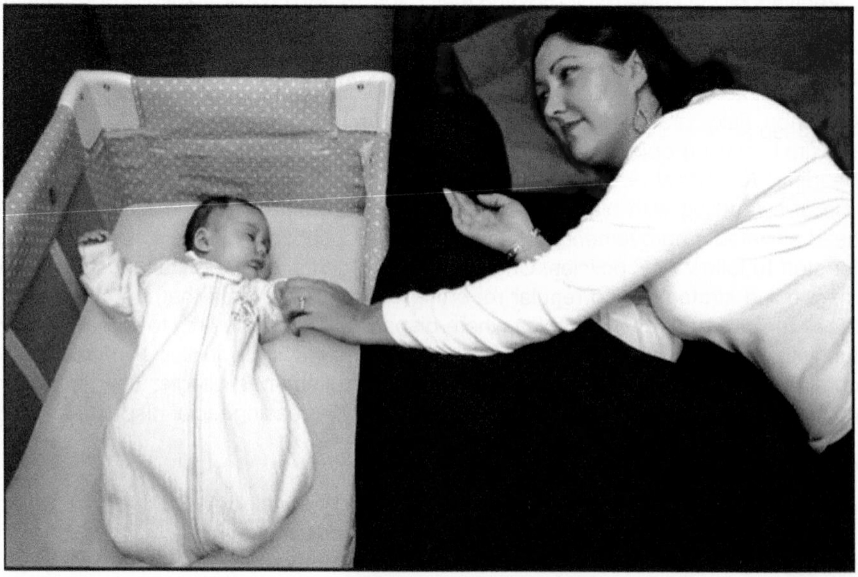

Fig. 1. Planned feeding spaces when at risk of falling asleep. (*Courtesy of* the Safe to Sleep® campaign, for educational purposes only.)

Key points

Planned Feeding Spaces When at Risk of Falling Asleep:
Flat, firm adult mattress/bed
Free of soft bedding/objects
Crib or bassinette nearby
NOT a couch, sofa, or padded chair

SPECIAL CIRCUMSTANCES

Other Caregivers

It is essential that all those who care for the infant in addition to the parents or primary caregivers are well versed in safe sleep practices. Whether the infant is asleep at night, or napping during the day, safe sleep is important for every sleep. Parents should be encouraged to share safe sleep information and recommendations with all of the infant caregivers and to seek childcare providers who will ensure safe sleep for their infants.

Travel and Crowded Living Situations

Portable cribs or play yards make great, safe sleep spaces for infants. Local organizations may have a mechanism to help parents obtain portable cribs or play yards to place their infants in for sleep. Although it seems strange, for situations in which a crib or bassinette is not available, a dresser drawer can be fashioned into an infant sleep space when traveling or in crowded living situations when space is a factor.

Ongoing Education

In addition to prenatal education and counseling about safe sleep and breastfeeding, and modeling and best practices in the hospital, new parents also need ongoing information and support once home. Innovative, creative solutions are needed to not only educate parents about the recommendations but also address common concerns and barriers and dispel myths. For example, a national, randomized controlled trial of mobile health video message delivered via email and text improved adherence to safe sleep practices.[28,38] The timing of the videos was designed to reach parents whose infants were at a certain developmental stage and age. More work is needed at the public health level to distribute information and affect attitudes and social norms about safe sleep and breastfeeding.

SUMMARY

Not all parents practice safe infant sleep practices or achieve the recommended breastfeeding durations. It is possible to help parents achieve both safe sleep and breastfeeding for their infants. Parents need to hear not only what the recommendations are but also about the reasoning behind the recommendations and receive assistance with troubleshooting barriers in order to make the healthiest and safest choices for their family. This education and support must start prenatally, be optimized and modeled in the hospital, and continue as the infant grows and develops.

Best practices

What is the current practice for SUID Prevention?

- Educating mothers about the benefits of breastfeeding
- Teaching families to always place their baby alone, on their back, and in a bassinette or crib for every sleep

What changes in practice are likely to improve outcomes?

- Instead of just stating the benefits and recommendations for breastfeeding, families need to receive counseling tailored to their knowledge and circumstances
- For safe sleep, a conversational approach that starts with what they know and believe about safe sleep and helping families and caregivers troubleshoot barriers may be more effective
- Modeling safe sleep practices and providing optimal support for breastfeeding in the hospital are critical for getting new parents off to a good start with their newborns

Clinical Algorithm for SUID Risk Reduction

Prenatal

- Start the conversation by asking questions such as "What have you heard about breastfeeding?" "Where do you plan to have your baby sleep?" "What do you and the people you trust to give you advice think about safe sleep for babies?" "What baby items do you have or are you possibly getting as you prepare for your baby?"
- Explore misconceptions and potential barriers and provide tailored education about the recommendations

In-Hospital

- Encourage safe skin-to-skin contact and 24-hour rooming-in
- Model safe infant sleep practices—supine, no objects in crib, flat surface, avoidance of bedsharing
- Provide optimal breastfeeding support—assisting with initiation and management of breastfeeding, encouraging feeding on cue, avoiding unnecessary supplementation, eliminating corporate advertising, and paying fair market price for infant formula
- Including safe sleep and breastfeeding conversations throughout the hospital stay and in discharge teaching
- Discuss strategies for safely feeding infants when parents are at risk of falling asleep

Ongoing

- Provide continued support, education, and counseling appropriate for the situation and infant's developmental stage
- Continue to inquire about and document feeding and infant sleep practices

CLINICS CARE POINTS

- Use a conversational approach.
- Discuss breastfeeding and safe sleep early and often, beginning during pregnancy and throughout infancy.
- Involve members of the support system.
- Engage community health workers to provide additional in-home or in-community support.
- Adopt evidence-based practices such as the Ten Steps for in-hospital care and peer support for discharge.

DISCLOSURE

The authors have no commercial or financial conflicts to disclose. Dr A. Kellams receives research funding from the NICHD. Dr L. Feldman-Winter receives grant support from NICHQ as national faculty co-chair for the HRSA-MCHB-funded NAPPSS-IIN Project.

REFERENCES

1. Shapiro-Mendoza CK, Parks S, Lambert AE, et al. The Epidemiology of Sudden Infant Death Syndrome and Sudden Unexpected Infant Deaths: Diagnostic Shift and other

Temporal Changes. In: Duncan JR, Byard RW, editors. SIDS Sudden Infant and Early Childhood Death: The Past, the Present and the Future. Adelaide (AU): 2018.

2. Shapiro-Mendoza CK, Tomashek KM, Anderson RN, et al. Recent national trends in sudden, unexpected infant deaths: more evidence supporting a change in classification or reporting. Am J Epidemiol 2006;163(8):762–9.
3. Moon RY, Darnall RA, Feldman-Winter L, et al, TASK FORCE ON SUDDEN INFANT DEATH SYNDROME. SIDS and other sleep-related infant deaths: evidence base for 2016 updated recommendations for a safe infant sleeping environment. Pediatrics 2016;138:e20162940.
4. Erck Lambert AB, Parks SE, Shapiro-Mendoza CK. National and state trends in sudden unexpected infant death: 1990-2015. Pediatrics 2018;141(3):e20173519.
5. Blackburn CM, Bonas S, Spencer NJ, et al. Parental smoking and passive smoking in infants: fathers matter too. Health Educ Res 2005;20(2):185–94.
6. Merritt TA, Philips R, Armstrong S, et al. When you smoke your baby smokes: advancing maternal and child health through an academic alliance to improve health of mothers and their infants. Przegl Lek 2010;67(10):821–3.
7. Rechtman LR, Colvin JD, Blair PS, et al. Sofas and infant mortality. Pediatrics 2014;134(5):e1293–300.
8. Carpenter R, McGarvey C, Mitchell EA, et al. Bed sharing when parents do not smoke: is there a risk of SIDS? An individual level analysis of five major case–control studies. BMJ Open 2013;3(5):e002299.
9. Blair PS, Sidebotham P, Pease A, et al. Bed-sharing in the absence of hazardous circumstances: is there a risk of sudden infant death syndrome? An analysis from two case-control studies conducted in the UK. PLoS One 2014;9(9):e107799.
10. Moon RY, Darnall RA, Feldman-Winter L, et al, TASK FORCE ON SUDDEN INFANT DEATH SYNDROME. SIDS and other sleep-related infant deaths: updated 2016 recommendations for a safe infant sleeping environment. Pediatrics 2016; 138(5):e20162938.
11. Thompson JM, Tanabe K, Moon RY, et al. Duration of breastfeeding and risk of SIDS: an individual participant data meta-analysis. J Pediatr 2017;140(5): e20171324.
12. Colson ER, Geller NL, Heeren T, et al. Factors associated with choice of infant sleep position. Pediatrics 2017;140(3):e20170596.
13. Kellams A, Hauck FR, Moon RY, et al. Factors associated with choice of infant sleep location. Pediatrics 2020;145(3):e20191523.
14. Centers for Disease Control. Breastfeeding Report card United States, 2020 2020. Available at: https://www.cdc.gov/breastfeeding/pdf/2020-Breastfeeding-Report-Card-H.pdf. Accessed November 29, 2020.
15. Colson ER, Willinger M, Rybin D, et al. Trends and factors associated with infant bed sharing, 1993-2010: the national infant sleep position study. JAMA Pediatr 2013;167(11):1032–7.
16. Centers for Disease Control. Safe sleep for babies: eliminating hazards. CDC vital signs 2018. Available at: https://www.cdc.gov/vitalsigns/pdf/2018-01-vitalsigns.pdf. Accessed November 25, 2020.
17. McCoy M, Heggie P. In-hospital formula feeding and breastfeeding duration: a propensity-score matched analysis. Pediatrics 2020;146(1). e20192946.
18. Feltner C, Weber RP, Stuebe A, et al. Breastfeeding programs and policies, breastfeeding uptake, and maternal health outcomes in developed countries. Rockville (MD): Agency for Healthcare Research and Quality (US); 2018.

19. Yamashita A, Isumi A, Fujiwara T. Online peer support and well-being of mothers and children: systematic scoping review. J Epidemiol 2020. https://doi.org/10.2188/jea.JE20200079.
20. Chepkirui D, Nzinga J, Jemutai J, et al. A scoping review of breastfeeding peer support models applied in hospital settings. Int Breastfeed J 2020;15(1):95.
21. Steurer LM. Maternity leave length and workplace policies' impact on the sustainment of breastfeeding: global perspectives. Public Health Nurs 2017;34(3):286–94.
22. Hauck FR, Thompson JM, Tanabe KO, et al. Breastfeeding and reduced risk of sudden infant death syndrome: a meta-analysis. Pediatrics 2011;128(1):103–10.
23. Beauregard JL, Hamner HC, Chen J, et al. Racial disparities in breastfeeding initiation and duration among U.S. Infants born in 2015. MMWR Morb Mortal Wkly Rep 2019;68(34):745–8.
24. Trachtenberg FL, Haas EA, Kinney HC, et al. Risk factor changes for sudden infant death syndrome after initiation of Back-to-Sleep campaign. Pediatrics 2012;129(4):630–8.
25. Lavista Ferres JM, Anderson TM, Johnston R, et al. Distinct populations of sudden unexpected infant death based on age. Pediatrics 2020;145(1):e20191637.
26. Smith LA, Geller NL, Kellams AL, et al. Infant sleep location and breastfeeding practices in the United States, 2011-2014. Acad Pediatr 2016;16(6):540–9.
27. Moon RY, Corwin MJ, Kerr S, et al. Mediators of improved adherence to infant safe sleep using a mobile health intervention. Pediatrics 2019;143(5):e20182799.
28. Moon RY, Hauck FR, Colson ER, et al. The effect of nursing quality improvement and mobile health interventions on infant sleep practices: a randomized clinical trial. Jama 2017;318(4):351–9.
29. Feldman-Winter L, Ustianov J, Anastasio J, et al. Best fed beginnings: a nationwide quality improvement initiative to increase breastfeeding. Pediatrics 2017;140:e20163121.
30. Bass JL, Gartley T, Kleinman R. Unintended consequences of current breastfeeding initiatives. JAMA Pediatr 2016;170(10):923–4.
31. Thach BT. Deaths and near deaths of healthy newborn infants while bed sharing on maternity wards. J Perinatol 2014;34:275–9.
32. World Health Organization and Unicef. Ten steps to successful breastfeeding 2018. Available at: https://www.who.int/activities/promoting-baby-friendly-hospitals/ten-steps-to-successful-breastfeeding. Accessed November 29, 2020.
33. Baby-Friendly USA Inc. Baby-friendly USA Releases Interim guidelines and evaluation criteria 2019. Available at: https://www.babyfriendlyusa.org/news/bfusa-releases-interim-guidelines-and-evaluation-criteria/. Accessed November 1, 2020.
34. Feldman-Winter L, Goldsmith JP. Committee on Fetus and newborn, Task Force on sudden infant death syndrome. Safe sleep and skin-to-skin care in the neonatal period for healthy term newborns. Pediatrics 2016;138(3):e20161889.
35. Bronheim S. Building on campaigns with conversations: an individualized approach to helping families embrace safe sleep and breastfeeding 2017. Available at: https://www.ncemch.org/learning/building/. Accessed November 1, 2020.
36. National Institute for children's health quality. National action Partnership to Promote safe sleep: improvement and Innovation Network (NAPPSS-IIN). Available at: https://www.nichq.org/project/national-action-partnership-promote-safe-sleep-improvement-and-innovation-network-nappss. Accessed June 14, 2021.
37. Merewood A, Bugg K, Burnham L, et al. Addressing racial Inequities in breastfeeding in the Southern United States. Pediatrics 2019;143(2):e20181897.
38. Moon RY, Mathews A, Joyner BL, et al. Impact of a randomized controlled trial to reduce Bedsharing on breastfeeding rates and duration for African-American infants. J Community Health 2017;42(4):707–15.

The Term Newborn

Prenatal Substance Exposure

Courtney Townsel, MD, MSc[a], Torri D. Metz, MD, MS[b],
Maya Bunik, MD, MPH[c,d,*]

KEYWORDS

• Substance use • Pregnancy • Neonatal withdrawal

KEY POINTS

- Current practice for maternal substance use is verbal screening early in pregnancy using a validated tool.
- Multidisciplinary team to support substance use treatment and comorbidities including mental health.
- Recognizing Neonatal Abstinence Syndrome (NAS).
- Adoption of standardized clinical assessments for NAS and prioritizing nonpharmacologic, family-centered care to improve hospital outcomes.
- Supporting safe breastfeeding Obstetric and pediatric practitioners collaborating to support mother and infant postpartum.

INTRODUCTION

Substance use disorder is common and has significant implications for both mothers and their neonates with increased risk of morbidity and mortality. Through education and training, obstetricians can become equipped to optimize care for pregnant patients with substance use disorder, optimizing outcomes. A recent review noted that overdose is a leading cause of maternal death in the United States.[1] Prevention of these deaths will require a multipronged approach with engagement at the health care practitioner, facility, community, and health care systems level. Importantly, maternal mortality is likely just the tip of the iceberg with a substantial number of cases of morbidity that go unrecognized. Appropriate screening and treatment of substance use disorder is needed.

[a] Department of Obstetrics and Gynecology, University of Michigan, 1540 East Hospital Drive SPC 4262, Ann Arbor, MI 48109, USA; [b] Department of Obstetrics and Gynecology, University of Utah Health, 30 North 1900 East, SOM 2B200, Salt Lake City, UT 84132, USA; [c] Department of Pediatrics, University of Colorado, Children's Hospital Colorado, 860 N Potomac Circle, Aurora, CO 80011, USA; [d] Pediatrics, Children's Hospital Colorado, Child Health Pavilion, 860 N Potomac Circle, Aurora, CO 80011, USA

* Corresponding author. Department of Pediatrics, University of Colorado Anschutz Medical Campus, Children's Hospital Colorado, 860 N Potomac Circle, Aurora, CO 80011.
E-mail address: Maya.bunik@childrenscolorado.org

Clin Perinatol 48 (2021) 631–646
https://doi.org/10.1016/j.clp.2021.05.011

Perhaps the most important principle of providing care for pregnant women with substance use disorder is recognition that addiction is a chronic medical disease. The biology of addiction is outside of the scope of this article; however, the importance of understanding an underlying neurophysiology that is responsible for addictive behaviors is critical. With this recognition comes an understanding of the importance of screening and treatment during pregnancy. Treatment must, therefore, be provided as it would for any other chronic medical conditions in a nonjudgmental way that optimizes a therapeutic alliance between the health care practitioner and the patient.

Over recent years, the most commonly used drugs in pregnancy are opioids, marijuana, and alcohol, which are covered in detail in this article. Opioid use disorder disproportionately affects women[2] and has been the focus of numerous interventions including the use of medication-assisted therapy in pregnancy to improve outcomes and reduce the risk of relapse.

This article describes screening for substance use in pregnancy, comorbidities that often accompany substance use disorder in pregnancy, prenatal and intrapartum care considerations, and care of the term newborn exposed to drugs in utero, including guidance on breastfeeding. The importance of multidisciplinary care for pregnant patients with substance use disorder and their neonates is emphasized.

SCREENING FOR SUBSTANCE USE DISORDERS DURING PREGNANCY

Several professional organizations recommend universal screening in pregnancy for both prior and current substance use including the American College of Obstetricians and Gynecologists (ACOG), the American Academy of Pediatrics, the United States Preventive Task Force, and the Centers for Disease Control and Prevention (CDC).[3] Screening for substance use disorders in pregnancy consists of maternal interviews or drug toxicology testing. Universal screening increases proper identification of exposures in pregnancy, allowing for the development of appropriate treatment plans, and provides practitioners the opportunity to observe for evidence of neonatal abstinence syndrome (NAS) in drug-exposed infants after delivery. Substance use screening based solely on factors such as lack of prenatal care, race/ethnicity, or prior adverse pregnancy outcomes can lead to significantly lower rates of diagnosis of substance use disorder and adds to the culture of mistrust and implicit bias health professionals should avoid.[4]

Obtaining a history using open-ended questions in a nonjudgmental fashion is more likely to result in patient disclosure of substance use. Several validated screening questionnaires are available for routine screening for substance use in pregnancy (**Table 1**). Substance use screening should occur at the initial prenatal appointment for all patients and then in the subsequent trimesters for women with risk factors such as a positive initial screen for current substance use or past substance use.[3]

Urine drug testing may be used as an adjunct to screening questionnaires and interviews. Some obstetric practices perform routine urine drug screening on all patients at the initial intake. However, urine drug testing should not be performed without first obtaining patient consent. Pregnant women may decline drug toxicology testing due to fears of reporting the positive test results to authorities, loss of child custody, and denial of welfare benefits after delivery.[5] Obstetric health care practitioners should prioritize the patient-practitioner relationship by using positive screening and toxicology test results as an opportunity for intervention and not to shame or criminalize patients. Women who continue to use substances in pregnancy have better maternal

Table 1
Substance use screening in pregnancy

Screening Test	Description	Substance
T-ACE • Positive screen ≥ 2 points	**Tolerance** (2 points) How many drinks does it take to feel first effect? **Annoyance** (1 point) Have people annoyed you by criticizing your drinking? **Cut down** (1 point) Have you felt you should cut down on your drinking? **Eye-opener** (1 point) Have you ever had a drink first thing in the morning to steady your nerves or relieve a hangover?	Alcohol
TWEAK • Positive screen ≥3 points	**Tolerance** (2 points) Requires 3 or more drinks to feel effect **Worry** (2 points) Has family or friends worried or complained about your drinking in the past year? **Eye-opener** (2 points) Do you sometimes take a drink in the morning when you first get up? **Amnesia** (1 point) Has a friend or family member told you about something you said or did while you were drinking that you could not remember? (blackout) **Cut down** (1 point) Do you sometimes feel the need to cut down on your drinking?	Alcohol
AUDIT-C • Maximum score is 12 • >2 positive screen	How often do you have a drink containing alcohol? Never (0), Monthly (1), 2–4x/mo (2), 2–3x/wk (3), ≥4x/wk (4) How many drinks containing alcohol do you have on a typical day when you drink? 1–2 (0), 3–4 (1), 5–6 (2), 7–9 (3), ≥10 (4) How often do you have 6 or more drinks on one occasion? Never (0), <Monthly (1), Monthly (2), 2–3x/mo (3), ≥4x/mo (4)	Alcohol
4P's Plus • Associated with a licensing fee • Positive screen if admission to use month before pregnancy	Problem with alcohol or drugs **Parents**? **Partner**? In the **Past** have you ever used alcohol? In the month before you knew you were **Pregnant** how many cigarettes did you smoke? How much alcohol did you drink?	Any substance
SURP-P	In the month before you knew you were Pregnant how much alcohol (beer, wine, liquor) did you drink? Never (0), Any (1) Have you ever felt you need to cut down on your drug or alcohol use? # of affirmative items = score 0 = low risk, 1 = moderate risk, 2–3 = high risk	Any substance

(*continued on next page*)

Table 1
(*continued*)

Screening Test	Description	Substance
CRAFFT	Ever ridden in a **Car** driven by you or someone else who was "high" or had been using drugs or alcohol? Do you ever use drugs or alcohol to **Relax**? Do you ever use drugs or alcohol **Alone**? Do you **Forget** things you did while using drugs or alcohol? Have **Friends/Family** ever told you to cut down on alcohol or drug use? Ever gotten in **Trouble** while using alcohol or drugs? (all positive answers = 1 point)	Any substance

1 AUDIT-C: Alcohol Use Disorders Identification Test-Consumption.
2 ASSIST: Alcohol Smoking and Substance Involvement Screening Test.
3 SURP-P: Substance Use Risk Profile-Pregnancy.

and infant outcomes if they attend routine prenatal appointments. Thus, the therapeutic relationship is critical.

Drug testing at the time of delivery typically is left to the discretion of the newborn medical provider team and consists of maternal and infant urine testing, neonatal meconium, or umbilical cord testing. Bogen and colleagues 2016[6] surveyed birth hospitals in the United States and reported the distribution of screening specimens in infants most commonly included urine (85%), and meconium (76%), but also umbilical cord tissue (10%). Testing of maternal urine is often performed if there is concern for a pregnancy complication that is associated with maternal drug use, which may influence care. For example, hypertension could be associated with recent stimulant use. In the past, there was a heavy reliance on meconium testing for the neonate. In more recent years, hospitals have moved to testing a segment of umbilical cord for drug use, as both are thought to reflect late pregnancy use,[7] and a segment of umbilical cord is much easier to collect than meconium.

MEDICAL COMORBIDITIES

Substance use disorder often occurs in patients with other mental health disorders such as depression, anxiety, and posttraumatic stress disorder.[8,9] A history of adverse childhood experiences is also common among people with substance use disorder.[10] Thus, the importance of trauma-informed care is emphasized in this population.

In addition to screening for mental health disorders, there are several other medical problems for which people with substance use disorders are at increased risk. These include blood-borne infections such as human immunodeficiency virus (HIV), hepatitis B, and hepatitis C. It is standard of care to screen for HIV and hepatitis B in pregnancy. However, in the past, hepatitis C was not typically part of routine prenatal laboratories. More recently the CDC has recommended that all pregnant patients be screened for hepatitis C unless the population prevalence in the region is less than 0.1%.[11] Repeat testing for these blood-borne viruses should be performed in the third trimester, as a new diagnosis would influence intrapartum management and postnatal care of the neonate.

There are a few other medical comorbidities that may arise in patients with substance use disorder that would benefit from multidisciplinary care. These include complications such as endocarditis from intravenous drug use or methamphetamine-induced cardiomyopathy. Often these comorbidities have a significant influence on overall pregnancy management.

SPECIFIC EFFECTS OF COMMONLY USED SUBSTANCES

Determining the potential effects of each individual substance on the mother or fetus can be difficult. Research is limited by underreporting of prenatal exposure, and polysubstance use is frequent. Furthermore, the risk of prenatal drug use depends not only on the type of substance but also on the timing of exposure and dose effects. Medication and substance use during the first trimester may increase the risk of congenital abnormalities or spontaneous abortion, whereas exposure during the second and third trimester, particularly if it is chronic, may increase the risk of fetal growth restriction, neurodevelopmental delay, placental abruption (a shearing of the placenta from the uterine wall), pregnancy loss, and NAS. Additional concerns include maternal malnutrition with poor weight gain, lack of adequate health care, increased risk of infectious diseases, and psychiatric illnesses, all of which can negatively affect perinatal outcomes.

Opioids

Opioids are a class of drugs that include illegal formulations such as heroin, synthetic forms such as fentanyl, and prescription forms such as hydromorphone. Opioids act by binding the opioid receptors (mu, delta, and kappa), which are responsible for mediating psychoactive and somatic effects. The central nervous system action of opioid drugs has led to its potential for misuse.

Drug withdrawal in newborns caused by exposure in utero is called neonatal abstinence syndrome (NAS) or neonatal opioid withdrawal syndrome (NOWS) when the maternal drug exposure is opioids. Opioid use in pregnancy has been associated with numerous poor outcomes for the fetus and infant. These conditions include, but are not limited to, preterm delivery, birth defects (eg, neural tube, cardiac, and gastroschisis), low birth weight, sudden infant death syndrome, and difficulty controlling maternal pain following cesarean birth.[4,12,13]

Medication-Assisted Therapy

Opioid agonist pharmacotherapy with either methadone (opioid receptor agonist) or buprenorphine (mixed opioid receptor agonist) is first-line therapy for patients with opioid use disorder. These agents are preferred to medication-assisted withdrawal because withdrawal has been associated with higher rates of relapse.[4]

Maternal methadone dosages usually require uptitration in pregnancy, due to the physiologic increased volume of distribution, to avoid withdrawal symptoms (eg, nausea, abdominal cramps, irritability, and anxiety).[4] Providers should counsel pregnant women on MAT that maternal dose and duration of MAT do not predict severity of NAS. Therefore, pregnant women on MAT should be maintained on the dose of medication that controls their withdrawal symptoms. Although methadone is currently the most common pharmacotherapy agent in pregnancy, buprenorphine has been shown to result in lower rates of NAS. Women who enter pregnancy on methadone should not be switched to buprenorphine because of the potential for withdrawal due to buprenorphine's partial agonist properties.

Buprenorphine is available as a monoproduct (Subutex) and in combination with naloxone (Suboxone), an opioid antagonist, to reduce diversion. Studies have found no adverse effects and similar outcomes when comparing buprenorphine alone with the combination of buprenorphine and naloxone. Patients who desire buprenorphine must have access to providers with prescribing privileges.

Marijuana

Marijuana is the substance most commonly used during pregnancy in the United States. The psychoactive compound tetrahydrocannabinol (THC) in marijuana binds the cannabinoid receptor CB1 to exhibit the drug's effects. There is consistent evidence of an effect of prenatal marijuana use on fetal growth[14]; this is biologically plausible, given the importance of the endocannabinoid system on placentation.[15] Evidence related to an increased risk of neonatal intensive care unit admission is also emerging. The literature regarding the effect of perinatal marijuana use on other outcomes such as preterm birth is mixed.[16,17]

There are 3 longitudinal cohorts that examine the association between marijuana use in pregnancy and long-term neurologic outcomes.[16,17] These data are limited by unmeasured confounding variables related to environmental differences during childhood between children exposed to marijuana in utero and those who were not. However, findings from these studies suggest that children exposed to cannabis in utero may have permanent neurobehavioral and cognitive impairments.

A longitudinal study of 648 mothers showed that at age 5 years children exposed to marijuana (at least 1 joint per day) in the first trimester had a mean IQ that was 6 points lower than youth not exposed.[18] The same cohort showed that at age 10 years, the youth exposed to marijuana were about twice as likely to have depression compared with youth not exposed.[19] Then, at age 14 years these youths were about 12 times more likely to have used marijuana compared with youth not exposed in utero and scored significantly lower on tests of school achievement.[18,20] This finding remained significant even after controlling for current parental use of marijuana.

ACOG recommends pregnant women or those considering pregnancy discontinue the use of marijuana secondary to the potential neonatal risks.[21] Consequences include potential negative effects on fetal brain development, low birth weight, and increased risk of stillbirth and preterm delivery. In addition, prenatal marijuana use has been associated with the potential for behavioral problems and attention-deficit/hyperactivity disorder (ADHD) in exposed school-age children.

There are no available medication-assisted treatments of marijuana use disorder in pregnancy. Similarly, there is no described neonatal withdrawal syndrome. For pregnant patients with marijuana use disorder, cognitive behavioral therapy is an option. In addition, given that most of the pregnant patients report using marijuana for "treatment" of nausea, anxiety, or depression or to help with insomnia,[22] exploration of other safe and effective options for the treatment of these disorders is warranted.

Tobacco

Although rates of smoking cigarettes in pregnancy have declined from 13.2% in 2006 to 7.2% in 2016, the actual prevalence of tobacco smoking varies and is influenced by many social factors such as race/ethnicity, age, and education.[23] Tobacco use in pregnancy is associated with orofacial clefts, placental abruption, placenta previa, preterm prelabor rupture of membranes, low birth weight, increased perinatal mortality, and sudden infant death syndrome.[23] After birth infants with in-utero exposure to tobacco have increased rates of asthma, upper respiratory infections, childhood obesity, and colic.[23]

In addition to traditional cigarette smoking there has been an increase in both nicotine and marijuana use through electronic cigarettes or e-cigarettes (also known as electronic nicotine delivery systems "ENDS"). Using an e-cigarette is commonly called "vaping." E-cigarettes work by heating a liquid to produce an aerosol that users inhale into their lungs. Liquids can contain nicotine, THC, cannabinoid oils, flavoring, and other additives. In 2019, 7% of pregnant women reported using e-cigarettes at any point around the time of pregnancy, and 1.4% reported use in the last 3 months of pregnancy.[24] E-cigarette use is thought to have the same risks as traditional smoking, including higher rates of low birth weight, stillbirth, and neonatal apnea.[25–27]

Alcohol

There is no amount of alcohol considered to be safe at any time in pregnancy. All women should be screened for and educated on the potential negative effects of alcohol use during pregnancy. In-utero exposure has been shown to increase the risk of fetal alcohol spectrum disorder (FASD). In 2010 the CDC estimated that 0.3 of every 1000 children aged 7 to 9 years were living with FASD in the United States.[28] However, the National Institutes of Health reports that rates could be as high as 1% to 5% of school-age children. Research and diagnosis can be clouded by the lack of confirmation of maternal alcohol use.

The signs of FASD include both physical and developmental conditions such as low birth weight, abnormal facial features, small head size, poor motor control, speech delay, hyperactive disorders, learning disabilities, and low IQ. Classic facial features include a flat upper lip, philtrum, and midface; smaller eye openings; and skin folds at the corner of the eyes.[29] Infants or children may also exhibit visual and hearing impairment, feeding difficulties, and poor eye-hand coordination skills. A variety of symptoms can occur secondary to alcohol exposure and can be classified within the fetal alcohol disorder spectrum; this includes not only FASD but also alcohol-related neurodevelopmental disorder and alcohol-related birth defects. Birth defects can include cardiac anomalies, renal agenesis, bone, abnormalities, and neural tube defects. Spontaneous abortions and stillbirths are increased in women who report moderate-to-heavy alcohol use in pregnancy.[30]

Management options for woman with alcohol use in pregnancy should be individualized. Behavioral therapy is a mainstay of treatment. Therapies such as disulfiram, acamprosate, and naltrexone are classified as category C medications in pregnancy.[31] In addition, women should be treated for potential nutritional deficiencies.

The diagnosis of alcohol withdrawal syndrome in pregnancy can be delayed in those who do not offer a history of alcohol use. The syndrome may appear as hypertension, tachycardia, headache, and delirium, and seizures can be mistaken for preeclampsia or eclampsia. Just as in the nonpregnant state, alcohol withdrawal can be life-threatening and should be treated. Pregnant women in withdrawal are at additional risk for placental abruption and hemorrhage. The data surrounding the potential risks of short-term benzodiazepines in pregnancy for the treatment of acute withdrawal are limited. Concern exists for the potential of teratogenic effects when used the first trimester as well as hypotonia and respiratory depression if used near the time of delivery. However, given the potentially fatal consequences of withdrawal, pregnant women should receive appropriate care in order to ensure their safety.[31]

Cocaine

Cocaine is an addictive stimulant, derived from coca plant leaves, that leads to dopamine release within the brain causing the characteristic "high" described by users. There are 2 chemical forms of cocaine: the water-soluble hydrochloride salt (white powder) and the water-insoluble form known as "crack" or "freebase." Intravenous drugs and risky sexual behavior that can be seen in cocaine users further increase the threat of contracting communicable diseases such as HIV and hepatitis C.[32]

Cocaine use in pregnancy is associated with significant negative maternal and neonatal outcomes. In addition to overdose, mothers are at risk of myocardial infarction, cardiac arrhythmias, stroke, and hypertensive crisis. The increased risk of placental abruption places the fetus at considerable jeopardy of stillbirth, preterm delivery, and prematurity. Other risks include precipitous delivery, premature rupture of membranes, and low birth weight.[32,33] Prenatal cocaine exposure can lead to poorer adolescent functioning, worse perceptual reasoning, impairment in procedural learning, higher rates of oppositional defiant disorder and attention-deficit disorder, diminished short-term memory, and impaired language development.[33]

Amphetamines

Classified as a stimulant, amphetamines are used to treat various conditions such as ADHD and narcolepsy. Often patients do not realize that prescription amphetamines, such as methylphenidate, have a high potential for tolerance and use disorder. Amphetamines and their byproducts readily cross the placenta and are concentrated in breast milk. Prenatal amphetamine exposure has been shown to increase the risk of fetal growth restriction, preterm delivery, and low birth weight.[34] Therefore, prescription use in pregnancy should be individualized to patients in whom the risks of discontinuing the medication to the mother outweighs the potential risks to the fetus.

The use of 3,4-methylenedioxymethamphetamine (MDMA), also known as "Ecstasy" or “Molly,” is increasing. Lower milestone and motor quality scores at 4 months of life were noted in infants born to women who used MDMA during pregnancy.[35] Severe hyperthermia can occur with MDMA intoxication. Exposure to high temperatures during the first trimester has been associated with neural tube defects. Other common side effects of acute MDMA intoxication include transient hypertension and tachycardia. Such symptoms could be particularly dangerous in a pregnant patient with preexisting hypertension, gestational hypertension, or underlying cardiac conditions.

Methamphetamines are a more potent version of amphetamines, and their use in the general population has been on the increase since the 1980s. Admission rates for treatment of methamphetamine use among pregnant women increased from 8% in 1994 to 28% in 2006.[36] In addition to the addictive potential, methamphetamine is associated with maternal seizures, arrhythmias, hyperthermia, and hypertension. These conditions can be especially concerning in a pregnant patient and use has been associated with placental abruption, preterm delivery as well as fetal and neonatal loss.[37] Fetal growth restriction has been shown to be 3.5 times more likely in women using methamphetamines during pregnancy, even after correcting for other confounding factors such as alcohol, maternal weight, and tobacco use.[38] Exposed infants are more likely to require admission to the neonatal intensive care unit (NICU), have a small head circumference, and suffer from poor feeding.[39] Women using methamphetamines are more likely to seek prenatal care later in the pregnancy or not at all. In addition, poor maternal weight gain is associated with active use.

General considerations for known substance use in the mother at birth

Health care practitioners should be concerned if mothers have relapsed to substance use (illicit or legal misuse) within 3 months of delivery of the infant or engaged later in pregnancy in prenatal care or treatment of sobriety.[40] Their infants are at higher risk of preterm birth and low birthweight, which are associated with adverse health outcomes later in life.[41–43] As part of the overall approach to managing the mother-infant dyad the health care practitioner should include the following:

- Screening of mother and/or infant as described earlier
- Careful review infectious disease status (HIV, hepatitis B, hepatitis C, tuberculosis) and any other health issues
- Verification of prescription medications and dosage

- Timing/frequency/duration of substance exposure but this can be difficult to determine
- Screening for behavioral health and psychosocial issues (social work, navigator)
- Lactation support, pumping as needed to maintain supply
- Decisions about safety of infant receiving mother's own milk
- History or evidence of polysubstance use and lack of appropriate maternal family and community support systems make for challenges in discharging the mother-infant home to a safe environment

The initial evaluation of the infant for withdrawal symptoms

Management of term infant with opioid exposure. Lower birth weight and NAS are the outcomes most commonly associated with opioid use in pregnancy. Some research indicates an association with adverse longer-term neurocognitive, behavioral, and developmental outcomes. As with other substance use disorders, these outcomes are complex, including genetic, environmental, and biological factors.[44]

Neonatal abstinence syndrome. The current opioid addiction crisis is affecting an increasing proportion of mother-infant pairs over time. NAS has increased to a prevalence rate of 4%.[45] NAS is a postnatal drug withdrawal syndrome exhibited by opioid-exposed infants that is characterized by hyperactivity of the central nervous system and gastrointestinal tract. Because most of the infants affected by withdrawal are opioid exposed the term "neonatal opioid withdrawal syndrome" (NOWS) is also being used.[46,47] Infants are fussy, irritable, and have trouble feeding and therefore may experience early weight loss. Treatment usually consists of pharmacologic and nonpharmacologic interventions with wide variability in approaches across the United States.[48] Creating an environment to decrease the dysregulation in the infant with NAS is key. Standardizing clinical assessment and prioritizing nonpharmacologic, family-centered care improves hospital outcomes.[49]

Formalized NAS Scoring Forms are available.[50] The Finnegan Neonatal Abstinence Scoring System[51] is a 31-item scale designed to quantify the severity of NAS and to guide treatment; it is the most comprehensive scale, but it is found to be too complex for routine use in nurseries. The Lipsitz Neonatal Drug-Withdrawal Scoring System[52] is an 11-item scale, with each symptom numerically scored (0–3) based on severity of symptoms; a score of 4 is a recommended cutoff for the institution of pharmacologic therapy. This is the system recommended by the American Academy of Pediatrics.[53]

Opioid-exposed newborns rooming-in with mother or other family members seem to be significantly less likely to be treated with pharmacotherapy and have substantial reductions in length of stay compared with those cared for in NICUs.[45,53] Although these nonpharmacologic approaches of rooming-in and breastfeeding seem promising, the interventions are heterogeneous and not yet standardized.[54]

In general, morphine is the most common first-line pharmacotherapy for NAS followed by methadone.[6] Yet, short-term outcomes seem better in infants receiving methadone compared with morphine. Observation periods for opioid-exposed newborns vary from 2 to 3 days to 1 week and usually require NICU stay when requiring medical treatment. More studies are needed to determine longer term neurodevelopmental outcomes, which are likely related to the need for phenobarbital, overall health of the infant, and postnatal caregiving environment.[55]

Breastfeeding Breastfed neonates exposed to opioid medication prenatally and methadone-exposed breastfed newborns have lower incidence of NAS and require shorter pharmacotherapy for NAS than infants who are not breastfed[56]; this adds to the evidence regarding the benefits of breastfeeding for neonates prenatally exposed to opioids.

Methadone maintenance treatment has been available since 1965 and should be encouraged for breastfeeding patients with opioid use disorder.[57] The concentrations in human milk are low. Assessment of longer-term outcomes is ongoing.[58] Mothers on stable doses of methadone maintenance should be encouraged to breastfeed irrespective of dose.[59]

Although buprenorphine is less commonly used in pregnancy, low levels of buprenorphine are found in breastmilk. Buprenorphine has poor oral bioavailability in infants with low levels found in their urine and serum, so it is thought to be acceptable, even preferable, in nursing mothers.[60,61]

Management of the term infant with alcohol exposure. Although prenatal alcohol exposure causes craniofacial anomalies, fetal growth restriction, neurologic abnormalities, cognitive impairment, and birth defects as described previously, FASD is underdiagnosed. Diagnosis of FASD is challenging because self-reported maternal drinking history is not reliable and diagnostic dysmorphic facial features are not always obvious in this disorder. Different diagnostic systems and disagreements over criteria have slowed progress in the diagnosis and management of FASD. Neuroimaging shows abnormalities in brain structure, which are associated with deficits in cognition, executive function, memory, vision, hearing, motor skills, and other behavioral issues.[62]

Breastfeeding Human milk alcohol levels parallel maternal blood alcohol levels. Alcohol interferes with the milk ejection reflex, which may reduce milk production through inadequate breast emptying. Mothers should limit alcohol intake to the equivalent of 5 ounces of wine or 8 ounce of beer and wait 2 hours after drinking to resume breastfeeding, just like the nomograms of drinking and driving.[63] Some mothers use milk test strips to assist in assessing levels of alcohol in their breastmilk. If breastfeeding mother ingests more than one drink the recommendations[64] are to instruct mother to "pump and dump" their breastmilk until feeling unaffected or about 8 hours.[65]

Management of infants exposed to tobacco. Only 40% of women quit smoking during pregnancy, with more than half relapsing within 6 months and up to 90% relapsing within 1 year.[66]

Prematurity risk is doubled, and low birth weight is increased 3-fold with maternal smoking in pregnancy.[67] Studies of infants within the first month who were born to mothers who smoked reported increased signs of irritability and hypertonicity compared with those of nonsmokers.

Maternal smoking approximately doubles the risk of sudden unexpected infant death (SUID), defined as infant death at an age younger than 1 year. Moreover, nicotine can augment the clinical manifestations of withdrawal for infants with prenatal exposure to opioids or alcohol.[64]

Breastfeeding Most breastfeeding women who previously smoked relapse, and mothers who smoke are less likely to breastfeed.[68,69] Nicotine transfers to the infant via milk and chemicals transfer via secondhand smoke when mothers smoke near their infants. Breastfeeding can help negate the risks of SUIDS and respiratory infections in neonates exposed to tobacco.[70] Breastfeeding should be encouraged and cessation assistance offered. Smoking cessation modalities such as the nicotine patch, nicotine gum, and bupropion are all compatible with breastfeeding.[71]

Management of infants exposed to marijuana. The infant exposed to marijuana in pregnancy does not usually present with withdrawal symptoms, although sedation, poor feeding, and weight loss have been described.[72,73] Longer term outcomes studies suggest that prenatal cannabis exposure is associated with greater risk neurodevelopmental effects in children older than 1 year and for psychopathology during middle childhood.[19,74] Concerns have been raised regarding mother's regulation and sensitivity to their infant and toddlers in terms of caregiving when using marijuana.

Breastfeeding THC, the psychoactive component of marijuana, is known to have a long half-life and to be lipophilic. Most of the previous research done was when marijuana potency was 4-fold less than in more contemporary products.[75]

Baker and colleagues (2018)[76] published a study of 8 anonymous women who smoked 0.1 g cannabis. They reported low levels of THC in breastmilk and obtained samples over a short period of 4 hours. From this they extrapolated that a breastfeeding infant would ingest a mean of 2.5% of the maternal dose or 8 μg per kilogram.

Bertrand and colleagues (2018)[77] in a cross-sectional study tested single milk samples from women who reported marijuana use to a milk research repository and found variable levels of THC and metabolites for up to 6 days.

Wymore and colleagues (2020)[78] found that in women who tested positive at birth, THC was persistent for more than 6 weeks in breastmilk. This study raised concern regarding guidance to pump and discard breastmilk because it may be unrealistic for the 6 weeks or longer time period.

Given these data, it appears that in order to promote safe breastfeeding and limit infant exposure to THC, it may be best to emphasize abstaining from marijuana early on in pregnancy and throughout the breastfeeding period. However, the difficulties in marijuana abstinence may be multifactorial ranging from perceived benefits related to mood stabilization or cannabis use disorder.

Postpartum depression. Postpartum depressive symptoms are most prevalent among postpartum substance users and those with a substance use history. The postpartum period is a critical time. Postpartum alcohol use (prevalence range 30%–49%) and drug use (5%–9%) tend to be higher than during pregnancy (5%–11%, 3%–4%, respectively). Being unemployed, unmarried, and a cigarette smoker puts new mothers at even higher risk of ongoing substance use.[79] Awareness and screening for postpartum depression with a validated tool at postpartum and newborn visits are important. Partnership and communication between obstetrician-gynecologists and primary care providers to reduce maternal substance use is paramount for the health and safety of both infant and family.

Breastfeeding Studies have shown that depression during pregnancy is one of the factors that may contribute to breastfeeding failure.[80] There is also an association between breastfeeding and postpartum depression. Breastfeeding can promote hormonal processes that protect mothers against postpartum depression by attenuating the cortisol response to stress. It can also reduce the risk of postpartum depression, by helping the regulation of sleep and wake patterns for mother and child, improving mother's self-efficacy and her emotional involvement with the child, reducing the child's temperamental difficulties, and promoting a better interaction between mother and child.[81] For mothers in recovery, breastfeeding may be a positive activity and motivator for continued sobriety.

TEAMING UP FOR POSTDISCHARGE CARE

As was reviewed in this article, this is a challenging and complex management issue that requires a cohesive multidisciplinary team.[82] The following is a summary of key points for continued maternal-infant success:

- Planned support for the mother that includes a treatment program for substance use disorder that will accept the infant and provide medication for opioid use disorder if needed, behavioral and psychiatric care when needed, and postpartum obstetric care, for example, contraceptives if desired.

- Family and others supporting the mother should receive overdose training and a naloxone prescription if opioid misuse is a concern.
- Safe housing and case management for both mother and infant.
- Provision of accessible care for the infant by a health care practitioner who is nonjudgmental and knowledgeable about withdrawal and treatment.
- Initiation of pediatric care before hospital discharge that is accessible to the mother if the infant is difficult to care for or develops any signs of late onset of withdrawal or illness.
- Pediatric follow-up should include frequent visits to provide ongoing support and developmental assessment for any emerging neurodevelopmental concerns.

Strong teamwork is necessary for the future success of the mother-infant pair—for the mother toward maintaining sobriety and for the infant to have an emotionally healthy family and safe home environment.

CLINICS CARE POINTS

- Use validated screening tool for maternal substance use.
- Consider universal screening of all mothers to avoid bias.
- Support breastfeeding whenever possible and safe.
- Engage multidisciplinary team for maternal-infant care during and after birth hospital stay.

DISCLOSURE

The authors have no relevant conflicts of interest to disclose.

Best practices

- Current practice for maternal substance use is verbal screening early in pregnancy using a validated tool
- Multidisciplinary team to support substance use treatment and comorbidities including mental health
- Recognizing NAS
- Adoption of standardized clinical assessments for NAS and prioritizing nonpharmacologic, family-centered care to improve hospital outcomes
- Supporting safe breastfeeding
- Obstetric and pediatric practitioners collaborating to support mother and infant postpartum

REFERENCES

1. Building US. Capacity to Review and Prevent Maternal Deaths. (2018). Report from nine maternal mortality review committees. 2020. Available at: https://reviewtoaction.org/Report_from_Nine_MMRCs. Accessed October 25, 2020.

2. SAMHSA. 2020. Available at: https://store.samhsa.gov/product/Behavioral-Health-Barometer-2015/SMA16-BARO-2015. Accessed October 25, 2020.

3. Wright TE, Terplan M, Ondersma SJ, et al. The role of screening, brief intervention, and referral to treatment in the perinatal period. Am J Obstet Gynecol 2016;215(5):539–47.
4. Committee Opinion No. Committee Opinion No. 711 summary: opioid use and opioid use disorder in pregnancy. Obstet Gynecol 2017;130(2):488–9.
5. Pulatie K. The legality of drug-testing procedures for pregnant women. Virtual Mentor 2008;10(1):41–4.
6. Bogen DL, Whalen BL, Kair LR, et al. Wide variation found in care of opioid-exposed newborns. Acad Pediatr 2017;17(4):374–80.
7. Montgomery D, Plate C, Alder SC, et al. Testing for fetal exposure to illicit drugs using umbilical cord tissue vs meconium. J Perinatol 2006;26(1):11–4.
8. Kelly TM, Daley DC. Integrated treatment of substance use and psychiatric disorders. Soc Work Public Health 2013;28(3–4):388–406.
9. Ross S, Peselow E. Co-occurring psychotic and addictive disorders: neurobiology and diagnosis. Clin Neuropharmacol 2012;35(5):235–43.
10. Dube SR, Felitti VJ, Dong M, et al. Childhood abuse, neglect, and household dysfunction and the risk of illicit drug use: the adverse childhood experiences study. Pediatrics 2003;111(3):564–72.
11. Centers for disease control and Prevention. Testing recommendations for Hepatitis C virus infection: CDC recommendations for Hepatitis C screening among Adults in the United States. Available at: https://www.cdc.gov/hepatitis/hcv/guidelinesc.htm#:~:text=CDC%20Recommendations%20for%20Hepatitis%20C,is%20less%20than%200.1%25* Accessed November 4, 2020.
12. Broussard CS, Rasmussen SA, Reefhuis J, et al. Maternal treatment with opioid analgesics and risk for birth defects. Am J Obstet Gynecol 2011;204(4):314.e1-11.
13. Yazdy MM, Mitchell AA, Tinker SC, et al. Periconceptional use of opioids and the risk of neural tube defects. Obstet Gynecol 2013;122(4):838–44.
14. Committee on the Health Effects of Marijuana: An Evidence Review and Research Agenda; Board on Population Health and Public Health Practice; Health and Medicine Division; National Academies of Sciences. The Health Effects of cannabis and cannabinoids: the current state of evidence and recommendations for research. 2020. Available at: http:www.nap.edu/246252017. Accessed October 29, 2020.
15. Correa F, Wolfson ML, Valchi P, et al. Endocannabinoid system and pregnancy. Reproduction 2016;152(6):R191–200.
16. Metz TD, Borgelt LM. Marijuana use in pregnancy and while breastfeeding. Obstet Gynecol 2018;132(5):1198–210.
17. Metz TD, Stickrath EH. Marijuana use in pregnancy and lactation: a review of the evidence. Am J Obstet Gynecol 2015;213(6):761–78.
18. Goldschmidt L, Richardson GA, Willford J, et al. Prenatal marijuana exposure and intelligence test performance at age 6. J Am Acad Child Adolesc Psychiatry 2008;47(3):254–63.
19. Paul SE, Hatoum AS, Fine JD, et al. Associations between prenatal cannabis exposure and childhood outcomes: results from the ABCD Study. JAMA Psychiatry 2021;78(1):64–76.
20. Day NL, Goldschmidt L, Thomas CA. Prenatal marijuana exposure contributes to the prediction of marijuana use at age 14. Addiction 2006;101(9):1313–22.
21. Marjiuana. 2020. Available at: https://www.acog.org/clinical/clinical-guidance/committee-opinion/articles/2017/10/marijuana-use-during-pregnancy-and-lactation. Accessed November 14, 2020.
22. Retail marijuana public health Advisory Committee. Monitoring health concerns related to marijuana in Colorado: 2016. Changes in marijuana use patterns,

systematic literature review, and Possible marijuana-related health effects. Colorado Department of Public Health and Environment; 2016. 2020. Available at: https://drive.google.com/file/d/0B0tmPQ67k3NVQlFnY3VzZGVmdFk/view. Accessed November 14, 2020.
23. Tobacco, Nicotine Cessation During Pregnancy: ACOG Committee Opinion Summary. Tobacco and nicotine cessation during pregnancy: ACOG Committee Opinion summary, number 807. Obstet Gynecol 2020;135(5):1244–6.
24. Kuehn B. Vaping and pregnancy. JAMA 2019;321(14):1344.
25. Hurt RD, Renner CC, Patten CA, et al. Iqmik–a form of smokeless tobacco used by pregnant Alaska natives: nicotine exposure in their neonates. J Matern Fetal Neonatal Med 2005;17(4):281–9.
26. Gupta PC, Subramoney S, Sreevidya S. Smokeless tobacco use, birth weight, and gestational age: population based, prospective cohort study of 1217 women in Mumbai, India. BMJ 2004;328(7455):1538.
27. Gunnerbeck A, Wikström AK, Bonamy AK, et al. Relationship of maternal snuff use and cigarette smoking with neonatal apnea. Pediatrics 2011;128(3):503–9.
28. Fasd. 2020. Available at: https://www.cdc.gov/ncbddd/fasd/data.html.
29. Warren KR, Foudin LL. Alcohol-related birth defects–the past, present, and future. Alcohol Res Health 2001;25(3):153–8. Accessed November 16, 2020.
30. Bellantuono C, Tofani S, Di Sciascio G, et al. Benzodiazepine exposure in pregnancy and risk of major malformations: a critical overview. Gen Hosp Psychiatry 2013;35(1):3–8.
31. DeVido J, Bogunovic O, Weiss RD. Alcohol use disorders in pregnancy. Harv Rev Psychiatry 2015;23(2):112–21.
32. Cain MA, Bornick P, Whiteman V. The maternal, fetal, and neonatal effects of cocaine exposure in pregnancy. Clin Obstet Gynecol 2013;56(1):124–32.
33. Cressman AM, Natekar A, Kim E, et al. Cocaine abuse during pregnancy. J Obstet Gynaecol Can 2014;36(7):628–31.
34. Wright TE, Schuetter R, Tellei J, et al. Methamphetamines and pregnancy outcomes. J Addict Med 2015;9(2):111–7.
35. Singer LT, Moore DG, Fulton S, et al. Neurobehavioral outcomes of infants exposed to MDMA (Ecstasy) and other recreational drugs during pregnancy. Neurotoxicol Teratol 2012;34(3):303–10.
36. Methamphetamine. 2020. Available at: https://www.acog.org/clinical/clinical-guidance/committee-opinion/articles/2011/03/methamphetamine-abuse-in-women-of-reproductive-age. Accessed November 16, 2020.
37. Gorman MC, Orme KS, Nguyen NT, et al. Outcomes in pregnancies complicated by methamphetamine use. Am J Obstet Gynecol 2014;211(4):429.e1-7.
38. Smith LM, LaGasse LL, Derauf C, et al. The infant development, environment, and lifestyle study: effects of prenatal methamphetamine exposure, polydrug exposure, and poverty on intrauterine growth. Pediatrics 2006;118(3):1149–56.
39. Shah R, Diaz SD, Arria A, et al. Prenatal methamphetamine exposure and short-term maternal and infant medical outcomes. Am J Perinatol 2012;29(5):391–400.
40. Reece-Stremtan S, Marinelli KA. ABM clinical protocol #21: guidelines for breastfeeding and substance use or substance use disorder, revised 2015. Breastfeed Med 2015;10(3):135–41.
41. Brogly S. Maternal and child health after prenatal opioid exposure. JAMA Netw Open 2019;2(6):e196428.
42. Azuine RE, Ji Y, Chang HY, et al. Prenatal risk factors and perinatal and postnatal outcomes associated with maternal opioid exposure in an urban, low-income, multiethnic US Population. JAMA Netw Open 2019;2(6):e196405.

43. Hack M, Schluchter M, Andreias L, et al. Change in prevalence of chronic conditions between childhood and adolescence among extremely low-birth-weight children. JAMA 2011;306(4):394–401.
44. Larson JJ, Graham DL, Singer LT, et al. Cognitive and behavioral impact on children exposed to opioids during pregnancy. Pediatrics 2019;144(2):e20190514.
45. MacMillan KDL, Rendon CP, Verma K, et al. Association of rooming-in with outcomes for neonatal abstinence syndrome: a systematic review and meta-analysis. JAMA Pediatr 2018;172(4):345–51.
46. Devlin LA, Davis JM. A practical approach to neonatal opiate withdrawal syndrome. Am J Perinatol 2018;35(4):324–30.
47. Piccotti L, Voigtman B, Vongsa R, et al. Neonatal opioid withdrawal syndrome: a developmental care approach. Neonatal Netw 2019;38(3):160–9.
48. O'Connor AB, Collett A, Alto WA, et al. Breastfeeding rates and the relationship between breastfeeding and neonatal abstinence syndrome in women maintained on buprenorphine during pregnancy. J Midwifery Womens Health 2013;58(4):383–8.
49. Whalen BL, Holmes AV, Blythe S. Models of care for neonatal abstinence syndrome: what works? Semin Fetal Neonatal Med 2019;24(2):121–32.
50. Jansson LM, Velez M, Harrow C. The opioid-exposed newborn: assessment and pharmacologic management. J Opioid Manag 2009;5(1):47–55.
51. Finnegan LP, Connaughton JF, Kron RE, et al. Neonatal abstinence syndrome: assessment and management. Addict Dis 1975;2(1–2):141–58.
52. Lipsitz PJ. A proposed narcotic withdrawal score for use with newborn infants. A pragmatic evaluation of its efficacy. Clin Pediatr (Phila) 1975;14(6):592–4.
53. Holmes AV, Atwood EC, Whalen B, et al. Rooming-in to treat neonatal abstinence syndrome: improved family-centered care at lower cost. Pediatrics 2016;137(6):e20152929.
54. Short VL, Gannon M, Abatemarco DJ. The association between breastfeeding and length of hospital stay among infants diagnosed with neonatal abstinence syndrome: a population-based study of in-hospital births. Breastfeed Med 2016;11:343–9.
55. Czynski AJ, Davis JM, Dansereau LM, et al. Neurodevelopmental outcomes of neonates randomized to morphine or methadone for treatment of neonatal abstinence syndrome. J Pediatr 2020;219:146.e1.
56. Welle-Strand GK, Skurtveit S, Jansson LM, et al. Breastfeeding reduces the need for withdrawal treatment in opioid-exposed infants. Acta Paediatr 2013;102(11):1060–6.
57. Wong S, Ordean A, Kahan M. SOGC clinical practice guidelines: substance use in pregnancy: no. 256, April 2011. Int J Gynaecol Obstet 2011;114(4):190–202.
58. Davis JM, Shenberger J, Terrin N, et al. Comparison of safety and efficacy of methadone vs morphine for treatment of neonatal abstinence syndrome: a randomized clinical trial. JAMA Pediatr 2018;172(8):741–8.
59. Demirci JR, Bogen DL, Klionsky Y. Breastfeeding and methadone therapy: the maternal experience. Subst Abus 2015;36(2):203–8.
60. Tolia VN, Murthy K, Bennett MM, et al. Antenatal methadone vs buprenorphine exposure and length of hospital stay in infants admitted to the intensive care unit with neonatal abstinence syndrome. J Perinatol 2018;38(1):75–9.
61. Jansson LM, Di Pietro JA, Elko A, et al. Pregnancies exposed to methadone, methadone and other illicit substances, and poly-drugs without methadone: a comparison of fetal neurobehaviors and infant outcomes. Drug Alcohol Depend 2012;122(3):213-9.
62. Wozniak JR, Riley EP, Charness ME. Clinical presentation, diagnosis, and management of fetal alcohol spectrum disorder. Lancet Neurol 2019;18(8):760–70.

63. Bunik M. The Pediatrician's role in encouraging exclusive breastfeeding. Pediatr Rev 2017;38(8):353–68.
64. Jansson LM, Di Pietro JA, Elko A, et al. Pregnancies exposed to methadone, methadone and other illicit substances, and poly-drugs without methadone: a comparison of fetal neurobehaviors and infant outcomes. Drug Alcohol Depend 2012;122(3):213–9.
65. Wilson J, Tay RY, McCormack C, et al. Alcohol consumption by breastfeeding mothers: frequency, correlates and infant outcomes. Drug Alcohol Rev 2017; 36(5):667–76.
66. Kia F, Tosun N, Carlson S, et al. Examining characteristics associated with quitting smoking during pregnancy and relapse postpartum. Addict Behav 2018;78:114–9.
67. Pereira PP, Da Mata FA, Figueiredo AC, et al. Maternal active smoking during pregnancy and low birth weight in the americas: a systematic review and meta-analysis. Nicotine Tob Res 2017;19(5):497–505.
68. Napierala M, Mazela J, Merritt TA, et al. Tobacco smoking and breastfeeding: effect on the lactation process, breast milk composition and infant development. A critical review. Environ Res 2016;151:321–38.
69. Cohen SS, Alexander DD, Krebs NF, et al. Factors associated with breastfeeding initiation and continuation: a meta-analysis. J Pediatr 2018;203:190.e21.
70. Carlin RF, Moon RY. Risk factors, protective factors, and current recommendations to reduce sudden infant death syndrome: a review. JAMA Pediatr 2017; 171(2):175–80.
71. Baraona LK, Lovelace D, Daniels JL, et al. Tobacco harms, nicotine pharmacology, and pharmacologic tobacco cessation interventions for women. J Midwifery Womens Health 2017;62(3):253–69.
72. Ryan SA, Ammerman SD, O'Connor ME. Marijuana use during pregnancy and breastfeeding: implications for neonatal and childhood outcomes. Pediatrics 2018;142(3):e20181889.
73. Eiden RD, Schuetze P, Shisler S, et al. Prenatal exposure to tobacco and cannabis: effects on autonomic and emotion regulation. Neurotoxicol Teratol 2018;68:47–56.
74. Campolongo P, Trezza V, Palmery M, et al. Developmental exposure to cannabinoids causes subtle and enduring neurofunctional alterations. Int Rev Neurobiol 2009;85:117–33.
75. Chandra S, Radwan MM, Majumdar CG, et al. New trends in cannabis potency in USA and Europe during the last decade (2008-2017). Eur Arch Psychiatry Clin Neurosci 2019;269(1):5–15.
76. Baker T, Datta P, Rewers-Felkins K, et al. Transfer of inhaled cannabis into human breast milk. Obstet Gynecol 2018;131(5):783–8.
77. Bertrand KA, Hanan NJ, Honerkamp-Smith G, et al. Marijuana use by breastfeeding mothers and cannabinoid concentrations in breast milk. Pediatrics 2018; 142(3):e20181076.
78. Wymore EM, Palmer C, Wang GS, et al. Persistence of Δ-9-Tetrahydrocannabinol in Human Breast Milk. JAMA Pediatr 2021;175(6):632–4.
79. Chapman SL, Wu LT. Postpartum substance use and depressive symptoms: a review. Women Health 2013;53(5):479–503.
80. Stewart DE, Vigod SN. Postpartum depression: pathophysiology, treatment, and emerging therapeutics. Annu Rev Med 2019;70:183–96.
81. Figueiredo B, Dias CC, Brandão S, et al. Breastfeeding and postpartum depression: state of the art review. J Pediatr (Rio J) 2013;89(4):332–8.
82. Jansson LM, Patrick SW. Neonatal abstinence syndrome. Pediatr Clin North Am 2019;66(2):353–67.

The Term Newborn

Alternative Birth Practices, Refusal, and Therapeutic Hesitancy

Michelle Leff, MD, IBCLC[a,*], Jaspreet Loyal, MD, MS[b]

KEYWORDS

- Routine recommendations • Alternative birth practices • Refusal
- Therapeutic hesitancy

KEY POINTS

- Refusal of various routine newborn care practices is uncommon but has increased over the past several years.
- It is important for clinicians to know what types of interventions may be refused by parents and why.
- Clinicians should be knowledgeable about current societal trends in newborn care and be able to speak about alternative practices and the evidence around these alternative practices.
- Physicians should meet parents where they are on the hesitancy spectrum and develop strategies to address specific concerns respectfully.

INTRODUCTION

Childbirth has evolved throughout history in many ways. In the United States, there is a strong cultural belief that childbirth should be a very personal, controlled, special experience. The general public has more access to medical information, and there has been a shift from paternalistic practices to a shared decision-making model. Patients regularly report doing their research and come to a visit with ideas about their diagnosis and treatment. It is not uncommon for expectant parents to spend hours deciding how and where to deliver their newborn. Expectant parents reach out to a wide circle for information including friends, family, books, the Internet, and social media. Although in-hospital births are still the norm in the United States, freestanding birthing centers and midwives offering home births are more prevalent than in the near past. In addition to choosing the ideal location to give birth, many Web sites,

[a] Department of Pediatrics, University of California San Diego; [b] Department of Pediatrics, Yale School of Medicine, 333 Cedar Street, New Haven, CT 06520, USA
* Corresponding author. 9300 Campus Point Drive, Mail Code 7774, La Jolla, CA 92037.
E-mail address: mleff@health.ucsd.edu

Clin Perinatol 48 (2021) 647–663
https://doi.org/10.1016/j.clp.2021.05.012 perinatology.theclinics.com

books, and instructors encourage families to develop a birth plan that sets out preferences for all aspects of the birth encounter. A quick Internet search yields an abundance of templates and preformatted birth plans with all sorts of ideas about how to direct this experience. In many ways, individuals taking ownership of their health and medical care is positive and patients should be their own advocates.

Some aspects of labor and delivery and newborn care can be personalized without harm, whereas other medical recommendations are there for a reason. The newborn hospital stay is designed to monitor the newborn during the first critical hours of transition from the in utero environment. Policies are in place to protect the newborn from infection and to detect issues while treatment is most effective. There is strong agreement among most health care clinicians and medical organizations about what is best practice during the birth stay. In addition to observation of vitals, ensuring voiding and stooling, and providing feeding support, the American Academy of Pediatrics (AAP) and others recommend specific interventions before hospital discharge. These interventions include the administration of intramuscular vitamin K for prevention of vitamin K deficiency bleeding of the newborn (VKDB), ocular prophylaxis for the prevention of gonococcal neonatal ophthalmia, hepatitis B (HepB) vaccination within 24 hours of birth, and universal screening for medical conditions such as metabolic disturbances, hearing loss, and critical congenital heart disease (CCHD).[1–3]

It is important for clinicians caring for newborns to be aware of different concerns and emerging trends around hesitancy and refusals by parents to better address them. Requested alternatives to common newborn interventions and screenings include complete refusal, delays, or substitution with a different intervention (**Table 1**). What follows is a discussion of birth practices, parent hesitancy regarding routine in-hospital newborn care, and recommendations for communicating with families.

HESITANCIES AND REFUSALS IN THE WELL NEWBORN UNIT

Vitamin K, Ocular Prophylaxis, and Hepatitis B Vaccine

Newborn clinicians most commonly encounter refusal of one or more of the following recommended interventions: vitamin K administration, ocular prophylaxis, and HepB vaccine. The reported frequency of refusal of intramuscular (IM) vitamin K by parents ranges from 0% to 3.2% in US hospitals, up to 14.5% in home births, and up to 31.0% in birthing centers.[4] It has been shown that parents who refuse IM vitamin K are more likely to refuse HepB immunization and ocular prophylaxis.[5] Reported reasons for IM vitamin K refusal are concern of harm from the injection, a desire to be natural, and a belief in alternative methods of prophylaxis.

Reasons for why parents refuse ocular prophylaxis are not reported in the literature. Anecdotally from the authors' experience, some parents believe that ocular prophylaxis is unnecessary if the mother's prenatal gonorrhea testing gives negative result. Other parents worry about the potential harmful effect of ocular prophylaxis on mother-newborn bonding and the newborn's microbiome. In a single-center study in Michigan, investigators reported that of 3758 newborns, 5.9% did not receive ocular prophylaxis.[6]

This same study revealed that 13.6% of newborns did not receive HepB vaccine at their institution.[6] National statistics show that approximately 25% of infants in the United States do not receive the birth dose of Hep B vaccine.[7] Vaccine refusal is complex, and there are many studies about parental attitudes toward childhood immunizations. In a review of qualitative studies on parents' attitudes toward childhood vaccinations, investigators reported that experiences, emotions, routine ways of thinking, information sources, peers/family, risk perceptions, and trust, among other

Table 1
Examples of refusals encountered in the newborn care setting

Refusal	Reasons for Refusal	Parent Requested Alternatives
Prenatal testing	Parent not wanting to know about a potential birth defect, not planning to terminate pregnancy	No prenatal testing Less-invasive forms of testing
GBS prophylaxis	Concern for disruption of newborn microbiome, perception that risk of GBS infection to the newborn is low	Vaginal Hibiclens, treat and retest, garlic cloves in vagina, yogurt in vagina
Intramuscular vitamin K	Concern for harm from injection and ingredients, thought to be unnecessary, parents seeking more "natural" approaches	No prophylaxis Oral vitamin K Increasing maternal dietary intake of vitamin K
Ocular prophylaxis	No prenatal exposure to gonorrhea, negatively affects bonding, chemical irritation	No prophylaxis Colostrum/breast milk in the eye as prophylaxis
Hepatitis B vaccine	No maternal exposure to hepatitis B, pain from injection, newborn is too young/immune system not strong enough yet	Delay Decline all together
Hypoglycemia screening	Unnecessary, pain from multiple heel sticks, interference with breastfeeding	No screening Ad lib feedings
Newborn screening	No known family genetic conditions, pain, concern that government is collecting newborn's DNA, concern for false-positive result and needless worry	No screening
Hearing screen	Belief that newborn's hearing is normal, fear of the machine and its effect on newborn's brain	No screening
Serum bilirubin	Pain from blood draw	No blood draws Wait for jaundice to be visible "Treat" with sunlight
TCB	Fear of the bilimeter	No screening Wait for jaundice to be visible

(*continued on next page*)

Table 1
(*continued*)

Refusal	Reasons for Refusal	Parent Requested Alternatives
Vital signs	Minimize interruptions to newborn, concern that crying is bad for newborn	Defer all or some vital signs
Hospital diapers	Concern that hospital diapers are bad for newborn's skin, concern for the environment	Use organic brand or cloth diapers only Keep newborn naked without a diaper
Supplementation	Perception that maternal breast milk is enough, fear of the supplement	No supplementation IV Fluids
Formula	Do not want standard hospital cow's milk-based formula because of concern for allergies or "substandard" ingredients	Prefer organic, soy, goat's milk, or European formulas
CCHD screen	Fear of the pulse oximeter	No screening
Birth certificate	Fear of government or agencies trying to track the newborn and/or family	None
Signing of waivers	Refuse to sign hospital IM vitamin K refusal form because of perception that by giving oral vitamin K, parents are complying with recommendations Want to maintain liability	None

Abbreviations: GBS, group B *Streptococcus*; IM, intramuscular; IV, intravenous; TCB, transcutaneous bilirubin.

factors, inform parents' attitudes and decision-making processes.[8] In a survey of parents in 2012 and 2014, investigators reported that clinician trust and communication, along with varying degrees of personal network influences, likely contribute to immunization decisions of parents.[9]

A review of state statutes in 2006 revealed that 32 states had laws mandating erythromycin ointment be applied as ocular prophylaxis.[10] Legislation around vitamin K administration in US states is not as robust. A few states require administration of IM vitamin K and others allow administration of oral vitamin K, a controversial alternative to IM vitamin K. Oral vitamin K is commonly used in parts of Europe as prophylaxis against VKDB but is not approved by the US Food and Drug Administration (FDA) for this use. Oral vitamin K is not as effective as the IM injection against VKDB, and there are several oral regimens to choose from, adding to the controversy.[4]

Routine Newborn Screening

Routine screenings recommended by the AAP during the hospital stay for an otherwise healthy late preterm or term newborn include screening for hyperbilirubinemia with a transcutaneous or serum bilirubin measurement, screening for a variety of conditions through collection of a dried blood spot, and screenings for hearing loss and CCHD via point-of-care testing before discharge.[1] These multiple screenings are completed per hospital protocol and state regulations. All 50 US states mandate newborn screening, but the conditions included vary state to state.[11] The Department of Health and Human Services currently recommends screening for 35 conditions including hearing loss and CCHD.[12] New conditions are added over time, and it is up to each state to decide which they will include in newborn screening. Most states screen for the entire list, a few do not, and a few states screen for additional conditions. Hearing and CCHD screenings are performed in all US states.[13,14] Nearly 13,000 newborns per year are diagnosed by newborn screening, about half of which are diagnosed with hearing loss.[15] Detection of hearing loss at an early age provides opportunities for early intervention to benefit a child's developmental outcomes. CCHD occurs in approximately 2 of every 1000 live births.[13] Information on what is tested for in each state in the United States, what conditions must be met for opting out, and what is done with the dried blood spots once the test is complete is readily available online for parents and clinicians.[16]

There is limited published information about the reasons for and frequency of refusal of dried blood spot collection, hearing screening, and CCHD screening. In a review of 40,440 live births in North Dakota, investigators found that 0.33% of newborns were not screened by blood spot due to refusal by a parent. Investigators reported that 97% of the refusals were among white women, 94% were home births, and 93% used state noncredentialed birth attendants.[17] The rate of parent refusal for dried blood spot collection in California is similar at approximately 0.30%. The refusal rate has been stable since about 2013 after having climbed from 0.11% in 2006 when refusal data were first collected (Jamie Matteson, MPH, California Department of Public Health, e-mail communication, July 22, 2020). The frequency of refusal of newborn hearing screening and CCHD screening by parents is not well known. In the authors' experience refusal of CCHD and newborn hearing screening is much less common because the procedures are not perceived as painful or invasive and do not result in the potential storage of genetic information.

Public health policy and practice implications of refusal of newborn screening by parents are complex and beyond the scope of this article.[18] There are also ethical questions around what components of newborn screening should be mandatory and when are parental exemptions permissible.[19,20] These complexities and variations across states makes it challenging for clinicians caring for newborns to have consistent messaging and know what to expect when parents push back against routine screening.

Risk-Based Screenings and Treatments

Additional screenings that may be performed on individual newborns based on specific risk factors include screening for hypoglycemia, infection, and car seat tolerance.[21,22] Treatments offered in the newborn unit may include phototherapy, intravenous antibiotics, glucose gel or supplemental feeds, and prolonged hospital stays for observation. Data on refusals of these screenings and treatments are not widely available. The authors have encountered refusals of all the aforementioned screenings and treatments by parents of newborns. Parents cite reasons such as their newborn appears healthy or that parents dislike their newborn getting poked. Parents may decline antibiotics because they have heard about how that can affect the newborn's microbiome. Parents may also worry about supplemental feeds to treat hypoglycemia and a potential negative affect on the success of breastfeeding.

Feeding

For parents who elect to feed their newborn with formula, most will select a standard US cow's milk-based formula, but there are increasing numbers of parents who are choosing other options such as homemade formula, goat's milk-based formula, or European formula. Homemade formula cannot meet the high standards of an FDA-approved commercially prepared newborn formula. Soy formula is medically acceptable for lactose intolerance and preferred by some vegan parents, but it is not considered the first choice by pediatricians and not recommended for preterm newborns.[23] European formulas are not approved for sale in the United States. Some families order online but should be cautioned about differences in iron content, measuring instructions, and language barriers. Anecdotally families choose these because they believe organic standards in Europe are higher than in the United States. There is no FDA-approved goat's milk-based formula yet for newborns, but there is a goat's milk toddler formula that is occasionally purchased by families. Most hospitals carry a limited option of formulas, which is usually based on purchasing contracts and may have strict guidelines on formula brought in by parents. Hospitals and newborn clinicians should be prepared to address families that bring their preferred formula to the hospital for use during the stay.

Even when newborn units strongly promote and support breastfeeding, some mothers will be unable or have an inadequate supply. Some of these parents turn to shared milk received from friends or purchased online from strangers. Risks and benefits need to be discussed in detail with families because shared milk has been found to carry bacteria and milk purchased online has been found to be contaminated with cow's milk.[24,25] An increasing number of newborn units are offering donor human milk from a certified milk bank. Pasteurized donor human milk (PDHM) from a certified milk bank is thought to be the next best option to mother's own milk.[26] Some families decline PDHM out of concerns over safety or feeling uncomfortable with the idea of giving another mother's milk to their child.[27] In some cultures, there is the idea of "milk kinship," defined as a relationship formed during nursing by a nonbiological mother, and this may affect a mother's acceptance of donor milk.

Bathing

Some alternatives that parents request may be reasonable and easy to accommodate even if the request is a variation from a unit's typical policy. For example, there is no set standard for bathing of the newborn unless the mother has positive test results for human immunodeficiency virus, and there is significant variation around timing of the newborn bath across the country. Historically it was standard practice in most well newborn units in the United States to immediately bathe the newborn, and this is still the case in many hospitals. Other units delay bathing by 4 to 6 hours to allow for maternal-newborn bonding and initiation of breastfeeding. The World Health Organization and Association of Women's Health, Obstetric and Neonatal Nurses recommend not removing vernix and delaying the bath for at least 6 to 24 hours.[28,29] Several studies have shown decreased hypothermia and hypoglycemia as well as increased rates of breastfeeding at discharge if this practice is followed. A recent review of the biology of vernix demonstrates its many beneficial properties.[30] The authors of this article focus on the challenges of differing parental preferences, whereas this is an example of patients perhaps leading improvements in health care.

Evolving Recommendations: Coronavirus Disease 2019 as an Example

Sometimes, recommendations from professional organizations can be difficult for clinicians to promote and refusal by parents is understandable. Specifically, in the spring of 2020, as the coronavirus disease 2019 (COVID-19) pandemic was beginning to ramp up in the United States, little was known about the effects of severe acute respiratory syndrome coronavirus 2 on newborns. With insufficient evidence and in an abundance of caution, the AAP initially recommended the temporary separation of mothers testing positive for COVID-19 and their newborn for the birth hospitalization. Negative impacts of this recommendation were seen on mother-newborn bonding and breastfeeding. In our experience, many mothers with COVID-19 refused to separate from their newborns citing lack of evidence for the practice and willingness to accept the risk to their newborn. In the summer of 2020, the AAP reversed their initial guidance to recommend rooming-in for these mother-newborn dyads.[31] In this case, refusal by parents to adhere to the initial recommendation was not without merit.

REFUSALS AND ALTERNATIVES IN LABOR AND DELIVERY

Out-of-Hospital Births and Elective Cesarean Delivery

Although the focus of this article is refusal of newborn interventions and screenings by parents, decisions made during pregnancy and the perinatal period influence what parents choose to do for their newborn. A study at one hospital in North Carolina showed that 72% of parents had made decisions about vaccination even before conception.[32] Unlike in many countries in the world, most US women deliver in a hospital; however, a small but growing number choose an out-of-hospital birth experience.[33,34] An out-of-hospital birth includes births occurring in a home, birthing center, clinic or doctor's office, or other location In 2012, 1.36% of US births were outside a hospital, up from 1.26% in 2011.[33] For context, in 2018, there were 3.79 million births in the United States.[35] As previously discussed, home births are often associated with refusal of routine newborn interventions such as vitamin K prophylaxis.[4]

A small proportion of pregnant women in the United States request to have an elective cesarean delivery (estimated 2.5% of all births). According to the American College of Obstetricians and Gynecologists (ACOG), a vaginal delivery should be recommended if there are no maternal or fetal indications for cesarean delivery. As long as a mother is properly counseled, however, her choice of cesarean delivery should be honored.[36]

Water Immersion

Immersion in water has been suggested by some as a beneficial alternative for labor, delivery, or both, and over the past few decades this practice has gained popularity in many parts of the world. The prevalence of water immersion in the United States is not well understood. The reported benefits include decreased pain or use of anesthesia and decreased duration of labor. According to the AAP and ACOG, there is no evidence that immersion in water during the first stage of labor otherwise improves perinatal outcomes, and it should not prevent or inhibit other elements of care. The safety and efficacy of immersion in water during the second stage of labor has not been established, and immersion in water during the second stage of labor has not been associated with maternal or fetal benefit. There have been case reports of rare but serious adverse effects in the newborn. Owing to insufficient evidence regarding the relative benefits and risks of immersion in water in the second stage of labor (underwater delivery), the ACOG recommends that birth occur on land, not water.[37] There are published studies in which investigators report that concerns against water birth are not evidence-based and that this practice is safe in low-risk pregnancies and that there is a high level of maternal satisfaction associated with water births.[38–40]

Umbilical Nonseverance

Although rare, some mothers practice "lotus birth" or umbilical cord nonseverance (UCNS), which is the practice of leaving the umbilical cord uncut so that it and the placenta remain connected to the newborn until they detach spontaneously. There is a plethora of information on the practice of UCNS on the Internet including a belief that UCNS is a spiritual practice and honors the relationship between the newborn and placenta. ACOG and the AAP do not recommend UCNS, but there are case reports of UCNS in the United States. In one case report of 6 mothers who chose UCNS, reasons given by mothers included wanting blood from the placenta to reach the newborn, concern for emotional trauma to the newborn, promotion of the newborn's development, and participation in a family cultural practice.[41] In this case series, 2 newborns developed hyperbilirubinemia, but there were no significant adverse outcomes. There was, however, a lower uptake of standard newborn interventions. In another case series of 3 newborns whose parents chose UCNS, investigators described complications associated with UCNS, specifically bacterial endocarditis, omphalitis, and bacteremia.[42]

Placenta Disposition

What to do with the placenta is a common question in some parts of the country. Options include disposal, use as fertilizer in one's garden, craft projects, and in some instances placentophagy or ingestion of the placenta. Placentophagy is common among mammals but not so among humans, although there appears to be a growing interest in the United States.[43] The placenta can be consumed raw, cooked, or encapsulated. There is no reported scientific evidence of clinical benefit of placentophagy.[44] Some of the purported benefits include positive influence on mood, iron status, and lactation. There has been a case report of a newborn who developed recurrent group B *Streptococcus* sepsis after the mother ingested placenta capsules contaminated with the bacteria.[45] In some facilities the request for the placenta is so common that policies exist to help with its disposition. Sometimes the parental request is at odds with the physician's desire for placental pathology, and this should be addressed with the family before its disposition.

STRATEGIES TO ADDRESS HESITANCY AND REFUSAL

Where to Start

When a clinician is confronted with medical hesitancy it can be hard to know how to address it. In medical training, clinicians are taught scientific principles, and generally they rely on these principles to educate their patients. Patients, however, may be coming from a place of emotion. Perhaps they have heard stories of children thought to be harmed by medical interventions. Giving families in this situation scientific data may not be the best strategy. Therefore, the most important first step for the clinician is to listen by engaging the family in a nonconfrontational conversation to try to determine the specific concern.

At the same time, it is helpful to try to gauge where the parents are on the spectrum of hesitancy/refusal (**Fig. 1**). Some families are truly undecided and want more information before making a choice. Others are adamantly against the recommendation and will not change their mind no matter what. Physicians with the Permanente Medical Group have recognized the difference in these groups of parents and developed a framework for vaccine discussions.[46] The same general principles can be used with any medical intervention. How a clinician addresses the family will need to vary based on where the family lies on this spectrum. For instance, pushing too hard with a family who is strongly opposed may alienate them further.

Another important starting point is for the clinician to develop rapport with the family before addressing refusals. Typically, a clinician will have been informed that a family has decided to refuse some aspect of their newborn's care before meeting the family on the well newborn unit. The clinician should not initiate the interaction by addressing the refusal immediately. Instead, clinicians should introduce themselves, congratulate the family, examine the newborn, and address any questions from the parents before entering a potentially difficult conversation.

Build Alliances

These discussions are made more difficult for the newborn clinician when they do not have a relationship with the family before their encounter on the postpartum unit. This is common when hospitalists staff a newborn unit instead of primary care clinicians who likely have a longer relationship with the family. Ideally, the obstetrician or midwife has begun the discussion of these important recommendations, but this may not always be the case. This becomes more problematic for the hospitalist if the parent perceives support for their viewpoint from their prenatal clinician with whom they have developed rapport and a trusting relationship. Newborn clinicians can be proactive and join committees that involve prenatal clinicians and help prepare or review educational materials for expecting parents. Clinicians working in ambulatory settings may

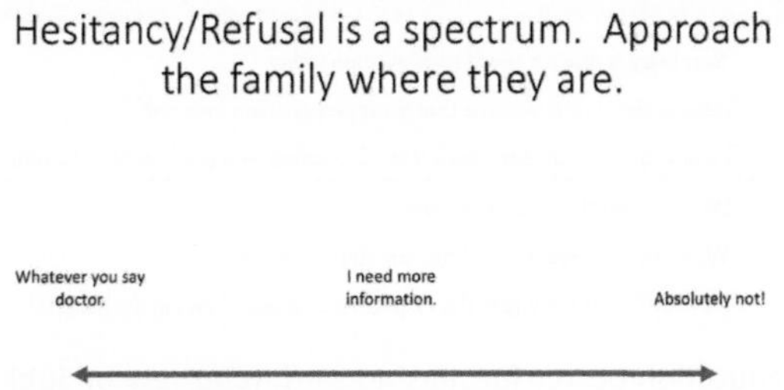
Hesitancy/Refusal is a spectrum. Approach the family where they are.
Whatever you say doctor.
I need more information.
Absolutely not!

Fig. 1. The spectrum of hesitancy and refusal.

offer prenatal consultations where routine newborn recommendations are discussed in preparation for the birth hospitalization.

Standard Scripting

The scripting of routine preventative newborn interventions is important. An example witnessed by one author involved the refusal of IM vitamin K by parents who had given it to their 2 previous children; they explained they refused it this time because the nurse asked them *if* they wanted it. With their previous children, no one had asked for their consent so they thought this must be something new. This example demonstrates the benefit of using a presumptive discussion, which has been studied by Opel et al.[47] in regard to vaccine discussions. The nurse should have said, "*it is now time for your child's vitamin K injection*" rather than "*would you like your child to have vitamin K*?" Educating the care team on scripting can be helpful, especially because usually a family has refused the intervention before the newborn clinician has seen the family, and the opportunity to re-engage the family may be lost. **Fig. 2** is an educational poster

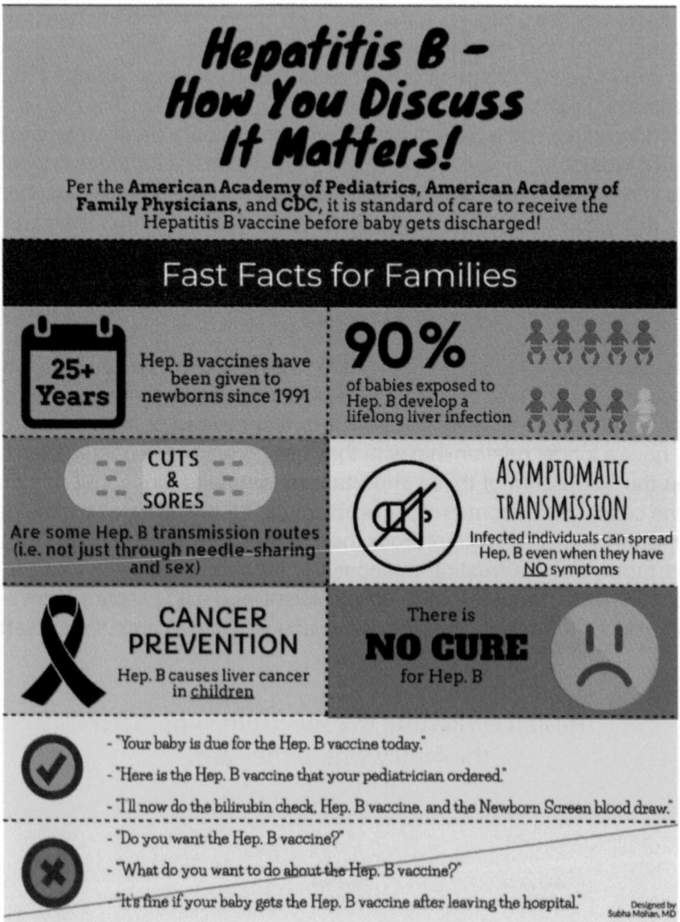
Hepatitis B - How You Discuss It Matters!
Per the American Academy of Pediatrics, American Academy of Family Physicians, and CDC, it is standard of care to receive the Hepatitis B vaccine before baby gets discharged!
Fast Facts for Families
25+ Years
Hep. B vaccines have been given to newborns since 1991
90%
of babies exposed to Hep. B develop a lifelong liver infection
CUTS & SORES
Are some Hep. B transmission routes (i.e. not just through needle-sharing and sex)
ASYMPTOMATIC TRANSMISSION
Infected individuals can spread Hep. B even when they have NO symptoms
CANCER PREVENTION
Hep. B causes liver cancer in children
There is NO CURE for Hep. B
- "Your baby is due for the Hep. B vaccine today."
- "Here is the Hep. B vaccine that your pediatrician ordered."
- "I'll now do the bilirubin check, Hep. B vaccine, and the Newborn Screen blood draw."
- "Do you want the Hep. B vaccine?"
- "What do you want to do about the Hep. B vaccine?"
- "It's fine if your baby gets the Hep. B vaccine after leaving the hospital."
Designed by Subha Mohan, MD

Fig. 2. Hepatitis B education poster for nursing staff. (*Courtesy of* Subha Mohan MD, University of California, San Diego, Department of Pediatrics.)

developed to help nurses discuss HepB vaccine and includes examples of presumptive statements.

Display Curiosity

During the discussion, the clinician should query the parents' sources of information. Are they relying on recommendations from a friend? Do they subscribe to a blog? Do they have an alternative medicine practitioner for themselves who gives them advice? Perhaps the information is coming from a religious organization. Recognize an individual's "religious belief" may differ from official religious teachings. Some families use the term "religious belief" to describe an opinion because it may carry more weight than a "personal belief." Ask about the family's origins. If they had a prior child in another country and experienced something different, they may be hesitant because of that difference.

An important cultural point is to determine who is the decision maker. In some families there may be a male head of household, so trying to persuade the mother will not work. In other families the mother is the medical decision maker for the children, so speaking with the father will not alter the situation (**Fig. 3**).

Making the Recommendation

Only after the clinician fully understands the parents' perspective should he or she then speak. The clinician should present their viewpoint in a calm manner. Some families will become angry when they feel challenged, but the clinician should avoid reciprocating the anger. There is evidence to suggest that some parents become more entrenched in their beliefs when challenged. If a clinician sees parents becoming

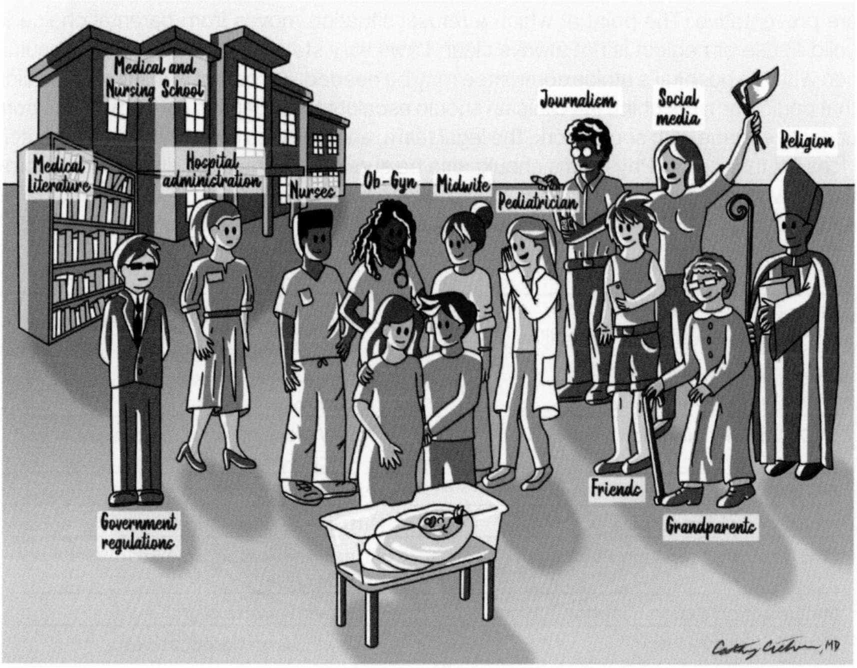
Medical and Nursing School
Medical literature
Hospital administration
Nurses
Ob-Gyn
Midwife
Pediatrician
Journalism
Social media
Religion
Friends
Grandparents
Government regulations

Fig. 3. Factors affecting medical decision making. (*Courtesy of* Catherine Cichon MD, MPH, University of California, San Diego, Departments of Medicine and Pediatrics.)

more adamant about their viewpoint during the conversation, it may be prudent to end the conversation for the time being. If possible, the clinician should leave information for the family to read, such as trusted Web sites or blogs that are backed by science (**Table 2**).

Meet the Family Where They Are

A clinician's method of discussion varies with the audience. A parent with a scientific background may respond best to facts and figures. A religious parent may do better with a religious argument. Statements from various religious organizations in regard to vaccines are available for clinicians to learn from (see **Table 2**). Another parent might do better with an emotional appeal. Remember to also speak to a family at their educational level. As scientists, clinicians are trained to think about incidence, prevalence, odds ratios, etc. Unless you are speaking to another physician or scientist, this is usually not the right language to use. In residency training, clinicians learn how to use layman's terms to discuss illness and treatment, and the same approach needs to be used when discussing these topics.

Be Persistent

Although a clinician may feel that a family who refused is a lost cause, evidence suggests that persistence pays off.[47] Most families will have a couple of interactions with hospital clinicians, so addressing the refusal again may be helpful. It is also important to not imply acceptance of their beliefs by not speaking up. Maintaining persistence without challenging parents takes practice. Sometimes using humor can help.

When a Refusal May Result in Harm

In the United States, parents have the right to decline most medical interventions that are preventative. The point at which a refusal situation moves from parental choice to child abuse or neglect is not always clear. Laws vary state by state. At times consultation with the hospital's ethics committee may be needed. If a parent is making a decision that could harm the child, the clinician should escalate to leadership on the well newborn unit and engage with social work, the legal team, and perhaps even child protective services for the region. Physicians should also be sure to document all discussions. Some well newborn units require parents to sign pertinent refusal forms. On occasion families refuse to sign such forms and the physician should document this refusal.

Table 2
Informational Web sites for families

American Academy of Pediatrics AAP-CA3's Natural Birth Plan	https://aapca3.org/aap-ca3s-natural-birth-plan-handout/
CHOP Vaccine Education Center	https://www.chop.edu/centers-programs/vaccine-education-center
The AAP Parenting Website	www.Healthychildren.org
What is Newborn Screening	https://www.babysfirsttest.org/
CDC Newborn Screening Portal	https://www.cdc.gov/newbornscreening/index.html
Immunization Action Coalition	https://immunize.org/
Evidence Based Birth	www.Evidencebasedbirth.com

Abbreviations: AAP, American Academy of Pediatrics; CDC, Centers for Disease Control and Prevention; CHOP, Children's Hospital of Philadephia.

Advocacy in the Community

Clinicians should consider working on health care refusals and hesitancy at higher levels. Ways to promote routine recommendations include outreach to community pediatric and prenatal clinicians. Specifically, as out-of-hospital births in the United States continue to rise, more pregnant women are seeking out midwifery care. Midwives' philosophy on counseling expectant parents begins with education, shared decision making, and ultimately a respect for the mother's decision. Pregnant women seek out midwives in the hopes for a delivery with minimal medical intervention for the mother and newborn. When these mothers seek out pediatric care for their newborn who may not have received common newborn interventions and screening following birth, there may be tension between the pediatrician and family and the midwifery practice. There is an opportunity here to bridge the gap, break down the silos between clinicians, and learn about how to collectively best take care of children.

Participation in local, city, or state medical societies is another way to get involved in the community. The AAP California Chapter developed a birth plan that promotes AAP recommendations that is posted on their Web site (see **Table 2**). There is a role for clinicians to advocate for journalists to not give time to nonscience. Clinicians can write letters to the editor for local newspapers or write for community bulletins, parenting magazines, or school newsletters. Clinicians can advocate at the state level for laws that promote scientific principles. Clinicians can use their social media accounts to counter science denial with science-backed posts. Some physicians have even run for state and national legislatures where they can sponsor laws that promote public health (**Box 1**).

Training the Next Generation

In this new era of informed health care consumers, clinicians also have a responsibility toward trainees (students, residents, fellows) to educate them on how to counsel parents who refuse common newborn interventions. The paternalistic type of physician whose word is considered the truth and final is no longer realistic. Today's pediatricians need to be aware of resources parents are using, need to be self-educated on the reasons for why newborn recommendations are the way they are, and need to be prepared to have sometimes challenging time-consuming conversations with

Box 1
Ways in which providers can promote evidence-based recommendations

- Develop parent handouts specific to your region or hospital
- Participate in hospital committees
- Help write hospital and clinic policies
- Perform prenatal consultations to educate expectant parents about newborn recommendations
- Form relationships with obstetric providers
- Join local and national medical organizations
- Write letters to the editor for local newspapers
- Write for community bulletins, parenting magazines, or school newsletters
- Lobby at the state and national levels
- Promote science-based information on social networks

informed parents in a respectful and nonjudgmental manner. Role playing is one strategy to help teach these skills.

SUMMARY

Although overall refusal of routine newborn interventions is uncommon, clinicians should be prepared to address the refusals appropriately. Refusals often do not occur in isolation. Refusals in the newborn period have been associated with delayed childhood vaccinations highlighting the larger public health implications of refusals that begin in the newborn nursery. The relationship between most pediatricians and a family begins in the newborn nursery, and trust has been shown to be correlated with factors such as acceptance of influenza vaccine, for example. The newborn period is a critical time for pediatricians to develop positive relationships with families who are hesitant or refuse routine newborn interventions. Clinicians should strive to form partnerships with parents. As with all relationships, flexibility on both sides is important. Perhaps if parents see that we are listening and flexible on some topics they will be more likely to listen to us on others. A physician should understand the science behind the recommendation to then know when to persist and when to yield. Most of all, the physician should have the skills to respectfully care for these families during their birth stay.

CLINICS CARE POINTS

- Educate yourself about why families are refusing newborn recommendations.
- Understand the spectrum of hesitancy and refusal.
- Develop and practice strategies to address refusals.

Best practices

What is the current practice?

Although uncommon, some parents of healthy newborns in the United States refuse various aspects of their newborn's care in the hospital, including but not limited to, refusal of hepatitis B vaccine, vitamin K prophylaxis, and newborn screening. In some cases, parents prefer alternatives that may not be evidence-based.

Best practice/guideline/care path objectives: Compliance of recommended routine interventions by parents of newborns following delivery. Tailored education and counseling of parents of newborns by clinicians.

What changes in current practice are likely to improve outcomes?

1. Clinician education and awareness of what recommendations parents of newborns may refuse and why
2. Understanding the spectrum of hesitancy and refusal
3. Developing and practicing strategies to address refusals beginning with multidisciplinary partnerships, displaying curiosity, and developing rapport with new parents.

Major recommendations

Summary statement: Refusal of routine newborn care by parents of newborns is uncommon, but clinicians need to be prepared to address these refusals because there are public health ramifications. A nonjudgmental family-centered approach to counseling around refusals is recommended.

DISCLOSURE

The authors have no commercial or financial conflicts of interest or any funding sources related to the content of this article to disclose.

REFERENCES

1. Benitz WE, Committee on Fetus and Newborn, American Academy of Pediatrics. Hospital stay for healthy term newborn infants. Pediatrics 2015;135(5):948–53.
2. American Academy of Pediatrics Committee on Fetus and Newborn. Controversies concerning vitamin K and the newborn. Pediatrics 2003;112(1 Pt 1): 191–2.
3. American Academy of Pediatrics. Prevention of neonatal ophthalmia. In: Kimberlin DW, Brady MT, Jackson MA, et al, editors. Red book: 2018 report of the committee on infectious diseases. 31st edition. Itasca (IL): American Academy of Pediatrics; 2018. p. 1046–50.
4. Loyal J, Shapiro ED. Refusal of intramuscular vitamin K by parents of newborns: a review. Hosp Pediatr 2020;10(3):286–94.
5. Loyal J, Taylor JA, Phillipi CA, et al. Factors associated with refusal of intramuscular vitamin K in normal newborns. Pediatrics 2018;142(2):e20173743.
6. Danziger P, Skoczylas M, Laventhal N. Parental refusal of standard-of-care prophylactic newborn practices: in one center's experience, many refuse one but few refuse all. Hosp Pediatr 2019;9(6):429–33.
7. Hill HA, Yankey D, Elam-Evans LS, et al. Vaccination coverage by age 24 months among children born in 2016 and 2017 – National immunization survey-child, United States, 2017-2019. MMWR Morb Mortal Wkly Rep 2020;69:1505–11.
8. Dubé E, Gagnon D, MacDonald N, et al. Underlying factors impacting vaccine hesitancy in high income countries: a review of qualitative studies. Expert Rev Vaccin 2018;17(11):989–1004.
9. Chung Y, Schamel J, Fisher A, et al. Influences on immunization decision-making among US parents of young children. Matern Child Health J 2017;21(12): 2178–87.
10. Burton T, Saini S, Maldonado L, et al. Parental refusal for treatments, procedures, and vaccines in the newborn nursery. Adv Pediatr 2018;65(1):89–104.
11. Centers for Disease Control and Prevention. Newborn screening portal. Available at: https://www.cdc.gov/newbornscreening/. Accessed June 2, 2020.
12. U.S. Health Resources and Services Administration. Recommended uniform screening panel. 2020. Available at: https://www.hrsa.gov/advisory-committees/heritable-disorders/rusp/index.html. Accessed November 10, 2020.
13. Glidewell J, Grosse SD, Riehle-Colarusso T, et al. Actions in support of newborn screening for critical congenital heart disease — United States, 2011–2018. MMWR Morb Mortal Wkly Rep 2019;68(5):107–11.
14. National Center for Hearing Assessment and Management. Sate EHDI information. Available at: https://www.infanthearing.org/states_home/. Accessed November 19, 2020.
15. Sontag MK, Yusuf C, Grosse SD, et al. Infants with congenital disorders identified through newborn screening — United States, 2015–2017. MMWR Morb Mortal Wkly Rep 2020;69(36):1265–8.
16. Baby's first test. Conditions screened by state. Available at: https://www.babysfirsttest.org/newborn-screening/states. Accessed November 19, 2020.
17. Njau G, Odoi A. Investigation of predictors of newborn screening refusal in a large birth cohort in North Dakota, USA. Matern Child Health J 2019;23(1):92–9.

18. Kraszewski J, Burke T, Rosenbaum S. Legal issues in newborn screening: implications for public health practice and policy. Public Health Rep 2006;121(1):92–4.
19. Hom LA, Silber TJ, Ennis-Durstine K, et al. Legal and ethical considerations in allowing parental exemptions from newborn critical congenital heart disease (CCHD) screening. Am J Bioeth 2016;16(1):11–7.
20. The President's Council on Bioethics. The changing moral focus of newborn screening: an ethical analysis by the president's council on bioethics. 2008. Available at: https://bioethicsarchive.georgetown.edu/pcbe/reports/newborn_screening/chapter4.html. Accessed November 10, 2020.
21. Committee on Fetus and Newborn, Adamkin DH. Postnatal glucose homeostasis in late-preterm and term infants. Pediatrics 2011;127(3):575–9.
22. Bull MJ, Engle WA, Committee on Injury, Violence, and Poison Prevention and Committee on Fetus and Newborn, American Academy of Pediatrics. Safe transportation of preterm and low birth weight infants at hospital discharge. Pediatrics 2009;123(5):1424–9.
23. Bhatia J, Greer F, American Academy of Pediatrics Committee on Nutrition. Use of soy protein-based formulas in infant feeding. Pediatrics 2008;121(5):1062–8.
24. Keim SA, Hogan JS, McNamara KA, et al. Microbial contamination of human milk purchased via the Internet. Pediatrics 2013;132(5):e1227–35.
25. Keim SA, Kulkarni MM, McNamara K, et al. Cow's milk contamination of human milk purchased via the internet. Pediatrics 2015;135(5):e1157–62.
26. Section on Breastfeeding. Breastfeeding and the use of human milk. Pediatrics 2012;129(3):e827–41.
27. Kair LR, Flaherman VJ. Donor milk or formula: a qualitative study of postpartum mothers of healthy newborns. J Hum Lact 2017;33(4):710–6.
28. World Health Organization. Recommendations on postnatal care of the mother and newborn 2013. Geneva (Switzerland): WHO Press; 2014. Available at: www.who.int. Accessed November 19, 2020.
29. AWHONN. Neonatal skin care: evidence-based clinical practice guideline. 4th edition. Washington, DC: AWHONN; 2018.
30. Nishijima K, Yoneda M, Hirai T, et al. Biology of the vernix caseosa: a review. J Obstet Gynaecol Res 2019;45(11):2145–9.
31. American Academy of Pediatrics. FAQs: management of infants born to mothers with suspected or confirmed COVID-19. 2020. Available at: https://services.aap.org/en/pages/2019-novel-coronavirus-covid-19-infections/clinical-guidance/faqs-management-of-infants-born-to-covid-19-mothers/. Accessed November 10, 2020.
32. Yarnall N, Knowles J, Lohr J. Development of vaccine preferences among parents of newborns. J Pediatr Infect Dis 2018;13(3):169–77.
33. MacDorman MF, Matthews TJ, Declercq E. Trends in out-of-hospital births in the United States, 1990–2012. NCHS Data Brief 2014;(144):1–8.
34. Watterberg K, Committee on Fetus and Newborn. Providing care for infants born at home. Pediatrics 2020;145(5):e20200626.
35. Martin JA, Hamilton BE, Osterman MJK, et al. Births: final data for 2018. Natl Vital Stat Rep 2019;68(13):1–47.
36. ACOG Committee Opinion No. 761: CESAREAN delivery on maternal request. Obstet Gynecol 2019;133(1):e73–7.
37. ACOG Committee on Obstetric Practice. Committee opinion No. 679: immersion in water during labor and delivery. Obstet Gynecol 2016;128(5):e231–6.

38. Young K, Kruske S. How valid are the common concerns raised against water birth? A focused review of the literature. Women Birth 2013;26(2):105–9.
39. Harper B. Birth, bath, and beyond: the science and safety of water immersion during labor and birth. J Perinat Educ 2014;23(3):124–34.
40. Neiman E, Austin E, Tan A, et al. Outcomes of waterbirth in a US hospital-based midwifery practice: a retrospective cohort study of water immersion during labor and birth. J Midwifery Womens Health 2020;65(2):216–23.
41. Monroe KK, Rubin A, Mychaliska KP, et al. Lotus birth: a case series report on umbilical nonseverance. Clin Pediatr (Phila) 2019;58(1):88–94.
42. Ittleman BR, German KR, Scott E, et al. Umbilical cord nonseverance and adverse neonatal outcomes. Clin Pediatr (Phila) 2019;58(2):238–40.
43. Farr A, Chervenak FA, McCullough LB, et al. Human placentophagy: a review. Am J Obstet Gynecol 2018;218(4):401.e1-11.
44. Marraccini ME, Gorman KS. Exploring placentophagy in humans: problems and recommendations. J Midwifery Womens Health 2015;60(4):371–9.
45. Buser GL, Mato S, Zhang AY, et al. Notes from the field: late-onset infant group B Streptococcus infection associated with maternal consumption of capsules containing dehydrated placenta – Oregon, 2016. MMWR Morb Mortal Wkly Rep 2017;66(25):677–8.
46. Craven J. Discussing immunization with vaccine-hesitant parents requires individualized approach. Pediatr News 2018. Available at: https://www.mdedge.com/pediatrics. Accessed November 17, 2020.
47. Opel DJ, Heritage J, Taylor JA, et al. The architecture of provider-parent vaccine discussions at health supervision visits. Pediatrics 2013;132(6):1037–46.

The Term Newborn
Hypoglycemia

Eustratia M. Hubbard, MD[a], William W. Hay Jr, MD[b,*]

KEYWORDS

- Oral dextrose gel • Glucose • Hyperinsulinism • Infant of diabetic mother
- Intrauterine growth restriction • Newborn

KEY POINTS

- Infants have lower glucose concentrations during the first few hours of life, which increase to levels similar to those of older children and adults by several days of age.
- Because severe and recurrent hypoglycemia has been associated with poor neurologic outcomes, close monitoring, and treatment of persistent hypoglycemia is recommended for at-risk infants and those with symptoms.
- Feeding is the optimal initial approach for transient, asymptomatic hyhpoglycemia; oral dextrose gel also may be used to augment feeding as an intervention for hypoglycemia.
- Intravenous dextrose infusion should be used to treat persistent or recurrent, severely low, markedly symptomatic (seizures, coma, hypotonia with apnea) glucose concentrations.
- Infants with persistent, recurrent low glucose concentrations despite appropriate treatment should not be discharged without a diagnosis and follow-up plan.

INTRODUCTION

Neonatal hypoglycemia is a common metabolic condition that continues to plague clinicians. Despite decades of clinical observations, basic and clinical research, and many scholarly efforts to define significant hypoglycemia in newborn infants, there still is no evidence-based definition of the severity and duration of low glucose concentrations that directly lead to adverse long-term neurodevelopmental sequelae and whether specific treatment of milder transient episodes of low glucose concentrations would improve outcomes. In this review, we summarize the recent literature regarding screening, diagnosis, prevention, treatment, and outcomes of hypoglycemia, focusing on the term infant.

FETAL AND NEONATAL GLUCOSE HOMEOSTASIS

Glucose is the primary metabolic fuel for fetal energy metabolism.[1] The fetal blood glucose concentration is typically 60% to 80% of the maternal level, the lowest value

[a] UC San Diego School of Medicine, UC San Diego Health, 9300 Campus Point Drive, La Jolla, CA 92037-7774, USA; [b] 401 Hudson Street, Denver, CO 80220, USA
* Correspondence author.
E-mail address: bill.hay@ucdenver.edu

Clin Perinatol 48 (2021) 665–679
https://doi.org/10.1016/j.clp.2021.05.013

during gestation being approximately 54 mg/dL. With the abrupt severing of the umbilical cord, exogenous glucose supply is terminated, and neonatal glucose levels fall, triggering a series of metabolic and hormonal adaptations that activate neonatal glucose production.[2]

The immediate postnatal fall in glucose concentrations reaches a nadir at about 1 to 2 hours of age, as low as 25 to 30 mg/dL, and most often without associated symptoms.[3] Glucose concentrations then stabilize at levels higher than 36 mg/dL by 4 to 6 hours of age, regardless of feeding. With ongoing milk feedings, glucose concentrations are relatively constant between 45 and 60 mg/dL and then gradually increase to those seen in children and adults, higher than 54 mg/dL after 2 to 3 days, achieving mean values >60 mg/dL after 72 hours.[4] Maintenance of glucose homeostasis depends on adequate feeding, carbohydrate content of nutrients, simultaneous supplies of lipids for energy production and protein for anabolic metabolism, digestive absorption, and gut incretin secretion that promotes pancreatic release of insulin. Despite the common sequence of metabolic adaptations to ensure adequate glucose production, it is not uncommon during this critical period for a physiologic imbalance to result in transiently low circulating glucose concentrations.

DEFINITIONS OF HYPOGLYCEMIA

Different methods have been used to determine glucose concentrations that should be considered normal or abnormal and potentially harmful.[5] Although contributing to a better understanding of neonatal glucose homeostasis, each of these has limitations.

Epidemiologic or Statistical

With this methodology, a hypoglycemia glucose concentration threshold is defined as two standard deviations below the population mean. When treating glucose concentrations as a continuum, the interquartile range may be considered as the normal range of glucose concentrations. Several studies of healthy, exclusively breastfed, term infants have documented a wide range of plasma glucose concentrations, from 18 to 166 mg/dL with a mean of ~54 mg/dL and an interquartile range of 41 to 60 mg/dL during 6 to 72 hours of life.[4,6–8] More than half of these seemingly normal infants have mean plasma glucose concentrations that are less than the lower limit for age as per guidelines from the American Academy of Pediatrics (AAP) and the Pediatric Endocrine Society (PES).[7]

Clinical

Assigning a low glucose concentration as a potential cause of clinically significant neurologic impairment should meet Whipple's triad: (1) measurement of low plasma glucose concentration is reliable, (2) signs and symptoms are consistent with hypoglycemia, and (3) abnormal findings resolve quickly after glucose concentration is normalized.[5] However, the plasma glucose value at which an infant demonstrates symptoms, even neurologic ones, may be much higher than that needed to cause brain injury. Basing the definition of critical glucose concentrations on the presence or absence of clinical signs is problematic because many newborns with very low glucose concentrations remain asymptomatic, and the symptoms associated with hypoglycemia are commonly seen with other conditions.

Physiological

The PES has suggested that the lower glucose concentrations that are common in infants during their first few days could be due to relative hyperinsulinemia.[9] The PES has defined the critical glucose concentration range for the first 48 hours of life as 55 to 65 mg/dL, representing values that in older children and adults would trigger neuroendocrine responses to increase glucose concentrations. Hence, they recommend that glucose concentrations should be >50 mg/dL in the first 48 hours and feedings should maintain glucose values >70 mg/dL after 72 hours.[9] However, there is no experimental evidence that this relative hyperinsulinemia causes significantly low glucose concentrations, leads to brain injury, or is in any way pathologic. Furthermore, there is no evidence that meeting the PES guidelines improves neurodevelopmental outcomes.

Neurodevelopmental

Most neurodevelopmental studies have varied considerably in terms of study populations, glucose screening methods, treatment protocols, and neurodevelopmental testing, and overall, they do not represent high-quality evidence.[10] Thus, they do not define the range of glucose concentrations that should be considered safe. The ongoing HypoEXIT trial (Current Controlled Trials number, ISRCTN79705768) is the first to compare neurodevelopmental outcomes using two different glucose thresholds for intervention. In this multicenter, noninferiority trial, asymptomatic at-risk infants—infants of diabetic mothers (IDMs), late preterm 35 to 37 weeks, or birthweight less than the 10th percentile or greater than the 90th percentile—with hypoglycemia were randomized into different protocols: a traditional threshold group with a plasma glucose less than 47 mg/dl as the cutoff for treatment and a low threshold group using less than 36 mg/dL.[11] Treatment options were the same in both and determined by providers. At 18 months of age, there were no significant differences in psychomotor test scores between the two groups; future follow-up when subjects are of school age is planned. Unfortunately, because only at-risk infants were included and those with severe initial hypoglycemia (<35 mg/dL) were excluded (5.2%), the study results have limited application.

Operational Thresholds

To date, the aforementioned methodologies have not identified a critical threshold of glucose below which deleterious consequences will occur. A single glucose value or specified range is unlikely to represent a cutoff that can be applied to all infants because many factors contribute to glucose homeostasis, including unmeasured alternate fuels that play an important role in neuroprotection during hypoglycemia. Normal ranges also need to account for differences in gestational age, weight, and clinical status. Recognizing this problem, operational thresholds have been recommended as indicators for intervention instead of relying on a definition of critical hypoglycemia.[12] The operational threshold is distinguished from a treatment target glucose concentration that is somewhat higher, for example, higher than 45 mg/dL in asymptomatic infants and higher than 60 mg/dL in severe cases that require intravenous (IV) glucose.

SCREENING AND MANAGEMENT GUIDELINES

The AAP and PES have provided different interpretations of the evidence available at the time of their recommendations, the AAP using the neurodevelopmental method and glucose nadirs from statistical models to determine the definition of hypoglycemia and the PES using an endocrine approach focusing on mean glucose values[13,14] (**Table 1**).

Several concerns about the application of the AAP or PES guidelines have been expressed. These recommendations are not firmly based on evidence from controlled

Table 1
Screening guidelines for glucose concentrations in at-risk infants

Organization	0–4 h[a]	4–24 h	24–48 h	>48 h
AAP	<25–40 mg/dL	<35–45 mg/dL	<45 mg/dL	<60 mg/dL
PES	<50 mg/dL	<50 mg/dL	<50 mg/dL	<60 mg/dL

Any symptomatic infant with glucose concentration less than 40 mg/dL should receive IV dextrose (AAP).

[a] Time includes the normal postnatal glucose nadir; asymptomatic infants with these low values do not require treatment beyond feeding, unless values remain low after 4 h of life.

studies, and they have not been compared in clinical trials to determine if either, or both, reduces adverse neurodevelopmental outcomes.[15,16] If nurseries follow the PES recommendation of a higher cutoff and longer observation period for hypoglycemia, significant increases in neonatal intensive care unit (NICU) admissions and length of hospital stay may occur.[17] With higher glucose thresholds and increased screening in the first 48 hours, more asymptomatic infants will be diagnosed with hypoglycemia. This could lead to overtreatment with formula feeding, costly NICU admissions, and IV fluids, all of which threaten successful breastfeeding.[16,18] Nevertheless, an advantage to following the PES guidelines after 48 hours is that infants with persistent hypoglycemia associated with hyperinsulinism will more likely be identified, although infants with intrauterine growth restriction (IUGR), whose relative hyperinsulinism is transient, may account for the majority of such cases.[19]

Most organizational guidelines recommend screening not only all symptomatic infants but also asymptomatic infants in the most common at-risk groups (**Table 2**). Infants who are born preterm (even by just 4–6 weeks), growth restricted, or exposed to perinatal stress are more likely to have abnormal neurodevelopmental testing later in childhood, and it remains possible, but not proven, that low glucose concentrations, common to all of them, may be partly responsible.

If one defines neonatal hypoglycemia as less than 47 mg/dL, the incidence in at-risk infants during the first 48 hours of life is high. In a study from Auckland, 51% of at-risk neonates had hypoglycemia and 19% had more than 1 episode.[20] Analysis of blood glucose concentrations using the glucose oxidase method included those occurring during the normal postnatal nadir; it is controversial whether infants, at-risk ones or not, should be screened during the expected nadir.[21] Extrapolating these data to the United States, more than half a million newborns would be screened with multiple blood draws, and hypoglycemia would be identified in about 12% if using the 47-mg/dL threshold.[22]

Most research has not robustly tested whether treating transient asymptomatic hypoglycemia, even in such at-risk infants, improves neurodevelopmental outcomes. Another study from Auckland showed that if at-risk newborns were screened for hypoglycemia and treated with the goal of maintaining blood glucose levels higher than 47 mg/dL, neonatal hypoglycemia was not associated with an increased risk of the primary outcomes of neurosensory impairment and processing difficulty at 2 years of age.[23] Risks were not increased among infants with unrecognized hypoglycemia captured on interstitial glucose monitoring. The lowest blood glucose concentration, number of hypoglycemic episodes, and negative interstitial increment (area above the interstitial glucose concentration curve and <47 mg/dL) also did not predict the outcome. When the infants were re-evaluated at 4.5 years of age, previous hypoglycemia was not associated with neurosensory impairment, but test scores for executive function and visual motor function were lower in those infants who had more severe

Table 2
Infants who should be considered for glucose screening

Asymptomatic Infants with Risk Factors	
Common	*Uncommon*
Prematurity (<37 0/7 wk)	Midline facial defects, microphallus (hypopituitarism)
Small-for-gestational age (SGA)[a]	Ambiguous genitalia (congenital adrenal hyperplasia)
Intrauterine growth restriction	Macroglossia, ear pits (Beckwith-Wiedemann)
Perinatal stress	Shock, acidosis, seizures (metabolic disorder)
Infant of diabetic mother (any type)	Family history of prolonged neonatal hypoglycemia
Large-for-gestational age (LGA)[b]	
Symptomatic Infants	
Neurogenic / autonomic	*Neuroglycopenic*
Hypothermia	Cyanosis
Sweating	Apnea
Pallor	Lethargy
Tachycardia	Stupor
Tachypnea	High-pitched cry
Vomiting	Hypotonia
Poor suck or refusal to feed	Seizure
Irritability	Coma
Jitteriness	

[a] <10th percentile on gestational-adjusted growth curves.
[b] >90th percentile on gestational-adjusted growth curves.

(<36 mg/dL) or recurrent episodes of hypoglycemia.[24] However, keeping blood glucose values higher than 47 mg/dL did not improve outcomes.

MEASUREMENT OF GLUCOSE

Blood glucose concentrations are up to 10% to 12% lower than plasma values. Sampling from an artery will obtain results 10% to 15% higher than from a vein, with capillary results in between. A higher hematocrit can lead to lower glucose concentrations, as does marked hyperbilirubinemia.

The gold standard technique for glucose measurement uses laboratory instruments, including blood gas analyzers, to analyze plasma glucose specimens using enzymes such as glucose oxidase, hexokinase, and glucose dehydrogenase.[25,26] These methods are less influenced by hematocrit and metabolites. Ongoing red cell glycolysis that can lead to false low glucose concentrations is reduced by using collection tubes containing glycolytic inhibitors and keeping the specimens on ice.

Point-of-care (POC) instruments can result in both higher and lower values (from ±5 mg/dL up to ±20 mg/dL) than standardized laboratory methods. Treatment thresholds for neonatal hypoglycemia are near the limits of accuracy for most POC devices. POC testing may be considered for glucose screening, but at least one reliable laboratory measurement should be promptly obtained to confirm the diagnosis of hypoglycemia, particularly if an infant has concerning symptoms or is requiring IV glucose infusion.[13] This result should be communicated directly to the ordering provider. Treatment in a markedly symptomatic infant should not be delayed until laboratory confirmation of hypoglycemia.

Continuous Glucose Monitoring

Continuous glucose monitoring (CGM) has been incorporated into many recent research studies evaluating the effectiveness of oral dextrose gel and feeding protocols in the management of neonatal hypoglycemia, as well as neurodevelopmental outcomes associated with low glucose levels.[8,23,24,27,28] However, whether CGM should be put into routine clinical practice remains controversial. Some investigators feel strongly that CGM is sufficiently accurate for current clinical use and can be more broadly applied, for example, in critically ill infants who are receiving IV nutrition and have abnormal or rapidly changing glucose concentrations.[29,30] CGM-guided glucose titration has shown to successfully increase the time spent in the euglycemic range, reduce hypoglycemia, and minimize glycemic variability in preterm infants during the first week of life.[31] Those who are skeptical cite the lack of information about the clinical significance of episodes of low interstitial glucose concentrations, what glucose value and duration signals intervention, and the uncertain benefits of treating these fluctuations. Premature adoption of CGM could lead to more treatment of more infants than would be necessary.[32]

PREVENTION AND TREATMENT OF NEONATAL HYPOGLYCEMIA

Prevention

Low glucose levels should be avoided in all neonates, particularly those at risk of aberrant glucose homeostasis. Prevention may begin prior to cutting the umbilical cord with initiation of skin-to-skin contact if the mother and infant are stable. Early and sustained skin-to-skin contact promotes successful breastfeeding, supports glucose homeostasis, and avoids cold stress.[33]

Oral feeding should be initiated as soon as possible, preferably within 1 hour for at-risk infants and all infants whose mothers intend to breastfeed.[34] Breastfeeding on demand has been shown to provide sufficient nutrition to term infants and to maintain normal glucose levels.[7,35] If the infant is not showing feeding progression by 12 to 24 hours from birth, supplementing breastfeeding with expressed breast milk (EBM), pasteurized donor breast milk (DBM), or formula may be considered. At-risk infants should be fed every 2 to 3 hours but more frequently if infants show hunger cues sooner. Formula-fed infants should also be observed for adequate feeding.

Treatment

Feeding

The key to all hypoglycemia management protocols is to optimize and advance feeding. Should initial efforts fail to raise glucose levels in the breastfed infant, then supplements with EBM, DBM, or formula may be considered. Bottle or gavage feeding may be necessary to assure adequate nutrition and avoid transfer to the NICU for IV fluids.

IV dextrose

The AAP recommends IV dextrose if glucose measurement is (1) less than 40 mg/dL at the time of symptoms consistent with hypoglycemia, (2) less than 25 mg/dL within

4 hours of life and *after* the first feeding, or (3) below the hour-specific threshold after feeding or other interventions have failed to raise glucose concentrations.[13] IV infusion should not be delayed while waiting for results of confirmatory laboratory glucose measurement. A minibolus consisting of 2 mL/kg of 10% dextrose (200 mg of glucose/kg) followed by a continuous infusion rate of 6 to 8 mg/kg/min may be considered for infants with serious clinical signs (seizures, coma, or marked hypotonia with apnea) and severe hypoglycemia (persistently <25 mg/dL).[36] For other situations, IV dextrose may be started at a rate of 3 to 5 mg/kg/min for IDMs, to avoid stimulating insulin secretion, and 4 to 6 mg/kg/min for late-preterm or term infants. The rate should be adjusted as per repeated glucose measurements obtained 30 minutes after IV infusion initiation and after every adjustment.[37] Previously, the minibolus followed by a continuous infusion rate of 6 to 8 mg/kg/min was recommended for very low glucose concentrations in all infants with hypoglycemia,[36] but this should be reconsidered after reports that rapid, prolonged, and unstable increases in glucose concentrations were associated with later abnormal neurodevelopmental outcomes.[24,37,38] Concurrent feeding is safe, achieves higher glucose concentrations at nearly all time points, and is associated with shorter duration of IV dextrose therapy and hospital stay.[39]

Oral dextrose gel

Numerous recent studies have documented successful use of oral dextrose gel for the treatment of neonatal hypoglycemia in at-risk infants, reporting increased blood glucose concentrations in combination with feeding (formula, EBM, or direct breastfeeding), reduced need for IV dextrose, decreased NICU admissions, less mother-infant separation, and increased breastfeeding.[40–45] The increase in glucose levels is higher after the infant is fed formula than after other feedings, but breastfeeding is associated with reduced requirement for repeat gel treatment.[27] At 2-year follow-up, no differences in neurosensory function have been detected between the dextrose gel and placebo groups.[46] More studies using CGM and long-term follow-up will be needed to determine if dextrose gel is similar to IV dextrose boluses in raising glucose concentrations too quickly and causing highly variable values, conditions which have been associated with neurosensory impairment.[24] Only one study to date has found that prophylactic use of dextrose gel did not reduce transient neonatal hypoglycemia or NICU admissions for hypoglycemia in at-risk infants. Possible explanations for this are that the high carbohydrate concentration of Insta-Glucose (77%) caused a hyperinsulinemic response or that oral dextrose minimally influences glucose homeostasis during the first few hours when counter-regulatory mechanisms are especially active.[47]

Not all commercially available dextrose gel products are equivalent and even within a brand, there is variation in dextrose concentrations; many contain preservatives, flavorings, and colorants.[48] Until recently, there has not been a preservative-free single-dose product specific for newborns. Many nurseries have incorporated oral dextrose gel into their hypoglycemia management protocols—see **Table 3** for an example.

IV medications

In cases of severe persistent hypoglycemia, pharmacotherapy may be required to achieve glucose stabilization. Options include glucagon, which stimulates hepatic glycogenolysis; hydrocortisone and dexamethasone, which promote gluconeogenesis and decrease insulin sensitivity; and diazoxide or octreotide, which suppress insulin secretion.

Table 3
Example of hypoglycemia protocol using dextrose gel

At-Risk Infant • IDM • LGA • SGA • <37 wk • Perinatal stress	• Feed by 60 min after birth • If the mother ill or unable to breastfeed by 60–90 min of life: provide colostrum, consider donor milk or formula • Check glucose 30–60 min after first feed • Feed on demand • Monitor for signs and symptoms of hypoglycemia • Recheck glucose before feeds
Asymptomatic Infant	<25 mg/dL 1 .Dextrose gel and feed; recheck glucose in 30 min 2 .Glucose remains <25 mg/dL, consider NICU and IV dextrose 25–44 mg/dL 1 .Dextrose gel and feed; recheck glucose in 30 min 2 .Repeat glucose <25 mg/dL, consider NICU and IV dextrose 3 .Repeat glucose 25–44, may repeat dextrose gel and feed >45 mg/dL 1 .Check glucose before feeds 2 .Add oral dextrose gel if the glucose level falls to <45 mg/dL

Symptomatic Infant	• Check glucose immediately
	• Mild to moderate symptoms and the infant can feed:
	  ○ <45 mg/dL: dextrose gel and feed
	  ○ Recheck glucose in 30 min
	  ○ Repeat glucose <35 mg/dL, transfer to the NICU; start IV dextrose if symptoms persist and laboratory glucose confirms <35 mg/dL
	• Severe symptoms:
	  ○ Urgent transfer to NICU for IV dextrose and further care
	  ○ While waiting transfer, consider dextrose gel ± gavaged milk, given slowly and cautiously, observing for emesis

Abbreviations: LGA, large-for-gestational age; SGA, small-for-gestational age.

SPECIAL POPULATIONS OF INFANTS WITH NEONATAL HYPOGLYCEMIA

Infants of Diabetic Mothers

Transient low glucose concentrations in the immediate postnatal period occur sooner, occur more frequently, and reach lower levels in IDMs, especially in those who had evidence of unstable maternal glucose concentrations during later gestation and labor.[49–51] IDMs should be fed as soon as possible after birth and as long as they are not exhibiting severe symptoms. Smaller and more frequent feedings or even constant nasogastric tube infusion of milk will help stabilize glucose concentrations. Milk is preferable over glucose-containing solutions because the milk sugar lactose contains 50% galactose. After intestinal absorption into the portal vein, galactose is cleared by the liver, is used for glycogen production, and does not stimulate pancreatic insulin secretion.

If an IDM is markedly symptomatic or unable to feed, a constant rate of IV dextrose should be started at 3 to 5 mg/kg/min *without* a preceding bolus. This slightly lower rate of infusion minimizes stimulation of insulin secretion and is consistent with glucose utilization rates of IDMs who are resting and have not had insulin stimulation.[52] Using the same dextrose infusion rate as other infants overestimates what IDMs need because the birth weight is exaggerated with excessive adipose tissue, whereas the brain, which accounts for most of whole-body glucose utilization, is not large for gestational age. With severe hypoglycemia complicated by seizures, coma, or marked hypotonia with apnea, the preferred therapy is a minibolus consisting of

200 mg/kg of glucose (2 mL of 10% glucose per kilogram of body weight) over 2 to 4 minutes, followed by a constant infusion of 6 mg/kg/min.[53] About 30 minutes after initiation of IV dextrose and after every rate adjustment, glucose levels should be checked, and if possible, the IV fluid rate should be reduced to maintain concentrations in the low normal range (45–55 mg/dL). This will avoid further hyperglycemia-induced insulin secretion, as well as rapid overcorrections and excessive time over the interquartile range. A common approach is to wean the dextrose infusion rate by 1 mg/kg/min for every plasma glucose concentration that is higher than 50 mg/dL, with measurements every 2 to 4 hours. CGM could prove to be useful in the management of an IDM, limiting the need for frequent glucose testing, enabling more timely adjustments in infusion rates, and determining when IV treatment could be safely and effectively discontinued as the infant nears full oral feeding, in addition to when glucose homeostasis is sufficient for safe discharge.

Infants with Intrauterine Growth Restriction

Recent clinical and observational research has focused on the unique problem of apparent persistent hyperinsulinemia–induced hypoglycemia in infants with IUGR.[9,54–56] Chronic placental insufficiency, and thus hypoxia, stimulates catecholamine release, leading to suppression of insulin secretion. In a nutrient-deficient environment, the expression of peripheral (eg, skeletal muscle) glucose transporters is increased or at least maintained, and the pancreas is programmed to be more susceptible to metabolic stimulation of insulin secretion.[57,58] After birth, when normal oxygenation is restored, catecholamine levels decrease and insulin suppression disappears. Normal increases in glucose levels from feeding may induce hypersecretion of insulin, leading to persistent hypoglycemia; a more exaggerated response may occur when IV dextrose is provided. An additional complicating factor is that many infants with IUGR have a higher head/body ratio and, thus, a higher weight-specific glucose utilization rate. All of these conditions place these infants at significant risk of severe and protracted hypoglycemia, which if unrecognized can lead to permanent neurologic damage.

Practical approaches to treat infants with IUGR and persistent hypoglycemia are controversial and not well established. Many of these infants require long NICU stays, after which they may need to be followed by endocrinology services.[56] IV dextrose should be used for severe, symptomatic hypoglycemia, but it is best to also encourage early and frequent breastfeeding, supplemented with DBM or formula as needed. Continuous enteral feeds may be considered. Diazoxide, plus a diuretic, can be used if the frequent feeding approach is not working after 1 to 2 weeks. Diazoxide carries a significant risk for producing pulmonary hypertension and hypoxia, and without diuretic treatment, it can lead to death. One must balance the risks, costs, and complications of longer hospital stays while waiting to establish normal glucose levels with interval breastfeeding or bottle feeding or diazoxide treatment with its added risks versus sending the infant home too early. These infants should not be discharged until normal glucose levels are maintained with a treatment plan that families are able to carry out. Caregivers and especially parents should be educated about the signs of hypoglycemia and to seek care if these are observed.

Infants with genetic hyperinsulinism or metabolic defects

Like the difficult but transient persistent hypoglycemia common in infants with IUGR, genetic disorders causing severe, recurrent, and protracted hypoglycemia, for example, congenital hyperinsulinism and fatty acid oxidation deficiency, need special attention.[59] These conditions can result in severe neurologic injury.[60] Two retrospective studies documented that more than 10% of neonates and older infants with a history of severe and persistent hypoglycemia went on to have significant developmental delay or epilepsy.[61,62]

Infants with repeated, marked, and prolonged, not just brief and transient, hypoglycemia should have diagnostic evaluations. These infants often have very low initial glucose concentrations that cannot be corrected easily with feeding and IV dextrose and require higher glucose infusion rates than other infants (up to 15–20 mg/kg/min). They should be treated with IV dextrose until stable, and glucose concentrations should be monitored frequently. Oral or enteral feeding should be continued, or started as soon as possible, with small, frequent, or even continuous feeding. CGM would likely benefit management of these infants if available. Signs of illness or hypoglycemia should be taken seriously because unrecognized progressive hypoglycemia can quickly lead to permanent neuronal injury and even death. Infants with genetic hyperinsulinism or metabolic defects should not be discharged without demonstrating for at least 2 days that they can maintain normal glucose concentrations for 4 to 6 hours between feedings.[63] A long-term management plan with endocrinology, gastroenterology, and often pediatric surgery services should also be finalized before discharge.

RISK OF ADVERSE NEURODEVELOPMENTAL OUTCOMES

Concurrence of associated conditions, particularly persistent hyperinsulinism or metabolic and hormonal defects with repeated episodes of severe hypoglycemia featuring seizures, flaccid hypotonia with apnea, and/or coma, should be avoided because these combined conditions are highly associated with permanent and serious neurologic injury.[10,24,64] Blood or plasma glucose concentrations lower than 18 mg/dL are definitely abnormal. However, if transient, lasting for minutes, and unaccompanied by severe clinical signs, there is no consistent evidence that they invariably lead to permanent neurologic damage or that treating with IV dextrose would prevent such injury. Low glucose concentrations should increase, and if they do not increase with feeding and perhaps oral dextrose gel, more aggressive management is indicated.

Early mild to moderate clinical signs (primarily those of increased epinephrine activity), such as jitteriness or poor feeding, that improve with effective treatment that restores glucose concentrations to the statistically normal range, higher than 45 mg/dL, are unlikely to cause later adverse neurodevelopmental conditions.[64] More serious clinical signs that are prolonged (many hours or longer) and refractory to short-term treatment, including flaccid hypotonia, coma, seizures, respiratory depression and/or apnea with cyanosis, high-pitched cry, hypothermia, and poor feeding after initially feeding well, are more likely to indicate potential for serious adverse and likely permanent neurologic impairment. It remains uncertain whether subclinical, but severe, hypoglycemic episodes also might be injurious; further research with CGM could help to document these episodes and whether immediate treatment would prevent adverse neurodevelopmental outcomes.

To date, however, there has been no convincing evidence that one or more brief episodes of low glucose concentrations below a specific value cause damage or what duration of extremely low glucose levels is dangerous. Therefore, one should be cautious about interpreting later neurodevelopmental disorders as caused by neonatal hypoglycemia.

LEARNING FROM MEDICAL LEGAL CLAIMS

A major concern for many clinicians regarding neonatal hypoglycemia is the history of medical legal claims filed against doctors and health-care professionals for possible causation of neurologic injury. A recent study from the United Kingdom documented a number of risks for such medical legal claims.[65] The most common risk factor was the failure to identify infants with low or borderline low birth weight (<2.5 kg). Failure to recognize presenting clinical signs also was noted, particularly those of hypothermia and abnormal feeding behavior, especially feeding poorly after initially feeding well. Clearly, clinicians can reduce risk of medical legal claims for infants with neonatal hypoglycemia by paying close attention to risk factors for hypoglycemia, developing both astute medical care and observation patterns, and establishing guidelines in their hospitals for prevention, diagnosis, and treatment.

SUMMARY

This review provides a rational background for what should be considered neonatal hypoglycemia in term newborn infants and a practical guide for screening, diagnosis, and management of low glucose concentrations. Early identification of the newborn infant at risk of hypoglycemia and institution of prophylactic measures to prevent neonatal hypoglycemia are recommended as a pragmatic approach despite the absence of a consistent definition of hypoglycemia in the literature. Current guidelines aimed at screening at-risk infants, early breastfeeding, monitoring prefeed glucose concentrations, treating symptomatic infants who have very low and recurrent low glucose concentrations, and identifying and aggressively managing infants with persistent hyperinsulinemia and metabolic defects may reduce the risk of brain injury from prolonged severe hypoglycemia. Further research is clearly needed. The major question remains: is there a specific low glucose concentration, a range of low concentrations, or a defined duration of such low values that defines pathologic hypoglycemia that causes brain damage in at-risk, or even normal, newborn infants?

CLINICS CARE POINTS

Neonatal hypoglycemia

Best practice/guideline/care path objectives

- Early identification of the at-risk infant
- Prophylactic measures to prevent neonatal hypoglycemia
- Treatments that prevent neurologic injury from severe and prolonged hypoglycemia

Changes in current practice are likely to improve outcomes

- Oral dextrose gel administered to an infant who has low glucose concentrations can raise glucose concentrations, prevent further low glucose values when combined with continued feeding, reduce need for NICU admission and intravenous dextrose treatment, and promote continued breastfeeding.

Major recommendations

- Screening at-risk infants
- Early and continued breastfeeding, supplemented with oral dextrose gel as needed
- Monitoring prefeed glucose concentrations while on oral or enteral feedings
- Treating symptomatic infants who have very low or recurrent low glucose concentrations
- Identifying and aggressively managing infants with persistent hyperinsulinemia and metabolic defects may help prevent neuronal injury.

Summary statements

- Current guidelines noted in this review provide reasonable approaches to identifying infants at risk and management that could prevent development of clinically significant hypoglycemia and help reduce the risk of brain injury from prolonged, recurrent, severely symptomatic hypoglycemia.

Best practices summary from references [3,5,8,13,14,22–24,40,41,46].

DISCLOSURE

E.M. Hubbard has received research support from Dexcom. W.W. Hay is a consultant for Astarte Medical, Inc., which has no commercial interests in neonatal hypoglycemia.

REFERENCES

1. Hay WW Jr, Sparks JW. Placental, fetal, and neonatal carbohydrate metabolism. Clin Obstet Gynecol 1985;28(3):473–85.
2. Güemes M, Rahman SA, Hussain K. What is a normal blood glucose? Arch Dis Child 2016;101(6):569–74.
3. Adamkin DH. Metabolic screening and postnatal glucose homeostasis in the newborn. Pediatr Clin North Am 2015;62(2):385–409.
4. Hoseth E, Joergensen A, Ebbesen F, et al. Blood glucose levels in a population of healthy, breast fed, term infants of appropriate size for gestational age. Arch Dis Child Fetal Neonatal Ed 2000;83(2):F117–9.
5. Cornblath M, Hawdon JM, Williams AF, et al. Controversies regarding definition of neonatal hypoglycemia: suggested operational thresholds. Pediatrics 2000; 105(5):1141–5.
6. Diwakar KK, Sasidhar MV. Plasma glucose levels in term infants who are appropriate size for gestation and exclusively breast fed. Arch Dis Child Fetal Neonatal Ed 2002;87:F46–8.
7. Wight NE. Hypoglycemia in breastfed neonates. Breastfeed Med 2006;1(4): 253–62.
8. Harris DL, Weston PJ, Gamble GD, et al. Glucose profiles in healthy term infants in the first 5 days: the glucose in well babies (GLOW) study. J Pediatr 2020;223: 34–41.e4.
9. Stanley CA, Rozance PJ, Thornton PS, et al. Re-evaluating "transitional neonatal hypoglycemia": mechanism and implications for management. J Pediatr 2015; 166(6):1520–5.e1.
10. Shah R, Harding J, Brown J, et al. Neonatal glycaemia and neurodevelopmental outcomes: a systematic review and meta-analysis. Neonatology 2019;115(2): 116–26.
11. Van Kempen AMW, Eskes PF, Nuytemans DHGM, et al. Lower versus traditional treatment threshold for neonatal hypoglycemia. N Engl J Med 2020;382(6): 534–44.
12. Cornblath M, Ichord R. Hypoglycemia in the neonate. Semin Perinatol 2000;24(2): 136–49.
13. Committee on Fetus and Newborn, Adamkin DH. Postnatal glucose homeostasis in late-preterm and term infants. Pediatrics 2011;127(3):575–9.
14. Thornton PS, Stanley CA, De Leon DD, et al. Recommendations from the pediatric endocrine society for evaluation and management of persistent hypoglycemia in neonates, infants, and children. J Pediatr 2015;167(2):238–45.
15. Adamkin DH, Polin R. Neonatal hypoglycemia: is 60 the new 40? The questions remain the same. J Perinatol 2016;36(1):10–2.
16. Rozance PJ, Hay WW Jr. Neonatal hypoglycemia–answers, but more questions. J Pediatr 2012;161(5):775–6.

17. Dani C, Corsini L. Guidelines for management of neonatal hypoglycemia—are they actually applicable? JAMA Pediatr 2020;174(7):638–9.
18. Mukhopadhyay S, Wade KC, Dhudasia MB, et al. Clinical impact of neonatal hypoglycemia screening in the well-baby care. J Perinatol 2020;40(9):1331–8.
19. Skovrlj R, Marks SD, Rodd C. Frequency and etiology of persistent neonatal hypoglycemia using the more stringent 2015 Pediatric Endocrine Society hypoglycemia guidelines. Paediatr Child Health 2019;24(4):263–9.
20. Harris DL, Weston PJ, Harding JE. Incidence of neonatal hypoglycemia in babies identified as at risk. J Pediatr 2012;161(5):787–91.
21. Hay WW Jr, Adamkin DH, Harding JE, et al. The postnatal glucose concentration nadir is not abnormal and does not need to Be treated. Neonatology 2018; 114(2):163.
22. Adamkin DH. Neonatal hypoglycemia. Semin Fetal Neonatal Med 2017;22(1): 36–41.
23. McKinlay CJ, Alsweiler JM, Ansell JM, et al. Neonatal glycemia and neurodevelopmental outcomes at 2 years. N Engl J Med 2015;373(16):1507–18.
24. McKinlay CJD, Alsweiler JM, Anstice NS, et al. Association of neonatal glycemia with neurodevelopmental outcomes at 4.5 years. JAMA Pediatr 2017;171(10): 972–83.
25. Roth-Kleiner M, Stadelmann Diaw C, Urfer J, et al. Evaluation of different POCT devices for glucose measurement in a clinical neonatal setting. Eur J Pediatr 2010;169(11):1387–95.
26. Beardsall K. Measurement of glucose levels in the newborn. Early Hum Dev 2010; 86(5):263–7.
27. Harris DL, Gamble GD, Weston PJ, et al. What happens to blood glucose concentrations after oral treatment for neonatal hypoglycemia? J Pediatr 2017;190: 136–41.
28. Harris DL, Battin MR, Weston PJ, et al. Continuous glucose monitoring in newborn babies at risk of hypoglycemia. J Pediatr 2010;157(2):198–202.e1.
29. Wackernagel D, Dube M, Blennow M, et al. Continuous subcutaneous glucose monitoring is accurate in term and near-term infants at risk of hypoglycaemia. Acta Paediatr 2016;105(8):917–23.
30. Perri A, Giordano L, Corsello M, et al. Continuous glucose monitoring (CGM) in very low birth weight newborns needing parenteral nutrition: validation and glycemic percentiles. Ital J Pediatr 2018;44(1):99.
31. Galderisi A, Facchinetti A, Steil GM, et al. Continuous glucose monitoring in very preterm infants: a randomized controlled trial. Pediatrics 2017;140(4):e20171162.
32. Hernandez TL, Hay WW Jr, Rozance PJ. Continuous glucose monitoring in the neonatal intensive care unit: not quite ready for 'plug and play. Arch Dis Child Fetal Neonatal Ed 2019;104(4):F344–5.
33. Moore ER, Bergman N, Anderson GC, et al. Early skin-to-skin contact for mothers and their healthy newborn infants. Cochrane Database Syst Rev 2016;11(11): CD003519.
34. Wight N, Marinelli KA, Academy of Breastfeeding Medicine. ABM clinical protocol# 1: guidelines for blood glucose monitoring and treatment of hypoglycemia in term and late-preterm neonates, revised 2014. Breastfeed Med 2014;9(4): 173–1799.
35. Eidelman AI. Hypoglycemia and the breastfed neonate. Pediatr Clin North Am 2001;48(2):377–87.
36. Lilien LD, Grajwer LA, Pildes RS. Treatment of neonatal hypoglycemia with continuous intravenous glucose infusion. J Pediatr 1977;91(5):779–82.

37. Rozance PJ, Hay WW Jr. New approaches to management of neonatal hypoglycemia. Matern Health Neonatol Perinatol 2016;2:3.
38. Suh SW, Gum ET, Hamby AM, et al. Hypoglycemic neuronal death is triggered by glucose reperfusion and activation of neuronal NADPH oxidase. J Clin Invest 2007;117(4):910–8.
39. Alsaleem M, Saadeh L, Kumar VHS, et al. Continued enteral feeding is beneficial in hypoglycemic infants admitted to intensive care for parenteral dextrose therapy. Glob Pediatr Health 2019;6. 2333794X19857415.
40. Harris DL, Weston PJ, Signal M, et al. Dextrose gel for neonatal hypoglycaemia (the Sugar Babies Study): a randomised, double-blind, placebo-controlled trial. Lancet 2013;382(9910):2077–83.
41. Hegarty JE, Harding JE, Gamble GD, et al. Prophylactic oral dextrose gel for newborn babies at risk of neonatal hypoglycaemia: a randomised controlled dose-finding trial (the pre-hPOD study). PLoS Med 2016;13(10):e1002155.
42. Rawat M, Chandrasekharan P, Turkovich S, et al. Oral dextrose gel reduces the need for intravenous dextrose therapy in neonatal hypoglycemia. Biomed Hub 2016;1(3):1–9.
43. Newnam KM, Bunch M. Glucose gel as a treatment strategy for transient neonatal hypoglycemia. Adv Neonatal Care 2017;17(6):470–7.
44. Makker K, Alissa R, Dudek C, et al. Glucose gel in infants at risk for transitional neonatal hypoglycemia. Am J Perinatol 2018;35(11):1050–6.
45. Gregory K, Turner D, Benjamin CN, et al. Incorporating dextrose gel and feeding in the treatment of neonatal hypoglycaemia. Arch Dis Child Fetal Neonatal Ed 2020;105(1):45–9.
46. Harris DL, Alsweiler JM, Ansell JM, et al. Outcome at 2 Years after dextrose gel treatment for neonatal hypoglycemia: follow-up of a randomized trial. J Pediatr 2016;170:54–9.e92.
47. Coors SM, Cousin JJ, Hagan JL, et al. Prophylactic dextrose gel does not prevent neonatal hypoglycemia: a Quasi-experimental Pilot study. J Pediatr 2018;198:156–61.
48. Solimano A, Kwan E, Osiovich H, et al. Dextrose gels for neonatal transitional hypoglycemia: what are we giving our babies? Paediatr Child Health 2019;24(2):115–8.
49. Hay WW Jr. Care of the infant of the diabetic mother. Curr Diab Rep 2012;12(1):4–15.
50. Persson B. Neonatal glucose metabolism in offspring of mothers with varying degrees of hyperglycemia during pregnancy. Semin Fetal Neonatal Med 2009;14(2):106–10.
51. Maayan-Metzger A, Lubin D, Kuint J. Hypoglycemia rates in the first days of life among term infants born to diabetic mothers. Neonatology 2009;96(2):80–5.
52. King KC, Tserng KY, Kalhan SC. Regulation of glucose production in newborn infants of diabetic mothers. Pediatr Res 1982;16(8):608–12.
53. Lilien LD, Pildes RS, Srinivasan G, et al. Treatment of neonatal hypoglycemia with minibolus and intraveous glucose infusion. J Pediatr 1980;97(2):295–8.
54. Hoe FM, Thornton PS, Wanner LA, et al. Clinical features and insulin regulation in infants with a syndrome of prolonged neonatal hyperinsulinism. J Pediatr 2006;148(2):207–12.
55. Hay W, Limesand S, Camacho L, et al. Persistent hypoglycemia in IUGR/SGA infants: an increasingly recognized and frustratingly difficult problem to diagnose and treat. Acta Paediatr 2017;106(S469):39.

56. Kozen K, Dassios T, Kametas N, et al. Transient neonatal hyperinsulinaemic hypoglycaemia: perinatal predictors of length and cost of stay. Eur J Pediatr 2018;177(12):1823–9.
57. Chen X, Green AS, Macko AR, et al. Enhanced insulin secretion responsiveness and islet adrenergic desensitization after chronic norepinephrine suppression is discontinued in fetal sheep. Am J Physiol Endocrinol Metab 2014;306(1):E58–64.
58. Camacho LE, Chen X, Hay WW Jr, et al. Enhanced insulin secretion and insulin sensitivity in young lambs with placental insufficiency-induced intrauterine growth restriction. Am J Physiol Regul Integr Comp Physiol 2017;313(2):R101–9.
59. Kostopoulou E, Shah P. Hyperinsulinaemic hypoglycaemia-an overview of a complex clinical condition. Eur J Pediatr 2019;178(8):1151–60.
60. Goel P, Choudhury SR. Persistent hyperinsulinemic hypoglycemia of infancy: an overview of current concepts. J Indian Assoc Pediatr Surg 2012;17(3):99–103.
61. Menni F, de Lonlay P, Sevin C, et al. Neurologic outcomes of 90 neonates and infants with persistent hyperinsulinemic hypoglycemia. Pediatrics 2001;107(3):476–9.
62. Meissner T, Wendel U, Burgard P, et al. Long-term follow-up of 114 patients with congenital hyperinsulinism. Eur J Endocrinol 2003;149(1):43–51.
63. Lord K, De León DD. Hyperinsulinism in the neonate. Clin Perinatol 2018;45(1):61–74.
64. Rozance PJ, Hay WW. Hypoglycemia in newborn infants: features associated with adverse outcomes. Biol Neonate 2006;90(2):74–86.
65. Hawdon JM, Beer J, Sharp D, et al. NHS improvement patient safety programme ‘reducing term admissions to neonatal units’. Neonatal hypoglycaemia: learning from claims. Arch Dis Child Fetal Neonatal Ed 2017;102(2):F110–5.

The Term Newborn

Evaluation for Hypoxic-Ischemic Encephalopathy

Sonia Lomeli Bonifacio, MD[a,*], Shandee Hutson, MD[b]

KEYWORDS

- Neonatal encephalopathy • Therapeutic hypothermia • Term infant
- Hypoxic-ischemic encephalopathy • Neurodevelopmental outcome
- Neuroprotection • Whole-body cooling • Head cooling

KEY POINTS

- Recognition of neonates with hypoxic-ischemic encephalopathy is a critical skill for all providers who attend deliveries or work in newborn nurseries.
- All such providers need to know how to perform the modified Sarnat examination and determine eligibility for therapeutic hypothermia, the standard-of-care neuroprotective treatment for moderate to severe HIE.
- The Sarnat examination should be performed at about an hour of age. If a newborn meets criteria for therapeutic hypothermia, the process of transferring to a treatment center should be started immediately and treatment should be initiated before 6 hours after birth.
- Once the decision is made to institute hypothermia, the therapy should be continued even if the examination improves.
- Serial Sarnat examinations should be performed and continued hourly until 6 hours for those who meet historical and biochemical criteria but not examination criteria at 1 hour.
- If a patient is passively cooled prior to transport, core temperature needs to be monitored every 15 minutes. Maintaining homeostasis should be the goal, with close attention paid to glucose levels, carbon dioxide levels, blood pressure, and avoidance of hyperoxia.

INTRODUCTION

Incidence of Neonatal Encephalopathy and Hypoxic-Ischemic Encephalopathy

Neonatal encephalopathy (NE) is a clinical syndrome of disordered neonatal brain function occurring in the first days after birth in babies born beyond 35 weeks of gestation.[1] The most common cause is hypoxic-ischemic encephalopathy (HIE) after perinatal asphyxia. HIE has an incidence of 1.5 per 1000 live births in developed countries

[a] NeuroNICU, Division of Neonatal and Developmental Medicine, 750 Welch Road, Suite 315, Palo Alto, CA, USA; [b] Department of Neonatology, NICN, Sharp Mary Birch Hospital for Women and Newborns, 8555 Aero Drive #104, San Diego, CA 92123, USA
* Corresponding author. Center for Academic Medicine, Division of Neonatology - MC: 5660 453 Quarry Road, Palo Alto, CA 94304-1419, USA
E-mail address: Soniab1@stanford.edu

Clin Perinatol 48 (2021) 681–695
https://doi.org/10.1016/j.clp.2021.05.014
0095-5108/21/

and up to 26 per 1000 live births in low-resource countries.[1,2] Worldwide, acute perinatal asphyxia is estimated to account for 23% of infant deaths.[2]

Recognition of Encephalopathy

NE is a clinically defined syndrome with multivariate etiologies characterized by abnormal levels of consciousness or seizures in an infant born at or beyond 35 weeks of gestation and often accompanied by difficulty in respiration and depression of tone and reflexes.[3]

Although HIE is estimated by some to account for up to 80% of cases of NE, perinatal infections, genetic and epigenetic abnormalities, placental abnormalities, metabolic disorders, coagulopathies, maternal risk factors, and neonatal vascular stroke have also been implicated. Evaluation of prenatal risk factors and postnatal testing can be helpful in determining causation; however, the cause remains undetermined in more than half of the cases.[4]

NE due to presumed perinatal hypoxia-ischemia can be differentiated from other etiologies by history of a sentinel event and consideration of fetal heart rate findings during labor and delivery, surrogate markers of hypoxia such as pH, evidence of multiorgan involvement, and patterns of brain injury on neuroimaging.[3] Additional clinical findings such as evolution of electroencephalography findings and the neurologic examination can help differentiate encephalopathy due to other potential etiologies.

Historical Outcomes

Historically, therapy for infants with HIE was limited to supportive care. The mortality rate for infants with moderate encephalopathy was 10%, and 30% of surviving infants went on to have disabilities. Outcomes in infants with severe encephalopathy were worse. Approximately 85% of infants with severe HIE died, and at least 75% of survivors had significant mental and physical impairment. These impairments included cerebral palsy, blindness, cognitive delay, seizure disorder, severe hearing loss, memory impairment, increased hyperactivity, and delayed school readiness.[5–8]

Pathophysiology of Hypoxic-Ischemic Encephalopathy

The brain injury that occurs after hypoxia-ischemia is commonly the result of both primary and secondary energy failure. The initial insult triggers a cascade of events, similar to the concept of falling dominos. During the initial phase, decreased cerebral blood flow leads to diminished oxygen and glucose energy substrates, decreased ATP production, and an increase in lactate levels. Lack of energy substrates results in a failure of Na^+/K^+ pumps and activation of an excitotoxic-oxidative cascade. Continuation of this cascade leads to an altered cell membrane, impaired cellular integrity, and cellular apoptosis and necrosis. Once blood flow is restored, there is a brief period of normal cerebral metabolism, followed by development of secondary energy failure. Continuation of the excitotoxic-oxidative cascade leads to secondary energy failure in the mitochondria. Lack of energy stores and inflammation, altered growth factors, and protein synthesis ultimately lead to brain cell apoptosis and necrosis over the next several days to week. The therapeutic window occurring between primary and secondary energy failure is approximately 6 hours. This was initially determined in animal studies and then supported in randomized controlled trials in infants.[5,8,9]

Randomized Control Trials of Hypoxic-Ischemic Encephalopathy

Multiple randomized trials have shown that when initiated within 6 hours of birth, either selective head cooling or whole-body cooling is associated with a reduction in mortality and long-term neurodevelopmental disability (NDD) for infants with moderate to severe HIE.[10–17] A systematic review and meta-analysis of 11 randomized trials including more than 1505 newborns with follow-up to at least 18 months showed that therapeutic hypothermia (TH) is associated with a significant risk reduction for death or moderate to severe neurodevelopmental disability (NDD) at 18 to 24 months (Relative Risk [RR] = 0.75; 95% confidence interval [CI] = 0.68–0.83), with the number needed to treat (NNT) of 7 (95% CI = 5–10).[15] Furthermore, survival without NDD was also increased (RR = 1.63; 95% CI = 1.36–1.95). When outcomes were analyzed based on the degree of encephalopathy at the time of randomization, pooled data from 5 trials showed infants with moderate encephalopathy who were treated with TH had a risk reduction of 0.68 (95% CI = 0.56–0.84) and an NNT of 6 (95% CI = 4–13) and those with severe encephalopathy had an RR of 0.82 (95% CI = 0.72–0.93) and an NNT of 7 (95% CI = 4–17). TH was shown to have a statistically and clinically significant effect on individual outcomes including cerebral palsy, neuromotor delay, and developmental delay.[15] The neuroprotective effect of TH carries through to early childhood.

Importance of Recognition of All Potentially Eligible Infants

Following these studies, TH has been recommended since 2010 as the standard of care for newborns with moderate to severe encephalopathy meeting inclusion criteria outlined in the studies. Recognition and early initiation of TH for all eligible infants is important because for every 7 infants treated, one infant will avoid death or moderate to severe disability compared with those who do not receive TH. There is ongoing debate about the impact of earlier initiation (<3 hours after birth) and later initiation (>3 hours) on the degree of neuroprotection. Every effort should be made to identify and initiate treatment within 6 hours after birth.

Tools to Recognize Encephalopathy

Any infant with perinatal depression or history of an acute perinatal event should receive prompt evaluation for HIE. This evaluation should include a detailed history, cord or infant blood gas sampling within 1 hour of birth, and physical examination, with particular attention to elements of the modified Sarnat examination. History should be examined for clues of an acute perinatal event capable of causing hypoxia-ischemia. Key features of the physical examination include alteration in the degree or quality of consciousness, activity, tone, posture, reflexes, and cardiorespiratory compromise.

Evaluation begins in the delivery room with assignment of Apgar scores. Apgar scores are commonly used as basic screening criteria for prequalification for TH therapy.[18]

The second common prequalification evaluation for TH includes laboratory tests to assess for metabolic acidosis. Severe metabolic acidosis at birth as seen on cord blood gas or early infant blood gas is thought to reflect the degree of fetal hypoxia-ischemia and is correlated with severity of brain injury.[18] Other laboratory evidence of end-organ damage secondary to perinatal asphyxia can include elevation of liver transaminase levels, coagulopathy, and elevated levels of cardiac troponin I.[19,20]

Examination tools commonly used as the entry criterion for TH include both the modified Sarnat examination and Thompson score. Benefits of these examination tools include allowing for standardization and requiring little additional training or equipment, allowing for use in both high- and low-resource settings. Although not originally intended for this use, the modified Sarnat examination has been used in NICHD studies, Cool Cap, TOBY, ICE, and other neuroprotective trials including NEATO and HEAL.[10,11,13,14,21,22] The Sarnat scale distinguishes 3 stages of encephalopathy: mild encephalopathy (stage 1) associated with sympathetic overdrive and hyperalterness, moderate encephalopathy (stage 2) marked by lethargy and hypotonia, and severe encephalopathy (stage 3), in which infants are obtunded and flaccid. It is important to note that an infant can have overlapping examination findings, with some categories scoring mild and others scoring as moderate or severe. In order to qualify for TH, an infant must have at least 3 of 6 categories identified as moderate or severe. Optimal timing of the examination is at about an hour of age, after initial resuscitation is completed. Providers should be aware that examination findings can change over time, even in the first 6 hours after birth, with some infants improving, whereas others may deteriorate. The current recommendation is that if infants have moderate to severe encephalopathy as per the Sarnat examination at about an hour of age and they meet the historical and biochemical criteria, they should receive TH.

The Thompson score has also been used to determine eligibility for TH.[23] It assigns a numerical value between 0 and 22 based on severity of neurologic condition in 9 different areas. It has been shown to have a high predictive value for adverse outcomes and high inter-rater reliability and offers a more precise numerical assessment of HIE than the mild, moderate, or severe categories assigned by the modified Sarnat examination.[24,25]

High-resource centers may benefit from the use of additional screening tools such as amplitude-integrated electroencephalogram (aEEG). Two clinical trials used aEEG screening as an entry criterion for TH.[10,13] Early aEEG has been shown to predict outcomes in normothermic infants, and evolution of the aEEG/EEG background during hypothermia has good prognostic accuracy for the outcome of death or NDD.[26,27] Early and continuous aEEG/EEG use is considered the standard of care in the era of TH.

Importance of a Standardized Approach and Tools to Help Determine Eligibility

TH remains the best evidence-based therapy for HIE. To achieve the greatest therapeutic benefit, infants with suspected HIE must be identified quickly and TH must be initiated within 6 hours of suspected hypoxic insult. Time is brain, with earlier initiation of TH associated with better motor outcomes.[28] The exact timing of the hypoxic-ischemic event may be difficult to ascertain. Depending on when the event occurred, infants at the time of screening may be experiencing worsening primary cerebral energy failure from hypoxia-ischemia, primary energy failure may be improving, or damage from secondary energy failure may be occurring. This is reflected in fluctuations seen in early physical examination and aEEG/EEG results. As some hypoxic-ischemic events may occur prior to delivery, rapid identification of infants with HIE followed by initiation of TH is necessary to try to ensure the therapeutic window is not missed.

Multiple barriers exist in both identifying newborns eligible for treatment and in reaching optimal neuroprotective core temperature prior to 6 hours of life. Infants born at centers not offering TH must be identified early in order to make referral and initiate treatment within the therapeutic window. Outborn infants referred for TH have been shown to have a greater delay in initiation of TH and more severe HIE than infants receiving TH who were born at TH centers.[29] The number of infants with HIE varies largely between centers, with small delivery services seeing only 1 to 2 cases per year. Neurologic examination findings can fluctuate, and providers may have variable skill levels in recognition of encephalopathy.

To overcome these barriers, a standardized approach must be taken to patient screening and tools must be put in place to determine eligibility (**Fig. 1**). Each institution that has a delivery service should be aware of TH criteria and have an established

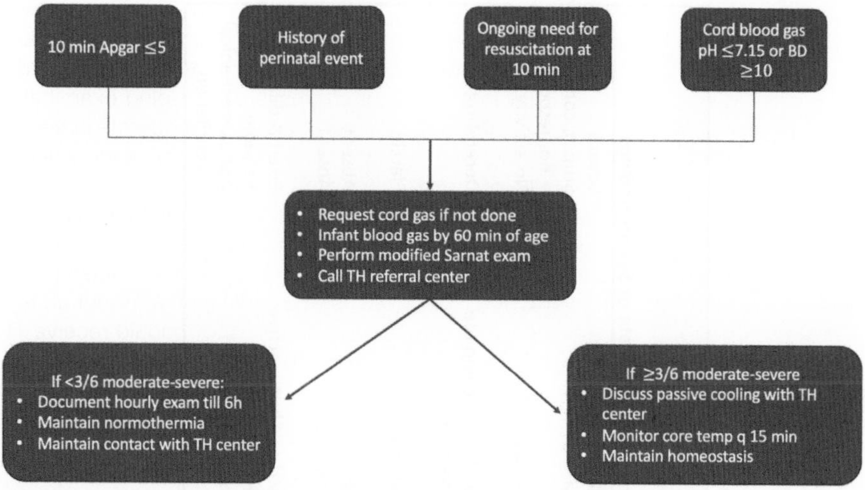
10 min Apgar ≤5
History of perinatal event
Ongoing need for resuscitation at 10 min
Cord blood gas pH ≤7.15 or BD ≥10
• Request cord gas if not done
• Infant blood gas by 60 min of age
• Perform modified Sarnat exam
• Call TH referral center
If <3/6 moderate-severe:
• Document hourly exam till 6h
• Maintain normothermia
• Maintain contact with TH center
If ≥3/6 moderate-severe
• Discuss passive cooling with TH center
• Monitor core temp q 15 min
• Maintain homeostasis

Fig. 1. HIE screening tool to identify potential candidates for TH.

relationship with a TH center. TH inclusion criteria should be posted in delivery and operating rooms. To aid in standardization and determination of eligibility, the American Academy of Pediatrics, International Liaison Committee on Resuscitation, and American Heart Association have released recommendations. Current guidelines suggest that TH be offered to infants born beyond 36 weeks of gestation with evolving moderate to severe HIE as per clearly defined protocols similar to those published in clinical trials[30,31] (**Table 1** with inclusion criteria).

Established protocols should include universal cord gas screening with automatic real-time notifications of cord blood gas results and mandatory reporting of pH less than 7.15 and base deficit (BD) higher than 10. All delivery room, well baby and neonatal intensive care unit (NICU) providers including nurses, physicians, and nurse practitioners, should undergo yearly training in identification of candidates for TH. Education should include initial management of infants with concern for HIE and resources for TH screening. Such resources available for TH screening include the CPQCC tool kit and mobile device apps including NeoCool. All infants who meet historical and laboratory criteria for HIE should have a standardized examination performed at 1 hour of age. If initial examination does not meet the criteria, serial neurologic examinations should be continued hourly until 6 hours of age. Smaller centers may benefit from tele examinations and should review the examination with neonatologists at their referral center. TH should be initiated after initial qualifying examination, and once an infant qualifies, they do not get additional time to unqualify for treatment even if examination improves.

When possible, infants with HIE should be transferred to the TH center with dedicated neonatal neurocritical care center. Infants with moderate to severe HIE receiving care in dedicated neonatal neurocritical care centers have been shown to have improved seizure detection, decreased antiseizure medication at discharge, and a reduction in abnormalities on brain MRI as compared with infants treated with TH in a standard NICU environment.[32,33]

Early Supportive Care of an Infant with Hypoxic-Ischemic Encephalopathy

Once infants with suspected HIE are identified, multiple supportive measures may be required to maintain homeostasis. Any hospital with a delivery center should be

Table 1
Therapeutic hypothermia inclusion criteria and modified Sarnat examination

Inclusion Criteria	Modified Sarnat Examination: Must Have 3 of 6 Categories with Moderate or Severe Findings			
• Term Infant	Category	Mild	Moderate	Severe
Pathway A • Cord or infant pH $\leq$ 7.0 or BD $\geq$ 16	Level of consciousness	Irritable, hyperalert	Lethargic	Stupor, coma, nonresponsive
• Perform examination	Spontaneous activity	Increased exaggerated movements, jittery	Decreased activity	No activity
Pathway B • No cord or infant blood gas, OR	Posture	Mild distal or arm flexion with leg abduction or slight extension	Distal flexion, complete extension	Decerebrate
• pH 7.01–7.15	Tone	Slightly increased	Hypotonia	Flaccid
• BD 10–15.9	Neonatal reflexes			
Must meet the following & Sarnat Examination Criteria:	• Suck	Uncoordinated	Weak	Absent
	• Moro	Exaggerated	Incomplete	Absent
• Perinatal event *AND*	ANS			
• Apgar at 10 minutes $\leq$ 5, **OR**	• Pupils	Dilated but reactive	Constricted but reactive	Fixed & dilated
• Assisted ventilation at 10 min	• Heart rate	Tachycardia	Bradycardia	Variable
	• Respiration	Irregular/tachypnea	Periodic breathing	Apnea/mechanical ventilation

Abbreviation: ANS, autonomic nervous system.

prepared to continue ongoing supportive care and provide timely, safe initiation of passive cooling.

Temperature

Temperature must be monitored closely from the start in the delivery room. The radiant warmer should not be turned off until after resuscitation and determination of eligibility for treatment. Asphyxiated newborns have decreased metabolism and poor endogenous heat generation. This may be associated with a rapid decline in temperature after birth.[34] If core temperature drops lower than 33°C, it may be accompanied by dangerous bradycardia. Hyperthermia should also be avoided because in both the NICHD NRN and CoolCap trials, elevated temperatures in the control group were associated with higher risk of death or disability.[35,36] The goal should be to maintain normothermia until determination of eligibility for treatment. If passive cooling is initiated, core temperature must be monitored closely.

Fluid, Electrolytes, Nutrition

Infants with HIE are at risk of labile glucose levels. Hyperglycemia and high glucose variability have been associated with poor neurodevelopmental outcomes.[37] Hypoxic-ischemic–induced changes can lead to poor glucose delivery, increased glucose utilization by the brain, and relative insulin resistance.[37,38] Hypoglycemia is also common in infants with perinatal asphyxia and may contribute to brain injury.[39] Therefore, glucose levels should be monitored closely and supplemental IV dextrose should be given as needed to maintain normoglycemia.

Fluid and electrolyte balance must be closely monitored in infants with HIE. Acute kidney injury and associated renal dysfunction are commonly seen. Hyponatremia, hypokalemia, and hypocalcemia are common, with an estimated 50% of infants with HIE having electrolyte abnormalities.[40] The initial metabolic acidosis seen in all infants with HIE is best slowly corrected with supportive measures. Sodium bicarbonate administration should be avoided because rapid changes in carbon dioxide may lead to alteration in cerebral perfusion.[41]

Hemodynamics

HIE is commonly associated with varying degrees of cardiac dysfunction, decreased cardiac output, pulmonary hypertension, and intravascular fluid shifts. Hypotension requiring inotrope support or evidence of transient myocardial ischemia is seen in approximately 60% of infants with HIE.[42] Inotropic and chronotropic support as well as fluid management should be individualized based on targeted neonatal echocardiography.[43] Blood pressure should be kept in the normal range to preserve cerebral perfusion pressure.

Coagulopathy

Both HIE and TH are associated with thrombocytopenia, platelet dysfunction, and disseminated intravascular coagulation. In the major TH trials, coagulopathy was reported in 12% to 43% of infants, with the incidence of bleeding ranging from 3% to 12%.[10,11,13] In one observational study of infants with HIE, the most common sites of bleeding were pulmonary, upper gastrointestinal, and umbilical, with 57% of infants requiring blood product transfusion within the first 12 hours.[44] Although there is limited consensus regarding levels at which to transfuse blood products, there is agreement that infants with suspected HIE should receive early evaluation for coagulopathy and close monitoring for clinically significant bleeding.

Infection

Owing to association of both chorioamnionitis and sepsis with hypoxia-ischemia and encephalopathy, initial blood culture and sepsis evaluation should be carried out for infants with suspected HIE and they should be treated with empiric antibiotics until sepsis can be ruled out.[45]

Respiratory

Both oxygenation and ventilation should be monitored closely, with special care taken to avoid hypocapnia and hyperoxia. Immediately after a perinatal asphyxial event, hypercapnea is common; however, it is frequently followed by hypocapnia in infants with HIE. This hypocapnia may be due to impaired energy metabolism leading to decreased carbon dioxide production or metabolic acidosis resulting in compensatory hyperventilation.[46] Hypocapnia may lead to cerebral vasoconstriction, decreased cerebral blood flow, and decreased cerebral oxygen supply due to the leftward shift of the oxyhemoglobin curve. For infants with HIE, early hypocapnia has been associated with increased injury on brain MRI and increased likelihood of adverse neurologic outcomes.[46,47] Therefore, especially in ventilated infants, P_{CO_2} levels should be monitored closely and efforts should be made to optimize frequency and tidal volumes to maintain P_{CO_2} levels of 40 to 50 mm Hg.[48]

Continuous pulse oximetry and arterial blood gas sampling are recommended to help avoid excessive use of oxygen. Early hyperoxia can lead to increased inflammation, free radical production, and impaired functional recovery after hypoxic brain injury. For infants with HIE, hyperoxia is associated with an increased risk of death or disability. For these infants, the risk of adverse outcome was greatest in infants with a combination of hyperoxia and hypocapnia.[49–53] Therefore, F_{IO_2} should be adjusted to the minimum level required to maintain SpO_2 higher than 92% and the P_{O_2} level of 50 to 100 mm Hg.[48,50]

Evaluation and Management of Seizures

Infants with HIE are at increased risk of clinical and electrographic seizures. Previous studies examining incidence of seizures in infants with moderate to severe HIE showed an incidence of 22% to 64%.[11,13,53,54] It is rare to have electrographic seizures in the first 1-2 hours after birth if the encephalopathy is due to an intrapartum hypoxic-ischemic insult. An observational study examining 26 infants with HIE treated with TH found the age of first seizure occurrence ranged from 6 to 95 hours, with a mean time of first seizure to be 35 hours.[54] Furthermore, many encephalopathic neonates display abnormal paroxysmal movements that appear to be suspicious for seizures but may not have EEG correlate. It has been well documented that health-care providers regardless of their level of training are uniformly poor at identifying true seizures by clinical observation alone.[55] Previous studies have suggested that only about one-third seizures in neonates are clinically visible and up to 80% of neonatal seizures may go undetected if relying on clinical signs alone.[53,56] It is therefore recommended that continuous EEG monitoring be initiated as soon as possible in infants with suspected HIE and that the decision to treat abnormal movements be based on correlation with EEG or aEEG monitoring. Prophylactic phenobarbital should not be administered. Antiepileptic medications can be considered when an infant displays recurrent paroxysmal movements consistent with seizures (eg, clonic movements that are not suppressible) when a patient is remote from transfer to a center with EEG monitoring. Although further studies are needed to determine the optimal pharmacologic agent for treatment of electrographic seizures in infants with HIE, phenobarbital is generally considered to be first-line therapy.[57]

Outpatient Follow-up of Infants with Hypoxic-Ischemic Encephalopathy After Therapeutic Hypothermia

Infants with history of moderate to severe HIE treated with TH require multidisciplinary follow-up to assess long-term motor, psychoeducational, auditory, and cognitive outcomes. Initial assessment by the multidisciplinary infant follow-up program may be carried out as early as 4 months of age. During the first year, infants should be monitored for motor or sensory deficits. Evidence of impaired cognition may become apparent during the second year. Fine and gross motor dysfunction usually presents during years two to four, followed by abnormalities in cognitive function and learning disabilities.[58]

Visual impairment at school age is seen in up to 41% of surviving infants with NE. Visual function is variably affected in infants with moderate HIE and often severely impaired in infants with severe HIE or abnormal MRI scans showing moderate or severe basal ganglia lesions or severe white matter changes.[59,60] Infants should have close monitoring of vision by a pediatrician and referral to pediatric ophthalmology in case of history of abnormal MRI with severe basal ganglia or white matter changes, severe HIE, moderate severe HIE with abnormal neurologic examination at discharge, or history of stroke associated with HIE.[61]

Hearing impairment is common in infants with history of moderate to severe HIE and has been documented in 10% to 18% of survivors.[62,63] Infants with history of moderate HIE should have repeated audiology evaluations included in ongoing developmental surveillance and early involvement of formal audiology and speech therapy as indicated.

Although many infants with moderate to severe HIE treated with TH will have seizure activity in the NICU, the number of these infants who go on to have childhood epilepsy is much smaller. One study reported 13% of infants with moderate to severe HIE treated with TH will have childhood epilepsy and 7% will continue to require antiepileptic medication at school age.[64] Infants with history of seizure activity during the NICU stay should be referred to neurology at discharge, whereas infants with history of HIE and no seizure activity can generally be seen by neurology within 1 to 3 months of discharge.

Difficulties in school are common in infants with history of moderate to severe HIE. School-age survivors with moderate to severe HIE have been shown to have intellectual, visual-motor integration, and receptive vocabulary scores significantly lower than their peers.[9] Difficulties with reading, spelling, and arithmetic are common, and in one study, they were seen in 30% to 50% of survivors.[6,65] A systematic review of 7 studies showed impairment of general cognitive abilities in up to 60% of infants with HIE without cerebral palsy (CP), including difficulties in attention, executive function, memory function, and language.[66] An increased incidence of autism spectrum disorders has been also been seen in infants with history of moderate to severe HIE.[67] Overall, infants with history of moderate to severe HIE at school age have been noted to have more emotional difficulties and to have increased academic special needs, need extra support in school, and frequently require individual learning plans.[7,68,69]

Predicting outcomes after hypoxic-ischemic encephalopathy

Predicting outcomes after perinatal asphyxia and HIE remains an active area of investigation. There are numerous studies on a variety of serum or cerebral spinal fluid biomarkers, although at this time, none are ready for real-time clinical application to help make decisions about which infants are likely to suffer HIE and thus would benefit from TH.[70] Metabolites such as lactate and alanine measured in cord blood at the time of birth in the setting of perinatal asphyxia by themselves perform poorly as a predictor of which infants will develop HIE, but when combined with clinical history, prediction is improved.[71] Clinical history, Sarnat stage, aEEG/EEG findings, and MRI severity of injury are important predictors of outcomes and readily available to clinicians. There is improved prediction when these factors are considered over the first several days of life.[72,73] For example, the need for chest compressions at delivery or presence of severe acidosis at birth while associated with outcomes perform poorly in prediction models when each is considered in isolation. Combining predictors measured at various time points improves prediction. This mimics the approach clinicians take when considering an individual patient. If we only consider factors identified at birth, we may have concern for poor outcomes (death or neurodevelopmental impairment), but our level of concern changes when we add in factors such as the aEEG/EEG background (normal vs burst suppression) at 24 or 36 hours after birth or MRI severity of injury (normal vs basal ganglia injury).

SUMMARY

HIE is a significant cause of neonatal morbidity and mortality. When initiated within 6 hours, TH has been shown to significantly improve survival and neurodevelopmental outcomes in infants with HIE. All providers who attend deliveries or care for newborns in the hospital should have the necessary training to identify HIE, determine infant eligibility for TH, and provide required supportive care to maintain homeostasis in infants after passive cooling has been initiated. After treatment of HIE with TH, multidisciplinary outpatient follow-up is needed to assess motor, psychoeducational, auditory, and cognitive outcomes and provide early intervention services as indicated.

CLINICS CARE POINTS

- Therapeutic hypothermia (TH) is standard of care for neonates with moderate-severe HIE and should be initiated within 6 hours after birth to optimize neuroprotecion.
- The modified Sarnat exam is the most commonly used tool to evaluate for encephalopathy.
- Evaluation of neonates who may qualify for TH should occur within the first hour after birth.
- Early communication (within 1 hour of birth) with a TH center can facilitate patient selection and expedite initiation of treatment and transfer.
- Close attention to temperature and levels of glucose, carbon dioxide and oxygen is needed to maximize neuroprotection.

Best Practices

What is the current practice?

Evaluation of the Term Newborn for HIE

Best Practice/Guideline/Care Path Objective(s)

- Consider HIE as a diagnosis in newborns with a history of fetal distress, sentinel events, or who require significant resuscitation at the time of birth.
- Be proficient in performing the modified Sarnat exam to identify newborns with encephalopathy.
- Use a screening algorithm to help identify patients with HIE who may qualify for therapeutic hypothermia (TH), standard of care treatment for moderate-severe HIE.
- Promptly call a TH center to discuss potential patients and arrange for timely transfer.

- Document serial Sarnat exams for the first 6 hours for newborns that meet historical and laboratory criteria for TH but do not meet exam criteria at one hour after birth.

What changes in current practice are likely to improve outcomes?

- Prompt identification and initiation of TH as early as possible within the first 6 hours after birth may optimize neuroprotection.
- Close attention to temperature, glucose and carbon dioxide levels, and oxygen exposure is needed. Hypoglycemia, hypocarbia, and hyperoxia are associated with brain injury and poor outcome.

Is there a Clinical Algorithm? If so, please include

- See **Fig. 1** and **Table 1**.

Major Recommendations

- Consider HIE and use of TH for newborns with encephalopathy.
- Follow criteria used in the randomized controlled trials to identify newborns with moderate-severe HIE who should receive TH.
- Perform hourly Sarnat exams for the first 6 hours in those who meet historical (perinatal event, fetal distress, need for resuscitation) and laboratory criteria (low pH, high base deficit) but do not have moderate-severe encephalopathy at 1 hour of age.
- Once a patient meets all criteria, start passive or active cooling with a goal temperature of 33.5C +/- 0.5C as soon as possible, with close attention to core temperature.
- Maintain homeostasis with regard to glucose, carbon dioxide, and oxygen levels, and blood pressure to minimize further brain injury.

Rating for the Strength of the Evidence

- Evidence for the use of TH to reduce morbidity and mortality in newborns with moderate-severe HIE is high. (level 1a – meta-analysis with numerous randomized controlled trials).

Bibliographic Source(s): Refs.[3,15]

DISCLOSURE

The authors have no conflicts of interest. S.L. Bonifacio is a recipient of the Thrasher Research Fund (TIME Study: A randomized controlled trial of Therapeutic Hypothermia for Infants with Mild Encephalopathy in California).

REFERENCES

1. Kurinczuk JJ, White-Koning M, Badawi N. Epidemiology of neonatal encephalopathy and hypoxic-ischaemic encephalopathy. Early Hum Dev 2010;86(6):329–38.
2. Lawn JE, Osrin D, Adler A, et al. Four million neonatal deaths: counting and attribution of cause of death. Paediatr Perinat Epidemiol 2008;22(5):410–6.
3. Executive summary: neonatal encephalopathy and neurologic outcome, second edition. Report of the American College of Obstetricians and Gynecologists' Task Force on neonatal encephalopathy. Obstet Gynecol 2014;123(4):896–901.
4. Aslam S, Strickland T, Molloy EJ. Neonatal encephalopathy: need for recognition of multiple etiologies for optimal management. Front Pediatr 2019;7:142.
5. Johnston MV, Fatemi A, Wilson MA, et al. Treatment advances in neonatal neuroprotection and neurointensive care. Lancet Neurol 2011;10(4):372–82.
6. Robertson CM, Finer NN, Grace MG. School performance of survivors of neonatal encephalopathy associated with birth asphyxia at term. J Pediatr 1989;114(5):753–60.

7. Marlow N, Rose AS, Rands CE, et al. Neuropsychological and educational problems at school age associated with neonatal encephalopathy. Arch Dis Child Fetal Neonatal Ed 2005;90(5):F380–7.
8. Shankaran S, Woldt E, Koepke T, et al. Acute neonatal morbidity and long-term central nervous system sequelae of perinatal asphyxia in term infants. Early Hum Dev 1991;25(2):135–48.
9. Ma H, Sinha B, Pandya RS, et al. Therapeutic hypothermia as a neuroprotective strategy in neonatal hypoxic-ischemic brain injury and traumatic brain injury. Curr Mol Med 2012;12(10):1282–96.
10. Azzopardi DV, Strohm B, Edwards AD, et al. Moderate hypothermia to treat perinatal asphyxial encephalopathy. N Engl J Med 2009;361(14):1349–58.
11. Shankaran S, Laptook AR, Ehrenkranz RA, et al. Whole-body hypothermia for neonates with hypoxic-ischemic encephalopathy. N Engl J Med 2005;353(15): 1574–84.
12. Simbruner G, Mittal RA, Rohlmann F, et al. Participants nnnT. Systemic hypothermia after neonatal encephalopathy: outcomes of neo.nEURO.network RCT. Pediatrics 2010;126(4):e771–8.
13. Gluckman PD, Wyatt JS, Azzopardi D, et al. Selective head cooling with mild systemic hypothermia after neonatal encephalopathy: multicentre randomised trial. Lancet 2005;365(9460):663–70.
14. Jacobs SE, Morley CJ, Inder TE, et al. Whole-body hypothermia for term and near-term newborns with hypoxic-ischemic encephalopathy: a randomized controlled trial. Arch Pediatr Adolesc Med 2011;165(8):692–700.
15. Jacobs SE, Berg M, Hunt R, et al. Cooling for newborns with hypoxic ischaemic encephalopathy. Cochrane Database Syst Rev 2013;(1):CD003311.
16. Tagin MA, Woolcott CG, Vincer MJ, et al. Hypothermia for neonatal hypoxic ischemic encephalopathy: an updated systematic review and meta-analysis. Arch Pediatr Adolesc Med 2012;166(6):558–66.
17. Zhou WH, Cheng GQ, Shao XM, et al. Selective head cooling with mild systemic hypothermia after neonatal hypoxic-ischemic encephalopathy: a multicenter randomized controlled trial in China. J Pediatr 2010;157(3):367–72, 372.e1-3.
18. Walas W, Wilińska M, Bekiesińska-Figatowska M, et al. Methods for assessing the severity of perinatal asphyxia and early prognostic tools in neonates with hypoxic-ischemic encephalopathy treated with therapeutic hypothermia. Adv Clin Exp Med 2020;29(8):1011–6.
19. Montaldo P, Rosso R, Chello G, et al. Cardiac troponin I concentrations as a marker of neurodevelopmental outcome at 18 months in newborns with perinatal asphyxia. J Perinatol 2014;34(4):292–5.
20. Muniraman H, Gardner D, Skinner J, et al. Biomarkers of hepatic injury and function in neonatal hypoxic ischemic encephalopathy and with therapeutic hypothermia. Eur J Pediatr 2017;176(10):1295–303.
21. Wu YW, Mathur AM, Chang T, et al. High-dose erythropoietin and hypothermia for hypoxic-ischemic encephalopathy: a phase II trial. Pediatrics 2016;137(6). https://doi.org/10.1542/peds.2016-0191.
22. Juul SE, Comstock BA, Heagerty PJ, et al. High-dose erythropoietin for asphyxia and encephalopathy (HEAL): a randomized controlled trial - background, aims, and study protocol. Neonatology 2018;113(4):331–8.
23. Groenendaal F, de Vries LS. Selection of babies for intervention after birth asphyxia. Semin Neonatol 2000;5(1):17–32.

24. Bhagwani DK, Sharma M, Dolker S, et al. To study the correlation of Thompson scoring in predicting early neonatal outcome in post asphyxiated term neonates. J Clin Diagn Res 2016;10(11):SC16–9.
25. Thorsen P, Jansen-van der Weide MC, Groenendaal F, et al. The Thompson encephalopathy score and short-term outcomes in asphyxiated newborns treated with therapeutic hypothermia. Pediatr Neurol 2016;60:49–53.
26. Hellstr√∂m-Westas L, Ros√©n I, Svenningsen NW. Predictive value of early continuous amplitude integrated EEG recordings on outcome after severe birth asphyxia in full term infants. Arch Dis Child Fetal Neonatal Ed 1995;72(1):F34–8.
27. Thoresen M, Hellstr√∂m-Westas L, Liu X, et al. Effect of hypothermia on amplitude-integrated electroencephalogram in infants with asphyxia. Pediatrics 2010;126(1):e131–9.
28. Thoresen M, Tooley J, Liu X, et al. Time is brain: starting therapeutic hypothermia within three hours after birth improves motor outcome in asphyxiated newborns. Neonatology 2013;104(3):228–33.
29. Natarajan G, Pappas A, Shankaran S, et al. Effect of inborn vs. outborn delivery on neurodevelopmental outcomes in infants with hypoxic-ischemic encephalopathy: secondary analyses of the NICHD whole-body cooling trial. Pediatr Res 2012;72(4):414–9.
30. Wyckoff MH, Aziz K, Escobedo MB, et al. Part 13: neonatal resuscitation: 2015 American heart association guidelines update for Cardiopulmonary resuscitation and emergency Cardiovascular care. Circulation 2015;132(18 Suppl 2):S543–60.
31. Wyckoff MH, Weiner GM, Collaborators NLS. 2020 International consensus on Cardiopulmonary resuscitation and emergency Cardiovascular care science with treatment recommendations. Pediatrics 2020. https://doi.org/10.1542/peds.2020-038505C.
32. Roychoudhury S, Esser MJ, Buchhalter J, et al. Implementation of neonatal neurocritical care program improved short-term outcomes in neonates with moderate-to-severe hypoxic ischemic encephalopathy. Pediatr Neurol 2019;101:64–70.
33. Bashir RA, Espinoza L, Vayalthrikkovil S, et al. Implementation of a neurocritical care program: improved seizure detection and decreased antiseizure medication at discharge in neonates with hypoxic-ischemic encephalopathy. Pediatr Neurol 2016;64:38–43.
34. BURNARD ED, CROSS KW. Rectal temperature in the newborn after birth asphyxia. Br Med J 1958;2(5106):1197–9.
35. Laptook A, Tyson J, Shankaran S, et al. Elevated temperature after hypoxic-ischemic encephalopathy: risk factor for adverse outcomes. Pediatrics 2008;122(3):491–9.
36. Wyatt JS, Gluckman PD, Liu PY, et al. Determinants of outcomes after head cooling for neonatal encephalopathy. Pediatrics 2007;119(5):912–21.
37. Pinchefsky EF, Hahn CD, Kamino D, et al. Hyperglycemia and glucose variability are associated with worse brain function and seizures in neonatal encephalopathy: a prospective Cohort study. J Pediatr 2019;209:23–32.
38. Curry DL, Curry KP. Hypothermia and insulin secretion. Endocrinology 1970;87(4):750–5.
39. Rozance PJ. Update on neonatal hypoglycemia. Curr Opin Endocrinol Diabetes Obes 2014;21(1):45–50.
40. Jacobs SE. Selective head cooling with mild systemic hypothermia after neonatal encephalopathy: multicentre randomised trial. J Pediatr 2005;147(1):122–3.

41. Lou HC, Lassen NA, Fris-Hansen B. Decreased cerebral blood flow after administration of sodium bicarbonate in the distressed newborn infant. Acta Neurol Scand 1978;57(3):239–47.
42. Shah P, Riphagen S, Beyene J, et al. Multiorgan dysfunction in infants with post-asphyxial hypoxic-ischaemic encephalopathy. Arch Dis Child Fetal Neonatal Ed 2004;89(2):F152–5.
43. Giesinger RE, Levy PT, Lauren Ruoss J, et al. Cardiovascular management following hypoxic-ischemic encephalopathy in North America: need for physiologic consideration. Pediatr Res 2020. https://doi.org/10.1038/s41390-020-01205-8.
44. Pakvasa MA, Winkler AM, Hamrick SE, et al. Observational study of haemostatic dysfunction and bleeding in neonates with hypoxic-ischaemic encephalopathy. BMJ Open 2017;7(2):e013787.
45. Grether JK, Nelson KB. Maternal infection and cerebral palsy in infants of normal birth weight. JAMA 1997;278(3):207–11.
46. Pappas A, Shankaran S, Laptook AR, et al. Hypocarbia and adverse outcome in neonatal hypoxic-ischemic encephalopathy. J Pediatr 2011;158(5):752–8.e1.
47. Lopez Laporte MA, Wang H, Sanon PN, et al. Association between hypocapnia and ventilation during the first days of life and brain injury in asphyxiated newborns treated with hypothermia. J Matern Fetal Neonatal Med 2019;32(8): 1312–20.
48. Thoresen M. Supportive care during neuroprotective hypothermia in the term newborn: adverse effects and their prevention. Clin Perinatol 2008;35(4): 749–63, vii.
49. Sabir H, Jary S, Tooley J, et al. Increased inspired oxygen in the first hours of life is associated with adverse outcome in newborns treated for perinatal asphyxia with therapeutic hypothermia. J Pediatr 2012;161(3):409–16.
50. Klinger G, Beyene J, Shah P, et al. Do hyperoxaemia and hypocapnia add to the risk of brain injury after intrapartum asphyxia? Arch Dis Child Fetal Neonatal Ed 2005;90(1):F49–52.
51. Vento M, Asensi M, Sastre J, et al. Oxidative stress in asphyxiated term infants resuscitated with 100% oxygen. J Pediatr 2003;142(3):240–6.
52. Koch JD, Miles DK, Gilley JA, et al. Brief exposure to hyperoxia depletes the glial progenitor pool and impairs functional recovery after hypoxic-ischemic brain injury. J Cereb Blood Flow Metab 2008;28(7):1294–306.
53. Murray DM, Ryan CA, Boylan GB, et al. Prediction of seizures in asphyxiated neonates: correlation with continuous video-electroencephalographic monitoring. Pediatrics 2006;118(1):41–6.
54. Wusthoff CJ, Dlugos DJ, Gutierrez-Colina A, et al. Electrographic seizures during therapeutic hypothermia for neonatal hypoxic-ischemic encephalopathy. J Child Neurol 2011;26(6):724–8.
55. Malone A, Ryan CA, Fitzgerald A, et al. Interobserver agreement in neonatal seizure identification. Epilepsia 2009;50(9):2097–101.
56. Clancy RR, Legido A, Lewis D. Occult neonatal seizures. Epilepsia 1988;29(3): 256–61.
57. Yozawitz E, Stacey A, Pressler RM. Pharmacotherapy for seizures in neonates with hypoxic ischemic encephalopathy. Paediatr Drugs 2017;19(6):553–67.
58. Amiel-Tison C, Ellison P. Birth asphyxia in the fullterm newborn: early assessment and outcome. Dev Med Child Neurol 1986;28(5):671–82.
59. Mercuri E, Atkinson J, Braddick O, et al. Visual function in full-term infants with hypoxic-ischaemic encephalopathy. Neuropediatrics 1997;28(3):155–61.

60. Mercuri E, Anker S, Guzzetta A, et al. Visual function at school age in children with neonatal encephalopathy and low Apgar scores. Arch Dis Child Fetal Neonatal Ed 2004;89(3):F258–62.
61. Robertson CM, Perlman M. Follow-up of the term infant after hypoxic-ischemic encephalopathy. Paediatr Child Health 2006;11(5):278–82.
62. Fitzgerald MP, Reynolds A, Garvey CM, et al. Hearing impairment and hypoxia ischaemic encephalopathy: incidence and associated factors. Eur J Paediatr Neurol 2019;23(1):81–6.
63. LindstràöàÇm K, Lagerroos P, Gillberg C, et al. Teenage outcome after being born at term with moderate neonatal encephalopathy. Pediatr Neurol 2006; 35(4):268–74.
64. Liu X, Jary S, Cowan F, et al. Reduced infancy and childhood epilepsy following hypothermia-treated neonatal encephalopathy. Epilepsia 2017;58(11):1902–11.
65. Dilenge ME, Majnemer A, Shevell MI. Long-term developmental outcome of asphyxiated term neonates. J Child Neurol 2001;16(11):781–92.
66. Schreglmann M, Ground A, Vollmer B, et al. Systematic review: long-term cognitive and behavioural outcomes of neonatal hypoxic-ischaemic encephalopathy in children without cerebral palsy. Acta Paediatr 2020;109(1):20–30.
67. Badawi N, Dixon G, Felix JF, et al. Autism following a history of newborn encephalopathy: more than a coincidence? Dev Med Child Neurol 2006;48(2):85–9.
68. Lee-Kelland R, Jary S, Tonks J, et al. School-age outcomes of children without cerebral palsy cooled for neonatal hypoxic-ischaemic encephalopathy in 2008-2010. Arch Dis Child Fetal Neonatal Ed 2020;105(1):8–13.
69. van Kooij BJ, van Handel M, Nievelstein RA, et al. Serial MRI and neurodevelopmental outcome in 9- to 10-year-old children with neonatal encephalopathy. J Pediatr 2010;157(2):221–7.e2.
70. Murray DM. Biomarkers in neonatal hypoxic-ischemic encephalopathy-Review of the literature to date and future directions for research. Handb Clin Neurol 2019; 162:281–93.
71. O'Boyle DS, Dunn WB, O'Neill D, et al. Improvement in the prediction of neonatal hypoxic-ischemic encephalopathy with the integration of umbilical cord metabolites and current clinical makers. J Pediatr 2021;229:175–81.e1.
72. Peeples ES, Rao R, Dizon MLV, et al. Predictive models of neurodevelopmental outcomes after neonatal hypoxic-ischemic encephalopathy. Pediatrics 2021; 147(2). https://doi.org/10.1542/peds.2020-022962.
73. Bonifacio SL, deVries LS, Groenendaal F. Impact of hypothermia on predictors of poor outcome: how do we decide to redirect care? Semin Fetal Neonatal Med 2015;20(2):122–7.

Printed and bound by CPI Group (UK) Ltd, Croydon, CR0 4YY
03/10/2024
01040477-0005